From Doctor to Healer

From Doctor to Healer

THE TRANSFORMATIVE JOURNEY

Robbie Davis-Floyd and
Gloria St. John

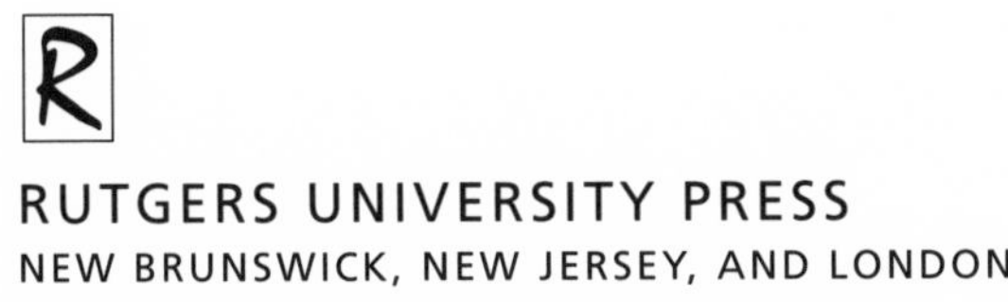

RUTGERS UNIVERSITY PRESS
NEW BRUNSWICK, NEW JERSEY, AND LONDON

Library of Congress Cataloging-in-Publication Data

Davis-Floyd, Robbie.
From doctor to healer : the transformative journey / Robbie Davis-Floyd and Gloria St. John.
p. cm.
Includes bibliographical references and index.
ISBN 0-8135-2519-5 (cloth : alk. paper). — ISBN 0-8135-2520-9 (pbk. : alk. paper)
1. Holistic medicine—Social aspects. 2. Medicine—Philosophy. I. St. John, Gloria, 1944– . II. Title.
R733.D38 1998
610'.1—dc21 97-39343
CIP

British Cataloging-in-Publication data for this book is available from the British Library

Manufactured in the United States of America

To the courageous healers we interviewed and their colleagues everywhere

Contents

Foreword

If someone had actually called me a healer when I was a young medical student, I would not have known if I was being damned or praised. After I began the practice of internal medicine, the first time a patient called me a healer I was actually embarrassed. I eventually recovered from my intellectual indigestion about being regarded as a healer, and I realize now that this is the ultimate compliment that can be paid a physician.

I came by my confusion honestly—because, oddly enough, healing is not something that is taught in medical school. Healing, we young doctors were instructed, is a process that happens automatically in wounds or surgical incisions; it has nothing to do with a physician's behavior or intentions (Dossey 1995).

The hemorrhage of healing from medicine begins early for doctors. The stage is set in college, when medical school–bound students have their first exposure to science courses. In lecture after lecture, the lesson that is subtly delivered is, There are two ways you can live your life. You can choose to be rational, analytical, objective, intellectual, and scientific; or you can choose to be irrational, intuitive, religious, or spiritual. A choice is mandatory; you cannot have it both ways. By the time most students wind up in medical school, their decision has been made. Although a few more padlocks are placed on the doors of emotion, intuition, and subjectivity during medical school, these portals have already been slammed shut, and may not open again during the physician's lifetime.

The divorce between the intellect and "the spiritual" comes at a profound cost to physicians. It demands that they live a divided, schizophrenic life, in which they place one vector of their psyche in opposition to another. This is an unnatural state of affairs, and it creates immense pain.

I often have the opportunity to discuss these issues at medical schools and hospitals. As a consequence, I receive feedback from physicians around the country about what they think and how they feel about the demands of their profession. One doctor, a faculty member at a prestigious medical school in the Northeast, wrote about the conflict he feels between his intellectual and spiritual inclinations. "This situation," he said with utmost sincerity, "is killing me."

Why are we forced to speak about "recovering" healing in medicine? How did we lose one of the most precious talents humans have ever possessed?

It's easy to make medical schools the whipping boy for these problems. Medical schools, however, do not exist in a vacuum. They arise *from* and *within* a culture, and they reflect the values of the society in which they are embedded. The loss of medicine's soul therefore reflects the spiritual emptiness of our culture as whole; medicine's problems are everyone's problems.

Consider, for example, the burdens our culture places on physicians in this emerging age of managed care. As physician John D. Lantos states in his book *Do We Still Need Doctors?*: "The doctor who must seek informed consent according to a legally defined protocol, in order to provide a treatment that the patient's insurance company has approved because it is the most cost effective, and who provides the treatment according to a practice guideline based on valid outcome studies is a very different creature than any doctor who has ever practiced before, since the beginning of time" (Abrams 1997).

The quest to recover healing in medicine reflects a virtual hunger for a spiritual dimension of life; it indicates a willingness to honor a transcendent, transpersonal aspect of existence.

This process, I am happy to say, seems to be going rather well. Today nearly thirty medical schools have courses that explore the role of religion and spirituality in health (Levin, Larson, and Puchalski 1997). National conferences at prestigious medical schools on spirituality and medicine have become routine. These developments would have been unthinkable a decade ago. They bespeak a new openness, and led one nationally known physician, Andrew Weil, to tell me in July 1996, "I'm a big fan of the health care crisis!"

Some professionals within medicine and science lament these developments. They view the transformation of physicians into healers as a descent into irrationality and a step backward in history. But the prediction that science will be ruinously contaminated by spirituality is an exaggeration. Science can exist, and has always existed, with the spiritual. According to a recent survey published in the prestigious science journal *Nature,* four out of ten U.S. scientists believe in God, a proportion that has not changed in eighty years (Larson 1997). Mathematicians, who are often regarded as representing the purest form of science, were the group of scientists most inclined to believe in a Supreme Being. These statistics suggest that the stereotypical view of the incompatibility of science and spirituality needs to be reconsidered.

In his book *A Sense of the Cosmos,* philosopher Jacob Needleman (1997:167) describes the earliest days of science. Four centuries ago, science arose in opposition to the teachings of the Church, which defined the workings of the world for everyone. What were these earliest scientists like? They were people, Needleman states, who above all wanted a direct, unmediated encounter with reality, a personal experience in which no authority or dogma blocked their approach. In Needleman's graphic metaphor, these early scientists *went to the wall of truth*, where they confronted the world alone and invited the universe to reveal itself through their primitive experiments. This is really the eternal quest of the mystic: to know the world as it actually is. This connection of science and spirituality was not fully appreciated, Needleman states, even by the founding fathers of science. It was quickly swamped by the rising emphasis on intellectuality and objectification. The spiritual essence of early science is precisely the quality that the physicians in the following pages have attempted to regain.

Reading Robbie Davis-Floyd and Gloria St.John's manuscript was a profoundly moving experience for me. The accounts of the transformational experiences of the physicians they interviewed reminded me of many past experiences, and brought tears. I saw my colleagues in these pages as participants in an archetypal hero's journey, in which a representative of a society ventures into unknown territory, risks immense dangers and death, and returns with a hard-won knowledge that is invaluable to those who stayed safely behind. I was reminded of a comment by psychologist C. G. Jung about pioneers. He said, "[H]ow great are the disadvantages of pioneer work: One stumbles through unknown regions . . . forever losing the Ariadne thread; one is overwhelmed by new impressions and new possibilities. . . . The second generation has the advantage of a clearer, if still incomplete picture; certain landmarks that at least lie on the frontiers of the essential have grown familiar, and one now knows what must be known if one is to explore the newly discovered territory" (quoted in Johnson 1997).

More and more heroes and heroines within medicine are making the journey of transformation. Their experiences will make it easier for physicians who come after them. In many instances, they risk everything; they seem to realize that a process that is not truly risky cannot be genuinely transformative. We are indebted to Davis-Floyd and St. John for telling their stories, and above all to the risk takers themselves.

"The dust of exploded beliefs may make a fine sunset," Geoffrey Madan said (quoted in Partington 1994:216)—and, one hopes, may set the stage for a fine sunrise as well. For a glimpse of modern medicine's sunrise of the soul, read on.

—Larry Dossey, M.D.

From Doctor to Healer

Introduction

At the age of twenty-three, Alex Cadoux graduated summa cum laude out of a class of thousands from the State University of New York at Stony Brook and entered medical school at the prestigious Johns Hopkins University in Baltimore, Maryland. Throughout most of his four years there, he was a model student: he worked hard, earned excellent grades, and never questioned the value of his training. But during the fourth year, in a rotation on the pediatric oncology ward, he began to have the uncomfortable feeling that he was, in his words, "torturing dying children. We all knew they were going to die. They had already been failing therapies, but were still undergoing very painful testing and treatments. These measures were barbaric, but we called them 'heroic.'"

During his first year of residency at Hopkins in internal medicine, Alex Cadoux found himself again on the oncology floor. "And I remember this day—so does my wife. I called her up and I said, 'I can't go on. I can't do this.' Which for me was big. I was tough. I could do anything. And I am tough. But at my core, I couldn't do this anymore." He left his residency and went into emergency medicine, where he felt he could make a positive difference. Years of heading the Emergency Medicine Department in a large city hospital made him even more aware of the limitations of Western medicine. Intrigued by the patients who sometimes refused the drugs he offered, preferring instead to use acupuncture or chiropractic, he began to explore alternative healing systems: "I started learning from my patients. I picked up my nose from the grindstone and realized that there's a larger world out there. There were other ways to approach these problems. I realized that the tools at my disposal were good tools, but they were very limited. I was fixing watches with a sledgehammer when what was required were small jeweler's tools."

He investigated the scientific literature on nutrition, and found that there were plenty of well-controlled studies published in reputable journals that demonstrated the value of healthy diets and nutritional supplements, and that mainstream physicians had ignored this whole body of research. Eventually he opened a wellness center staffed by a variety of alternative practitioners. There he began to practice nutritional medicine. He treated patients with chronic conditions that conventional medicine could not cure—headaches, gastrointestinal problems, irritable bowel, ulcerative colitis, Crohn's disease, food allergies, hypertension, hypoglycemia, diabetes, chronic fatigue syndrome, back and leg pain. Most of his clients came to him not because they believed in holistic medicine but because they were desperate. They had tried all the drugs and treatments conventional medicine had to offer and nothing had worked. Most such patients found that their conditions improved dramatically or disappeared completely under Cadoux's care.

One patient, the wife of a psychiatrist, had been in the hospital for two months because she was dying from a severe case of ulcerative colitis. Unable to eat anything by mouth, and bleeding from her rectum, she was scheduled to have her colon removed the next day. Called in as a last resort, Cadoux prescribed a special diet of organic food. Within twenty-four hours her bleeding and diarrhea stopped. Today she is an active and healthy mother of three, with her colon intact. And Cadoux's conventional colleagues, originally highly skeptical, now often refer patients to him.

Alex Cadoux, M.D., underwent what is typically referred to these days as a "paradigm shift." At first thoroughly imbued with the worldview of conventional medicine, he ended up leaving it almost completely behind. While he still prescribes conventional pharmaceuticals on rare occasions, he treats most of those who come to see him by recommending organic food, nutritional supplements, and various lifestyle modifications, from exercise to meditation. In other words, he has moved into the exciting and emergent realm of holistic healing.

This book is about the paradigm shifts of Alex Cadoux and many others like him. For the first time, we bring together in print the stories, told in their own words, of this new breed of healer: the holistic physician. You can find one in almost every American city or town. Some of them work in holistic clinics or wellness centers like the one founded by Alex Cadoux, where they can participate in a community of like-minded people. But often they practice in relative isolation, sometimes concealing from their medical colleagues the unconventional things that they do. Most earn far less money than they might if they had not made this paradigm shift. Like their more conventional colleagues, they paid their dues to the profession—four arduous years of medical school, followed by three or four even more arduous years of residency. Those who successfully pass through this grueling process usually feel that they are more than entitled to reap its long-promised financial and social rewards.

Why then do some physicians reject the technomedical paradigm under which they are trained? Why would they willingly give up high salaries and professional prestige to pursue this ephemeral thing called holistic healing, which is practically guaranteed to earn them less money, lowered status, and often even downright ostracism from other members of their profession? What compensates for these losses? And what can their choices tell us about the profound changes taking place in Western medicine as we move into the twenty-first century? Through individual tape-recorded interviews with forty holistic physicians, and stories recorded during group discussions from many more, we seek in this book to answer these questions, and to allow the hearts, minds, and voices of these physicians-in-transition to be heard.

Buddy, Can You Paradigm?

A paradigm, most simply, is both a model of and a template for reality. Complementary terms include "belief system" and "worldview." Just as a fish cannot breathe outside of the water it swims in, so an individual operating within a paradigm is subject to the illusion that the paradigm represents the whole of reality. But no paradigm does. All models of reality, no matter how complex, are bound to leave out some aspects of the "reality" they are attempting to model. Many paradigms come to constitute relatively closed conceptual systems that discount or exclude incompatible information, regardless of its potential validity within another paradigm. In the *Structure of Scientific Revolutions* (1970), philosopher Thomas Kuhn demonstrated that, far from being an accurate model of reality, the most a paradigm can be is a set of beliefs about the nature of an ultimately unknowable universe.

The limitations of paradigms are counterbalanced by their advantages: paradigms provide clear conceptual models that facilitate one's movement in the world. In acting not only as models of—but also as templates for—reality, paradigms enable us to behave in organized ways, to take actions that make sense under a given set of principles. "To paradigm," if you will, is to create the world through the story we tell about it. We then can live as cultural beings in the organized and coherent paradigmatic world we have created. We cannot live without paradigms. But we can learn to be conscious and aware of how they influence our thoughts and shape our experience, to understand that they open some possibilities while closing others. That awareness can bring a rare kind of freedom—the freedom to "think beyond."

In this book we will primarily be concerned with the three principal paradigms that currently shape medical practice in the United States, which we label the technocratic, humanistic, and holistic models. We stress throughout the book that these models are not graven in stone, but simply focal points on the American spectrum of beliefs about health care. A given physician may practice completely within one or may range among all three. Understanding the nature of these three paradigms is essential to understanding the paradigm shifts made by the physicians who are the subjects of this book. As they begin their journey away from the limitations, the emotional coldness, and the high-tech focus of technocratic medicine, they may find their comfort zone in the relationship-oriented warmth of the humanistic approach. Or they may choose to embrace holism and, in so doing, find themselves transformed.

Their journeys of transformation and their motivations for undertaking those journeys have profound implications for the direction of medical care in this country. Physicians are the standard-bearers of the values American society has invested in one of its primary institutions—its health care system. As physicians change their beliefs and practices, a quiet revolution is occurring not only across the desk of the consulting room but also within the halls of hospitals and in medical classrooms. One-third of the medical schools in this country now offer some courses in alternative medicine, and a recent survey by the National Institutes of Health revealed that 71 percent of medical students want to learn about such practices.

But let us not get ahead of the story. In what remains of this Introduction, we will introduce ourselves to our readers and briefly tell of our own engagement with the paradigm shifts of holistic physicians. We will describe our methods of data collection, and provide an overview of the chapters in this book. Throughout the book we will speak collectively as "we." Here, for the first and only time, you will hear our individual voices.

About the Authors

ROBBIE DAVIS-FLOYD, PH.D.

I am a cultural anthropologist with abiding and passionate interests in the realms of myth, ritual, and story, of gender, and of cross-cultural systems of healing and health care. My special focus has been in the anthropology of reproduction, a field in which my interest was sparked by the births of my own two children. For my first book, *Birth as an American Rite of Passage* (1992), I interviewed one hundred women about their pregnancy and childbirth experiences. At first confused by the standardized medical ways of treating these unique and individual events, I eventually came to interpret standard obstetrical procedures such as IVs, electronic fetal monitoring, pitocin, and episiotomy as rituals that convey the core values of American technocratic society to birthing women and their families. I analyzed these rituals as emergent from a paradigm that I labeled "the technocratic model of birth." Cumulatively, these ritual procedures work to convince the birthing woman of the inherent defectiveness of her body-machine, and of the inherent superiority of the technologies used to correct its deficiencies and improve its performance. I came to understand that the routine use of high technologies like the electronic fetal monitor (shown in study after study not to improve the outcome of birth, but only to raise the cesarean rate) serves a far deeper purpose than producing healthier babies. It counteracts our profound cultural fear of chaotic and uncontrollable natural processes by making it appear that these processes can in fact be culturally manipulated and controlled. So attached are we as a culture to this myth of technological transcendence of nature's limitations that we enact it every day, in almost every hospital across the county, in almost every birth, at an entirely unnecessary cost of billions of dollars, millions of unnecessary cesareans, and thousands of unnecessarily damaged babies. In my book, and in a series of articles (Davis-Floyd 1987, 1990, 1993, 1994), I have chronicled this cultural saga.

Against this backdrop, the midwives and physicians who resisted the technocratic approach, who sought to tell another story about birth and the female body—a story of wholeness, relationship, patience, and trust—stood out. I began to investigate the ways in which home-birth midwives relied on intuition—body knowing—to support women's desires for self-empowering and safe home births (Davis-Floyd and Davis 1996). For a study on obstetrical training, I interviewed twelve obstetricians, three of whom were beginning to consider themselves "holistic." Their practices in some ways resembled and in some ways differed radically from those of their conventional colleagues. The most telling difference was in their cesarean rates: at a time when the cesarean rates of conventional physicians were averaging almost 25 percent, each of these doctors had a rate of 17 percent or lower. And if you subtracted the women in their practices who were requesting repeat cesareans, their rates went down to under 10 percent (Davis-Floyd 1987). Clearly something was different here, and I wanted to know more about this new kind of doctor.

In the spring of 1993, I was invited to speak about ritual and about childbirth at the annual meetings of the American Holistic Medical Association (AHMA); it was there that my interest in holistic physicians took a quantum leap, and I spontaneously began to conduct my first set of interviews. I think I knew that I had to write this book when, on Saturday night during the musical entertainment, I personally witnessed two hundred and fifty medical doctors dancing ecstatically with their arms held up in the air, singing "I got the healin' spirit / Way down deep in my soul" at the top of their lungs!

But I had several other projects in line, a teaching job to do, and two children to raise, and I despaired of finding the time. Serendipitously, a flyer arrived in the mail inviting me to participate in a conference about holistic physicians. I wrote back that I could not attend, but was deeply interested in the topic. And that is how I found Gloria St. John.

GLORIA ST. JOHN, M.B.A.

I have been a professional in the health care field for twenty-five years. During this time I have actively participated, as an administrator or consultant, in nearly every type of setting where health care is delivered. I know intimately the goals, frustrations, vision, personnel, and procedures of clinics, financing programs, and hospitals. I have managed an outpatient clinic, been responsible for planning and marketing hospital services, and provided technical assistance to virtually every type of federally funded health program in this country. I have spent countless hours in discussions with managers, doctors, other health personnel, and patients about the health services they either provided or received. During this time I met thousands of well-intentioned, deeply committed individuals who devoted themselves to providing services to the ill and disadvantaged. Despite the fact that health care is a multibillion-dollar industry, it is my experience that very few individuals operating at the service delivery level are motivated by money alone. The talents, determination, and genius that most doctors, in particular, possess, could be used to create fortunes in the private business sector.

For many years I was satisfied to operate within the confines of orthodox medicine, and enjoyed the prestige and financial rewards this realm can provide. However, like many of the doctors in our study, I underwent a major shift in my personal values that prompted me to pursue my longstanding curiosity about the realm of alternative health care. As a result of the combination of my temperament with the pressures of the career and lifestyle I had chosen, I was diagnosed with chronic fatigue syndrome in 1987. Knowing that conventional medicine had little to offer, I went immediately to a classical homeopath and recovered very quickly. The deep healing brought on by the remedy I was given prompted other changes in lifestyle, among them a search for the unity and integration of work aligned with my beliefs.

Eventually I became the executive director of an organization known as the MetaPhysicians, a hundred or so M.D.'s, mostly from the San Francisco Bay Area, who came together as an association in 1988 with a unifying belief in their experience that spirit informed the practice of medicine. Terry Tyler, a psychiatrist, founded the organization out of a disillusion with medicine so complete that at one point he allowed his medical license to expire. I worked closely with him for years, and owe a great deal to his inspiration and his ability to articulate the wounds experienced by doctors. This organization and the impulses and contributions of its members sowed the seeds of my involvement in this book. As we recorded the stories of the MetaPhysicians, I recognized their journeys as more than personal adventures. I saw the embryo of what would be born, possibly not until the next century, as the medicine of the future.

To the general public, the psyche of the physician is a mystery. Trained to have answers, save lives, respond to emergencies, and process information at lightning speed, doctors tend to avoid unnecessary questions, intimacy, or even engagement with their patients. They often feel imprisoned in the ivory tower of their training and conditioning; when they want to break out, they have a great deal of difficulty finding the key. I was privileged to be part of that process for many physicians who began to tell the truth to each other through informal meetings and support groups. Over and over again the themes of dedication, compassion, disappointment, and hope emerged. I interviewed several MetaPhysicians for this book (see the appendix), and the reflections of Terry Tyler are incorporated throughout. I have been awed by the capacity for learning, for suffering, and for feeling evident in them and the other physicians I have known. It is my hope that this book will encourage doctors who are awakening to the limits of their training in Western medicine to feel supported by those who have responded to the call to become the healers they were born to be. The pathfinders whose experiences and voices are shared in the following pages have become a potent force in the evolution of medicine to a system open to the empowered patient and the conscious practitioner, both of whom bow to life itself.

Methods of Data Collection

Each of us conducted formal, tape-recorded interviews with twenty physicians whom we or others identified as "holistic physicians." Of these forty physicians, thirty-four turned out to also consider themselves holistic, meaning that they espouse a philosophy based on the idea of healing the whole person in whole life context, and incorporate alternative techniques such as homeopathy or acupuncture into their medical practices. Six can more accurately be described as "humanistic"; although for the most part they practice conventionally, they base their treatment style on a compassionate connection with their patients. These six helped us to recognize the differences between the humanistic and holistic paradigms of medicine.

Davis-Floyd conducted most of her interviews at the first three AHMA meetings she attended, in Kansas City in 1993, in Seattle in 1994, and in Phoenix in 1995. St. John conducted most of her interviews in the San Francisco Bay Area and in Chicago. Most interviewees readily agreed to the use of their real names. For the few who asked for anonymity, pseudonyms have been substituted. A complete list of interviewees and their medical specialties appears in the appendix. All interview material has been edited for grammar, clarity, and flow.

In addition to these forty interviews, which form our primary data source, we draw liberally in this book on the stories of seventeen Meta-Physicians collected by St. John and Terry Tyler in 1989; on Davis-Floyd's 1987 interviews with twelve obstetricians; on a set of interviews conducted in 1996 with five physicians in Houston, Texas, by Davis-Floyd's medical anthropology students at Rice University, Michelle Garza and Janna Flint; and on a series of thirty stories that appeared in *Holistic Medicine*, the AHMA journal, in a regular column called "Physician in Transition," initiated by editor Bill Manahan, M.D., in 1989. In this column, individual physicians share with their colleagues their own stories of professional and personal transformation. Bill Manahan, whose original intent was to publish as a book a number of the stories that appeared in this column between 1989 and 1993, instead generously sent them to us. (A list of the thirty authors of these columns, along with full referencing information, can be found in the appendix.) Together these resources constitute a collective database of information on the practices and the philosophies of more than one hundred physicians. Throughout this book, quotes from the authors' forty interviews will simply cite the interviewee's name. All other quotations from the sources described here will carry identifying citations. A special typeface will be used for all indented quotes from the primary sources described here, so that the reader may easily recognize them as such.

From Doctor to Healer: An Overview

What does this shift from doctor to healer entail? The root of the word "doctor" is the Latin *docere*, "to teach"; of "healer," the Old English *hal*, "to restore to health, soundness, or spiritual wholeness, to rid of sin, anxiety or the like." Teachers are not on the same level as their students; the teacher has the information that is regarded as important and authoritative. Concomitantly, the underlying premise of medical education and practice is that patients are in some way inferior to doctors, if only because they know less. Healing takes a different approach, as holistic physician Bethany Hays explained:

> In the conventional view, "healing" is something that happens outside of the patient's body and outside of their mind. You come in, you get a diagnosis, you get a treatment modality. In Western medicine it's usually a drug or surgery, and then that drug or surgery solves the problem, and you go away without any sense of relationship to the illness or to the person who

> solves the problem, and without any knowledge of what the illness meant in your life. In the holistic view, "healing" requires the active participation of the sick person. It requires that they address where they are in their lives, why the illness has occurred at this time, and what's going on that their bodies are asking them to address or evolve into a new way of thinking. In this system, the healer is a facilitator and doesn't address the illness as much as he addresses the patient and what the illness means to the patient.

Why do physicians decide to make this move from doctor to healer? What catalysts spark this transformational journey, this paradigm shift? What form does this journey take? What beliefs do they abandon, and which do they embrace? These questions and others like them form the subject matter of the body of this book. We see this journey as taking place along the spectrum of care constituted by the three primary paradigms of care available in the United States today: the technocratic, humanistic, and holistic models. The technocratic model defines one end of the spectrum, the holistic model falls on the opposite end, and the humanistic model can usefully be thought of as lying somewhere between these two. This book focuses on the radical paradigm shift from one end of the spectrum to the other—from technocratic to holistic—made by most of our interviewees. But many American physicians find this full paradigm shift far too threatening, and content themselves with a transition to the humanistic approach, which brings many satisfactions and does not demand nearly as radical a shift in practice or worldview. This humanistic model, while not the whole story, does hold rich promise for positive change in American medicine, and has far more possibilities for widespread mainstream acceptance than does the holistic model.

The book is divided into four sections. The two chapters in part I explicate the technocratic model of medicine and the process through which students absorb that model in medical school and residency. Chapter 1 describes the rise to dominance of the technomedical model, delineates its characteristics, and examines the principle of separation that underlies it and the linear, left-brained thinking it reflects. Physicians tell of the limitations that have caused so many patients and practitioners to strive to "think beyond" the narrow boundaries of this technocratic worldview. Chapter 2 interprets the seven years of medical school and residency as an initiatory rite of passage that imbues student-initiates with the core values and behavioral patterns of technocratic medicine. Current and former students relate both their awe and wonder at what they learn in medical school and their frustrations with the dehumanizing aspects of their training. Some of them successfully resisted their technomedical socialization; we will hear their stories too, and we take up the issue of gender, examining the particular challenges presented to women during medical training.

The chapters in part II describe the history and tenets of the two major paradigms that are working to expand technomedicine beyond its present narrow limits—the humanistic and holistic models of medicine. We begin in chapter 3 with the spectrum's middle range: the relationship-oriented humanistic model of medicine, the principles of balance and connection that underlie it, and the balanced, empathetic mode of thinking that fosters it. This more conservative model does not demand radical alterations in the technocratic approach, but rather softens its hard edges, adding warmth, compassion, conversation, and individualized treatment to patient care. (These are elements of holism as well—in fact, as we will explore in the book's final chapter, the holistic paradigm both encompasses and transcends the other two.) Chapter 4 explores that holistic paradigm, which defines the far end of the spectrum of care and constitutes the focal point for thought and practice that most of our interviewees have reached or toward which they aspire. Its underlying principles are connection and integration, and it emerges from a type of multimodal, right-brained type of thinking so fluid and integrative that it is difficult to explain many holistic principles in language that linear thinkers can make sense of; it thereby presents a revolutionary challenge to the technocratic worldview.

These three paradigms—the technocratic, humanistic, and holistic—define the conceptual and practical range of movement we discuss in this book. While the boundaries between them are blurry, it has been helpful to us as researchers and to our interviewees to identify their essential elements so that we can better understand the transformational journeys of physicians who choose to move across the spectrum these paradigms constitute, making the "paradigm shift" from doctor to healer that is the primary subject of this book. We trace these journeys in part III. Chapter 5 describes the primary catalysts that motivate physicians to move beyond the limitations of technomedicine into the wider world of holistic healing. From generalized frustration with the limits of techomedicine to the individual challenges of personal illness, we learn why physicians choose to make this journey and where they find the courage to take the first steps. Through retelling many of their stories, chapter 6 explores the myriad unique forms this transformational journey takes as well as the structural similarities these individual experiences share.

Part IV, "Living Holism," looks at the present and the future of holistic medicine. In chapter 7 we explore the practical repercussions of the full paradigm shift, with a focus on the specifics of medical practice within the holistic paradigm, including day-to-day realities such as job satisfaction, income, legal issues, and peer acceptance. Chapter 8 allows us to understand how the transformation of these physicians relates to the future of the vast American institution known as the health care system.

It has been a privilege to give cohesion in these pages to what may have appeared as idiosyncratic or isolated phenomena within the medical profession. The stories we tell and journeys we describe are the stories and journeys, not just of the hundred or so physicians we cite, but of countless doctors who have quietly undergone the profound transformation from doctor to healer. To all of them, we dedicate this book.

Acknowledgments

We wish to express our gratitude to several organizations and individuals who contributed to this book. First, we thank the Institute for Noetic Sciences for its financial support of the interviewing process, which allowed us to hear and, later, tell the actual stories of physicians. Second, we thank the American Holistic Medical Association for allowing us access to its members at conferences to conduct interviews for five consecutive years, for waiving conference registration fees to support our research, and for placing one of us on the conference program for three years to share this work when it was in process. Third, the MetaPhysicians, although no longer an organization in its own right, lent its spirit.

Individuals who must be mentioned include Terry Tyler, M.D., who founded the MetaPhysicians; he was the first to realize that his experience of transition was not an isolated one. We are deeply grateful to Bill Manahan, editor of *Holistic Medicine*, the magazine of the American Holistic Medical Association, for sending us the "Physician in Transition" stories and for his kind words and loving heart. We thank our editor, Martha Heller of Rutgers University Press, for her skills and for her unflagging enthusiasm and support. David Hess, Marilyn Schlitz, Peter Johnson, Alan Gaby, Bethany Hays, Barry Elson, and an anonymous reviewer also provided helpful editorial feedback.

Robbie Davis-Floyd expresses special thanks to her students at Rice University, Michelle Garza and Janna Flint, for the interview material they graciously allowed her to use, and to all of the premedical students in her medical anthropology classes at Rice for their open-mindedness and strong commitment to becoming healers. She also wishes to express her deep appreciation to her daughter, Peyton Floyd, for the consciousness and self-responsibility she brings to her own health care.

PART I

The Technocratic Paradigm

1 *The Technocratic Model of Medicine*

I do not recognize any difference between the machines made by craftsmen and the various bodies that nature alone composes.
—RENÉ DESCARTES

In the American mind, technology and evolutionary progress go hand in hand. When technology is combined with medicine, it assumes immense power and importance as the mediator between life and death, health and illness. American society's core value system is strongly oriented toward science, high technology, economic profit, and patriarchally governed institutions (Davis-Floyd 1992). Our medical system reflects that core value system: its successes are founded in science, effected by technology, and carried out through large institutions governed by patriarchal ideologies in a profit-driven economic context. Among these core values, in both medicine and the wider society, technology reigns supreme.

Doctors, in the course of discharging their responsibilities, often indoctrinate patients with the basic tenets of this technologically oriented system of values and beliefs. Formerly, the transmission of core societal values was vested in religious or spiritual institutions and their representatives. But by now the worship of science and technology has become the new American religion, and the priestly mantle of responsibility for transmitting these values has been laid in large part on physicians. It is no cultural accident that doctors must undergo a grueling seven-year-long training period, an initiatory rite of passage that thoroughly imbues them with the core values of the technocracy, enabling them to become not only physicians but also the representatives of Western society's deepest values and beliefs.

Of course, valuing technology does not require devaluing people; technology increasingly serves individuals in countless empowering ways. But the technology of a society is embedded in and created out of its dominant belief system, its worldview. The way a society conceives of and uses technology cannot help but reflect and perpetuate that worldview and the paradigm that underlies it. We label that paradigm "the technocratic model" because it is removed by decades of astonishingly sophisticated developments from its predecessor, the mechanistic model (Merchant 1983). These technologies have developed in a social context that privileges them and the individuals who control them, including M.D.'s. Despite its pretenses to scientific rigor, the American medical system is less grounded in science than in its wider cultural context. Like the medical systems of every other culture, technomedicine embodies the biases and beliefs of the society that created it.

A *technocracy* is a society that is hierarchical, bureaucratic, and organized around an ideology of technological progress. Undergirding modern medicine—with its specialized knowledge, technical procedures, and rules of behavior—is a paradigm that we label the technocratic model of medicine (or the technomedical model, for short). American physicians are steeped in this model throughout their training; it provides the underlying rationale for standard medical practice. We identify the basic tenets of the technomedical model as follows:

(1) Mind/body separation
(2) The body as machine
(3) The patient as object
(4) Alienation of practitioner from patient
(5) Diagnosis and treatment from the outside in (curing disease, repairing dysfunction)
(6) Hierarchical organization and standardization of care
(7) Authority and responsibility inherent in practitioner, not patient
(8) Supervaluation of science and technology
(9) Aggressive intervention with emphasis on short-term results
(10) Death as defeat
(11) A profit-driven system
(12) Intolerance of other modalities

These twelve interlinked tenets compose the skeleton of the technomedical model, its bare bones. In practice, this paradigm has many permutations that we do not treat here, and even within this model of medicine there is a great deal of variation between medical specialties and subspecialties and among individual practitioners. We acknowledge that such variations are rendered invisible by the approach we take.[1] Nevertheless, it is our conviction, as well as that of our forty interviewees, that biomedicine—or technomedicine, as we prefer to call it—exists in the United States as a hegemonic ideology that spawns an identifiable set of practices, is undergirded by a specific set of values and a style of thinking, and can be characterized in specific ways that are readily recognizable to both its adherents and its dissenters. All practicing physicians, whether they conform to this model or not, feel its pressure in myriad ways and will recognize that the standards by which they are evaluated come out of this paradigm and the view of reality it encodes.

Separation and Linearity

The main value underlying the technocratic paradigm of medicine is separation. The *principle of separation* states that things are better understood outside of their context, that is, divorced from related objects or persons. The impact of this divisive approach is profound and far-reaching in what it emphasizes as well as what it excludes. Various historians of science (Berman 1988, 1990; Grossinger 1982) have suggested that modern science itself is actually a product of a major separation, a choice to pursue the mechanical and measurable and leave the unquantifiable—the magic—behind.

This principle of separation arises from the left-brained, single-track, and overwhelmingly linear mode of thinking that has dominated Western science from its earliest codification. Although the whole brain is involved in all brain functions, the left hemisphere is predominantly involved in conceptually segmenting the flow of reality and classifying its parts.[2] We in the West achieve this classification in a linear fashion: we establish imaginary boundaries, which we often see as lines, between phenomena that are in fact connected. When we see connections, we see them too as lines. Anthropologist Dorothy Lee explains:

> In our own culture, the line is so basic that we take it for granted, as given in reality. We see it in visible nature, between material points, and between metaphorical points such as days or acts. . . . It is present in the induction and deduction of our science and logic. . . . Our statistical facts are presented lineally as a graph or reduced to a normal curve. . . . I have seen lineal pictures of nervous impulses and heartbeats, and with them I have seen pictured lineally a second of time. These were photographs, you will say, of existing fact, of reality—a proof that the line is present in reality. But I am not convinced . . . that we have not created our recording instruments in such a way that they have to picture time and motion, light and sound, heartbeats and nerve impulses lineally, on the unquestioned assumption of the line as axiomatic. [In Western culture] the line is omnipresent and inescapable, and so we are incapable of questioning the reality of its presence. (Lee 1950:92)

Conscious deductive reasoning, which can be logically explained and replicated, takes place in a linear fashion, with one idea leading to the next. Thus, this type of thinking is supervalued in the West and often couched in terms of normalizing rules; such rules insist that logical linear thinking (also known as "ratiocination") is the right way, indeed the only way, to arrive at a valid conclusion. Such logical progression from idea to idea and phenomenon to phenomenon presupposes the separateness of these ideas and things. This drive toward separation and classification can, if carried to an extreme, obscure the many meanings in the nonlinear, nonlogical interconnections and relationships between entities. Technomedicine continually runs this risk. For good or ill, it separates the individual into component parts, the disease into constituent elements, the treatment into measurable segments, the practice of medicine into multiple specialties, and the experience of illness from the flow of life.

Origins of the Technocratic Model of Medicine

In the twelfth and thirteenth centuries, the trade with the Arab world that developed as a result of the Crusades brought a wealth of new information about health and healing into Europe. Greek Hippocratic and Aristotelian traditions had been kept alive in Islamic cultural centers throughout the Middle East even as, in Europe, the medical legacy of the pagan Greeks and Romans was suppressed and forgotten. Flowing back into Europe from the 1100s on, this knowledge became the basis for the establishment of the first medical schools, which based their curricula on the Greek theory of the humors. Despite this institutionalization of medical training, the most effective practitioners of this time—and the main competition for physicians—tended to be female folk healers who worked empirically, gathering and experimenting with wild herbs. Four centuries of witch hunts and witch-burning effectively eliminated this class of healers; physicians often testified against them at their trials (Kors and Peters 1972). The witch hunts ended as Cartesian rationalism spread, relegating the fear of witches to the realm of quasi-religious superstition and ultimately separating religion from secular life. This cultural vivisection set the stage for the full acceptance of the mechanistic model that ultimately dominated the economic realm—which itself came to predominate, relegating religion and spirituality to the cultural margins.

Historically, the technomedical model derives from this mechanistic model of reality, which we inherited from the Scientific Revolution in Europe. As Carolyn Merchant demonstrates in *The Death of Nature* (1983), during the seventeenth century, when Western society experienced rapid commercial expansion, the machine replaced the organism as the underlying metaphor for the organization of the human universe. Prior to that, from the time of the druids to the time of Descartes, the European folk view saw the earth as a living organism infused with a feminine "world-soul" that interacted with humankind and all of nature in a vibrant, fully participatory way. Fourteen centuries of Christianity had weakened but not destroyed this folk conceptualization. But within the span of one century, Descartes, Bacon, Hobbes, and others developed and widely disseminated a philosophy that ultimately severed this sense of interconnection between humans and the planet they inhabit. This philosophy held that the world is not sentient but mechanistic, not participatory but inert. As a result of this switch in base metaphors, nature, society, and the human body came to be viewed as an assemblage of interchangeable parts that could be repaired or replaced from the outside. Under this model, God became the supreme clockmaker who set in motion a chain of events. Because nature was now viewed as a system of dead, inert particles moved by external, rather than inherent forces, the mechanical framework itself could legitimize the manipulation of nature. Those who freed themselves from the limitations of medieval superstition, this philosophy assumed, would discover these laws through science and manipulate them through technology. Power was thus to be "derived from active and immediate intervention in a secularized world" (Merchant 1983:193).

In the seventeenth century, applying this mechanical metaphor to the human body began the process of removing the body from the purviews of religion and philosophy and turning it over to science. To conceive of the body as a machine was to open it up to scientific investigation and get on with research, leaving all bothersome questions of spirituality and the integrity of the individual to the priests and philosophers. Phenomena such as feelings, social context, spiritual belief, and personality defied measurement and manipulation and thus had to be discounted. This view has characterized the technomedical approach right up to the present.

The Twelve Tenets of the Technomedical Model

(1) MIND-BODY SEPARATION

The human body presents a profound conceptual paradox to our society, for it is simultaneously a creation of nature and the focal point of culture. How can we be separate from nature when we are part of it? Descartes, Bacon, and others neatly resolved this problem in the 1600s when they established the philosophical separation of mind and body upon which the metaphor of the body-as-machine depends. This idea meant that the superior cultural essence of man, his mind—as well as the superior spiritual essence, his soul—could remain unaffected while the body, as a mere part of mechanical nature, could be taken apart, studied, and repaired.

Proponents of this approach have always been challenged to explain the origins and whereabouts of the mind, which stubbornly refuses to be reduced to the sum of its constituent parts. The technomedical model seems to assume that the mind does not actually reside in the body, but somehow transcends it.* Questions of spirit and soul also go unexplained in this model. Indeed, all nonquantifiable phenomena must be dismissed; often these are relegated to the marginalized realm of religion. During our interview with Larry Dossey, he put it this way:

> Western medicine is based on a reductionist, physically oriented view of human beings. Basically it says that everything that happens in the body is the result of what atoms and molecules are doing. There isn't any meaning to health and illness. Whether you're sick or if you're well, it's just a matter of the atoms and molecules following the blind order of nature. No meaning, no purpose, no goals, nothing of that sort. No real place for consciousness, attitudes, emotions, feelings, thoughts, because all that is just brain stuff, and therefore, more atoms and molecules and so on. So the whole thing leads to the conclusion that all therapies need to be physical in order to really work.

Prior to the development of this mechanistic model, religion was responsible for both the tangible body and the intangible soul. As the mechanistic approach took root in the Western world, body and soul were split asunder; the soul remained in the realm of religion, while primary responsibility for the human body was assigned to the medical profession. With the mechanistic model as its philosophical foundation, medicine could take on the challenging conceptual task of transforming the organic human body into a machine. This transformation was crucial to the development of Western society because the elaboration of an intelligible conceptual universe is an essential step in the formation of any society. Social cohesion and continuity are enhanced when a society's founding metaphors for cosmos, culture, and individual self are consistent with each other—when each element becomes a scaled-down version of the other. The body—the basic vehicle of human, and thus social, existence—officially had to reflect society's vision of itself. If a society chooses to see itself and the universe it inhabits as mechanistic, then it will need to see as equally mechanistic the human bodies that comprise it.

The problem here, of course, is that bodies are not machines, and therefore the human body represented a great challenge to this new mechanistic view. Thus it became both the cultural mission and the vested interest of Western medicine to prove the ultimate truth and viability of this

*Of course, models do not assume; people do! Occasionally throughout this book we will use phrases like "this paradigm assumes" or "the technocratic model insists" as shorthand for "proponents of the technocratic model insist." Use of this form of shorthand should not be interpreted as any indication that we are reifying paradigms into thinking systems. People think; paradigms provide templates for thought.

model by making the body *appear to be* as mechanistic as possible. American medicine's eventual success in this mission helped embed the machine metaphor in every aspect of American life, at the same time further enforcing the separation of body, mind, and soul.

(2) THE BODY AS MACHINE

In the mechanical world, taking things apart is the way to both learn how they work and fix them if they are broken. Why not use the same approach with the human body, which in addition to larger parts has molecules and cells to manipulate?

> The Cartesian model of the body-as-machine operates to make the physician a technician, or mechanic. The body breaks down and needs repair; it can be repaired in the hospital as a car is in the shop; once fixed, a person can be returned to the community. The earliest models in medicine were largely mechanical; later models worked more with chemistry, and newer, more sophisticated medical writing describes computer-like programming, but the basic point remains the same. Problems in the body are technical problems requiring technical solutions, whether it is a mechanical repair, a chemical rebalancing, or a "debugging" of the system. (Rothman 1982:34)

The February 1989 issue of *Life* suggests carrying this approach into the twenty-first century: "If we think of the human body as a kind of machine, doctors of the future will be like mechanics, simply replacing those parts that can't be fixed." Even physicians who stress the centrality of the soul have no problem maintaining a mechanistic view of the body as a "vessel," a "physical structure":

> It's very easy as a neurologist to deceive yourself into believing that we are nothing more than the compilation of our synapses . . . that free will and everything else is an illusion, and we are preprogrammed genetically by birth, by virtue of our neural programming. I don't believe that. I believe, actually, that human beings have a soul, and that the soul transcends the physical frame that we have. . . . I think the essence of who we are is the soul. . . . The body is this physical vessel that we exist in—a physical structure. (Peter Grote)

Physicians who treat patients as if their minds and bodies were separate often treat themselves the same way. Abuse of their bodies begins during medical school and intensifies during residency. Sleep-deprived and always on the run, medical students and residents cram their bodies with junk food and their brains with a surfeit of information (see chapter 2).

Once in private practice, trying to repay huge student loans and perhaps supporting a family, the physician who believes that the mind is not the body is all too likely to continue this pattern. In a system that rewards workaholism with money, status, and respect, M.D.'s turn their body-machines into tools for success. If they have to abuse that tool to make it continue to function in spite of overwork and high stress, and cut themselves off from their emotions, that behavior seems appropriate within this separatist worldview. As Jack Mansberger put it in our interview with him:

> Three or four years out in private practice, I stopped and looked at it, and what I saw was this tremendous box that I had built around my emotions. And it continued, because you just continue doing it and you just keep working and you just keep doing the same thing, and I wasn't feeling anything anymore. I used to be a kind of fun-loving guy, you know, have a good time and all those things. [People say you should] never go to a party that's all doctors because they're boring as hell. They don't have any outside interests, because they're stuck. And that's basically what's happened to me. I began to realize that I had shut off my emotions and couldn't even enjoy my wife and children or anything else. You ask yourself, What the hell are you doing here? But you're so busy doing it, you don't stop.

Many years of this sort of detached, self-abusive behavior deeply ingrain its patterns; it is hardly surprising that medical doctors have more problems than their patients with drugs and alcohol and have a higher suicide rate. Fritjof Capra (1988:279–280) sees this statistic as part of a schizoid trend in modern society; he notes that "our priests are not very spiritual, our lawyers are not beyond reproach . . . and our physicians are not very healthy." Bill Manahan, one of the physicians we interviewed, offered a rare glimpse at the emotional burden felt but rarely expressed by physicians in practice:

> It is so much pressure! The final decision is always mine. It is so much responsibility. From a deep and pleasant sleep I get ripped awake to learn that I soon may be responsible for the death of two previously healthy young women. How do I ever know which febrile child has meningitis? Am I doing an unnecessary spinal tap? Which forty-two-year-old man with chest pain has an MI [myocardial infarction—a heart attack]? Which thirty-one-year-old woman with a headache has a brain tumor? Which sixty-four-year-old man with fatigue is really depressed and will commit suicide within the next week? How many people did I see this week who were sexually or physically abused, but I was unable to "hear" what they were trying to tell me? Even if I do a perfect job and never miss a diagnosis, what about all the emotionally charged events that occur so frequently? How do I di-

> vorce myself from the pain of a child dying of cancer? From a seventy-four-year-old woman with painful arthritis who just wants to die? From the screaming agony of a mother whose seventeen-year-old has just been killed by a drunk driver while thoughts of my own seventeen-year-old pound in my head? We are expected to keep ourselves separated from not only our patients, but from our own pain, anger, and sadness.

Manahan's words illustrate the trauma and the contradiction that result from the mechanistic and separatist approach of the technomedical model, which seeks to separate not only doctor from patient, but also individuals from their emotions—an impossible task.

(3) THE PATIENT AS OBJECT

Mechanizing the human body and defining the body-machine as the proper object of medical treatment frees technomedical practitioners from any sense of responsibility for the patient's mind or spirit. Thus, practitioners often see no need to engage with the individual who inhabits that body-machine, preferring instead to think of and talk about their patient as "the gallbladder in 223": "[Listening to my coworkers excitedly explain] that an 'interesting case'—a child nearing a diabetic coma—had just been admitted, I realized with a shock what a distance that attitude puts between the doctors and their 'case,' who happened to be a very sick, frightened child with distraught parents" (Siegel 1986:4).

In *Birth in Four Cultures* (1993:70), anthropologist Brigitte Jordan demonstrates how this tendency to objectify patients as cases extends to refusal to discuss any details of that case with the patient who embodies it. A resident who had just performed a vaginal exam had the following conversation with an intern while standing at the foot of the laboring woman's bed:

> Resident: I think you're right. It's LOA.
> Intern: That's what I figured.
> Woman: What's LOA?
> Resident: It's loa, dear. You ever been to Hawaii? (Walks out with intern)
> Woman to anthropologist: I wish they wouldn't treat me like an idiot. It takes three of them to figure out that it's LOA and then they won't even tell me what it means. So what's LOA?
> (LOA stands for left, occipital, anterior—specifying the position relative to the pelvis of the baby's head.) (Jordan 1993:70)

As this scene indicates, the objectification of the patient can extend beyond discourse to objectifying the patient's body, discounting the patient's own ideas and feelings, and dismissing the patient's desire to be intellectually included in the conversation about her condition.

Medical interviews are cases in point. Typically, the physician attempts to elicit relevant information from the patient by asking a series of closed, rapid-fire questions that allow the patient little or no freedom to express personal opinions or concerns. The doctor does most of the talking; Beckman and Frankel (1984) showed that physicians interrupted patients after a mean time of eighteen seconds, and in 69 percent of visits did not allow them to complete their opening statements of symptoms and problems. Another study (Burack and Carpenter 1983) found that this type of interview uncovered only 6 percent of primary psychosocial problems. Physicians' lack of interest in the patient's views, fostered during medical training, is rooted in their underlying conceptualization of the patient not as a whole person but as the object of their treatment.

(4) ALIENATION OF PRACTITIONER FROM PATIENT

Susan DiGiacomo was a Ph.D. candidate in anthropology when she was diagnosed with Hodgkin's disease, a potentially fatal form of cancer. She describes her ordeal with the medical care system in "An Anthropologist in the Kingdom of the Sick." A trained researcher, she spent many hours reading up on all that was known about her condition and its treatment. When she discovered no consensus in the medical literature about how many chemotherapy sessions were required for a cure, she realized that her physicians were making experimental treatment decisions. She desired a collegial relationship with her physicians in which knowledge and information would be shared and treatment decisions mutually decided upon, while they sought to enforce a strict hierarchy in which she would follow the treatments they prescribed without asking too many questions. It took four years before these physicians came to fully understand and respect DiGiacomo's need for participation in her treatment decisions. She writes:

> Biomedicine as commonly practiced in the U.S. simultaneously individualizes its treatment of disease symptoms and routinizes dealings with the patient, so that the afflicted person is transformed from an integrated and fully functioning adult to a collection of diseased body parts. Further, biomedical opinion holds that sick people are less than fully competent adults simply by virtue of being physically unwell. The first difficulty of the patient, then, is not getting a fair hearing for his or her point of view concerning the illness and its treatment; it is getting the doctor to recognize that the patient, has, in fact, a point of view at all. . . . [F]rom the outset, the afflicted person is required to accept a reduced and defective patient self constructed for him or her by the doctor. (DiGiacomo 1987:4)

This kind of alienation from their patients is trained into physicians during medical school and residency, as they are taught to protect themselves by avoiding emotional involvement. Since their model of healing does not recognize any role for the emotions in illness and disease, it logically follows that there is no reason to deal with the patient's emotions at all. Thus they are free to protect their own feelings from the pain of caring too much about people who may die or whom they may never see again. In addition, as Melvin Konner points out in *Becoming a Doctor*:

> It is obvious . . . that the stress of clinical training alienates the doctor from the patient, that in a real sense, the patient becomes the enemy. (*Goddammit, did she blow her I.V. again? Jesus Christ, did he spike a temp?*) At first I believed that this was an inadvertent and unfortunate concomitant of medical training, but now I think that it is intrinsic. Not only stress and sleeplessness, but the sense of the patient as the cause of one's distress, contribute to the doctor's detachment. This detachment is not just objective but downright negative. To cut and puncture a person, to take his or her life in your hands, to pound the chest until ribs break, to decide upon drastic action without being able to ask permission . . . these and a thousand other things may require something stronger than objectivity. They may actually require a measure of dislike. (1987:373; italics in original)

As Arthur Kleinman notes in *The Illness Narratives*, at the heart of healing lies the potential for a powerful dialogue that can draw the practitioner into the patient's experience and so can make of illness and treatment a rare opportunity for moral education. But instead, the modern medical care system "does just about everything to drive the practitioner's attention away from the experience of illness. The system thereby contributes importantly to the alienation of the chronically ill from their professional care givers and, paradoxically, to the relinquishment by the practitioner of that aspect of the healer's art that is most ancient, most powerful, and most existentially rewarding" (1988:xiv).

(5) DIAGNOSIS AND TREATMENT FROM THE OUTSIDE IN

Perhaps the most revealing characteristic of the technomedical paradigm, the idea of diagnosing and treating patients from the outside in, speaks directly to the relationships among doctor, patient, illness, and cure. Only the rare physician is conscious that most medical practice is based on this principle or that alternatives to it exist.

The concept can best be understood in historical context. The American Medical Association, founded in 1848, coexisted over the next fifty years with a rich and diverse set of healing traditions and techniques. These included the medical and herbal lore of Native Americans, Appalachian and other Anglo folk traditions (see Kirkland et al. 1992), and the folk medicines of various immigrant groups. Homeopathy grew from European roots, while naturopathy, with its origins in native traditions reworked through European practice, and American regional developments like chiropractic and osteopathy gave healing a grass-roots flavor.

In the early 1800s, a large-scale health movement that today we would recognize as holistic began when one Samuel Thompson became profoundly disillusioned with the "regular doctors" of his time. Thompson developed a treatment regimen based on the belief that healing takes place not from the outside in, but from the inside out. In other words, the proper approach involves strengthening the body's ability to heal itself through nutrition, exercise, cleanliness, and right living. Thomsonianism swept the nation, for a time achieving equal status in a number of states with the medicine of the "regular doctors." In 1839, Thomsonianism boasted 3 million adherents out of an estimated U.S. population of 17 million (Grossinger 1982:224). Its success was a measure of popular dissatisfaction with "regular medicine." Descendants of the European barber-surgeons, the "regular doctors" were trained in the European medical tradition, which held that the job of the healer was to intervene in the disease process. The tools and techniques they had available for that intervention were rudimentary; their treatments consisted of bloodletting and administering toxic substances like mercury, which often killed their patients faster than the disease they were supposed to treat.

Perhaps not unfortunately, the role of the regular doctor was severely restricted in preindustrial American society by the limitations, not just of medical technology, but also of rural life. Most doctors practiced another trade such as farming, and many rarely saw their patients. A further limitation to the growth of professional medicine was the self-sufficiency of the rural population. As industrialization shifted the population to urban areas, the increase in communicable diseases along with labor specialization created a captive market for the medical profession. It was within this framework that the rationalists and the empiricists, whose philosophies are the forerunners of the technocratic and holistic models we describe in this book, squared off.

In brief, the rationalists took a mechanistic, materialist, and interventionist approach to medicine and based it on the cause-and-effect of Newtonian science. The empiricists based their treatments on respect for nature and the healing properties of herbs and other natural remedies that work with the body to strengthen it and support its life force. Two empirically based approaches to healing popular at the turn of the century were homeopathy and naturopathy. "Homeopathy" means treatment with the similar and "naturopathy" means treatment with nature; both of these healing systems involve supporting the body to heal itself and preventing illness by maintaining good health. "Allopathy," the work of the rationalists, means treatment with "the other" and involves introducing external agents to block the spread of disease once it has started.

The founding of the American Medical Association in 1848 gave the allopathic rationalists, the regular doctors, a strong organizational edge, and the introduction of the germ theory of disease in the late 1800s gave them, for the first time, a scientific basis on which to build their profession. Nevertheless, as many contemporary historians have noted, medicine's rise to dominance was not the straightforward result of scientific progress but had a great deal to do with physicians' publicity and organizational skills and their relationship with the American government. A medical monopoly was born after the publication of the Flexner Report, a study of medical training instituted and jointly funded by the Carnegie Foundation and the government in 1910, and supported by the AMA. It stands as the only systematic attempt at medical reform ever undertaken in this country.

The Flexner Report took as its standard the allopathic program that had been started at Johns Hopkins in Baltimore. The Report documented the variety of curricula used in the medical schools of the time, many of which taught homeopathy or naturopathy. Immediately following publication of the Flexner Report, all such schools were forced to adopt allopathic curricula or close. The nation witnessed an incredible level of harrassment aimed at eliminating nonallopathic practitioners. This approach was justified by the development and dissemination of the germ theory of disease, which aligned medicine with science in the public mind. Early results, which included the prevention of infections through sterilization and eventually (in the late 1930s) the healing of infections with antibiotics, were so dramatic that the allopathic model, with its focus on the aggressive use of symptom-suppressing substances, became the standard in the United States. The benefits of all other systems, which tended to focus on the inner resources of the individual and the powers of the immune system, were ignored. The result was the near-total dominance of the allopathic outside-in approach in American medicine from 1910 to the present, and the suppression of other modalities.[3]

For the individual physician, this outside-in approach often leads to a fascination with diagnosis and disease divorced from their human context, as a conventional technocratic physician describes:

> I took a hematology/oncology rotation when I was a senior medical student. I don't know why I was particularly struck by it except that it was

> exciting medicine. You could make diagnoses right away just by looking at blood films. . . . Hemologic malignancies: it's intellectually challenging. There are obscure diseases like certain kinds of anemias—interesting. Sickle cell disease is the best-defined genetic disease there is. . . . So that is scientifically pure to some degree. Some of the hereditary anemias and some of the clotting disorders are almost pure science. You can see a defect and you know what the molecular effect is and you can follow it all the way up to what happens on the physiological level. So that's fun . . . I enjoy it. (quoted in Biesele and Davis-Floyd 1996:306)

As this oncologist illustrates, conventional physicians often speak with delight of the fun of tracking a disease like a detective, the fascination of the "scientific purity" of sickle-cell anemia, the intellectual excitement sparked by a hemologic malignancy. While this outside-in approach has obvious benefits for the practitioner, it renders invisible the personality and the experiences of the patient who must live and perhaps die with these diseases.

(6) HIERARCHY AND STANDARDIZATION OF CARE

Hierarchy. In *Birth as an American Rite of Passage*, Davis-Floyd identifies science, technology, patriarchy, and institutions as primary components of the American core-value constellation. Hospitals display and perpetuate these core values especially well, because their hierarchies allow responsibility to be so generalized and diffused that few individuals have the power to fundamentally alter how things are done. Physicians and nurses who try to change the system often find themselves thwarted and stymied by other physicians, by hospital administrators, and ultimately by the combined forces of the legal and business systems of the technocracy.

Like its industrial predecessor, the technocracy is a hierarchically organized society. The term "technocracy" implies use of an ideology of technological progress as a source of political power (Reynolds 1991). It thus expresses not only the technological but also the hierarchical, bureaucratic, and autocratic dimensions of this culturally dominant reality model. As many businesses seek to make their own paradigm shift by busily transforming themselves into "organizational networks" and "flat corporations," our medical system remains true to its role as society's microcosm, rigidly hierarchical in three primary ways.

(1) The most basic kind of medical hierarchy is the subordination of the individual to the institution—many hospital routines, for example, operate in ways convenient for the medical staff but not for the patient.[4] Middle-of-the-night ministrations—weighing patients, taking blood pressure, drawing blood—may be an efficient use of staff time when not much

else is likely to be going on, but seem like harassment from the point of view of patients whose sleep cycles are constantly disrupted.

(2) A second type of medical hierarchy applies to physicians as a group, positioned over all other medical practitioners and far more powerful socially and politically than practitioners of other healing modalities. Health care workers bristle at the power of M.D.'s to define their responsibilities and circumscribe their authority. Subordinate practitioners such as nurses, physicians' assistants, nurse-practitioners, nurse-midwives, and physical therapists operate within strictly controlled scopes of practice determined by physicians. Refusing to license certain practitioners such as naturopaths (who are licensed in only eleven states), and restricting referral to others such as chiropractors, effectively consign many healing modalities to the medical margins. This treatment of health care workers and non-M.D. professionals contributes to the system's runaway costs and the uncontrolled proliferation of technology, which, in turn, produces moral and ethical dilemmas that the technomedical model is ill equipped to address.

(3) Finally, technomedicine's emphasis on specialty over primary care generates a hierarchy among physicians with powerful ramifications for economics and patient care. Primary care doctors, including family practitioners, internists, pediatricians, and obstetrician/gynecologists, have opportunities to become acquainted with their patients and to develop a sense of the patient's disease pattern and medical history. Strong patient-practitioner relationships often emerge; indeed, family practice is recognized as being one of the most caring and empathetic branches of medicine. Within the medical hierarchy, it has traditionally also been the most devalued. This devaluation reflected the overall trend in medicine toward devaluating generalists and privileging specialists, along with the high technology they command. Many experts believe that our country would be best served if at least half of our six hundred thousand doctors were primary care physicians, to whom about 80 percent of doctor visits are made. But two-thirds of American doctors are specialists, and up until recently medical graduates were choosing high-tech specialties at a rate of four to one—a trend that shows some signs of changing since HMOs around the country have begun to stress the importance of primary care.[5]

At least three forces contribute to the preference medical graduates have shown for becoming specialists. First is their training. Most medical school clinical training takes place within a hospital—the cathedral of specialists, where students observe the power and effectiveness of specialized techniques and are supervised by instructors who have mastered them. Most patients in hospitals need highly invasive care. They are there for testing, emergency treatment, or surgery. When the question is, Did the patient live or die? these techniques seem inordinately successful. Students are rarely exposed to the long-term, or even short-term, downside effects of such invasive care, which can range from infection to permanent disability, and thus they are often unduly prejudiced in its favor.

A second reason why students choose specialization is economic. Many medical graduates have staggering debt and are entering their careers several years behind their cohorts in other professions. Salaries for generalists range from $80,000 to $125,000. To earn this income, primary care doctors assume a great deal of responsibility for keeping abreast of technical developments in many, many areas. For example, family doctors must keep in mind prescribing levels as well as new drug developments for infant, adult, and aged patients. They maintain referral networks with every type of specialist, visit hospitalized patients, and take calls on nights and weekends. Specialists can work less and earn a great deal more.[6]

A third reason for choosing specialty care is the opportunity to practice solely through technique, leaving aside matters of social and interactional skills. Specialists are not expected to be overly concerned with the emotional status of their patients. They are expected to shine the light of their expertise on the problem, fix it if possible, and move on. They often participate directly in research, thereby linking themselves to the "pure science" that underlies medicine and sparing themselves the social science side of medical care. The more specialized a physician, the less is expected in terms of interpersonal skills, communication, and empathic expression. Wendell Berry speculates that specialization is a "way of institutionalizing, justifying, and paying highly for a calamitous disintegration . . . of the various functions of character [such as] workmanship, care, conscience, and responsibility" (1996:10). Specialists' social chilliness may be overlooked or borne by the patient, since interaction with them is usually limited; often the primary care doctor is enlisted to interpret results and provide guidance. One family practitioner, Glenn Masterson, expressed their differences in this way:

> A patient came in today who had been to the cardiologist, who is mad at her because she quit taking her drug because she didn't feel well with it. The cardiologist said he couldn't help her unless she went back on the medicine, so she did. I'd never tell a patient that. I'd tell them that I think this will help and there are reasons for taking it, there is a downside, but if it doesn't help, you're not happy with it, we can make a choice, try something else. . . . I never make a particular treatment a condition for a patient.

In the past three decades, the proliferation of chronic conditions has transferred many patients into the ongoing care of a specialist. Cancer is now considered a chronic disease, with patients undergoing years of treatment before succumbing, or, in less than half the cases, being cured. Rheumatologists and endocrinologists as well as oncologists are likely to follow patients through many episodes of their illness, juggling drugs and therapies anew each time.

The economic impact of the growth of specialties is staggering. Patients have become powerless to assess the relative value of diagnostic and treatment options. Typically, persons with a complex or unresponsive conditions are handed around from one specialist to another with little coordination of care until they either give up or succumb to the ill effects of the pharmacological disaster that follows. Managed care has attempted to control costs by imposing new behaviors on both doctors and patients without, in most cases, examining the underlying greediness of the technocratic behemoth driving the system—a situation exacerbated by technomedicine's hierarchical structure and continuing attempts to standardize care.

Standardization. As in other realms of social life, in medicine, hierarchy and standardization go hand in hand. Those at the top of a hierarchy, considered more important, are granted the authority to determine the rules by which others must live. As we have seen, medical care in this country flows through hierarchical channels. Traditionally these have been headed by doctors who use techniques and therapeutics approved by regulatory bodies within licensed institutions; today the head of a given medical hierarchy is more likely to be the CEO of the managed care or insurance company. In both cases, the leader will set up the system to enforce standardization of care, as deviation from the norm can result in litigation or punitive action against the physician or the institution or both.

Physicians' acceptance and approval of the standardization of care derives from the value the technocratic model of medicine places on separation. If patients can be separated from their environment and community, the body isolated from the mind and emotions, and the limb, tissue, or organ isolated from the rest of the body, it is possible to predict with some accuracy how the body-machine will respond to a given therapy. Western medicine isolates in order to standardize, and in turn, standardization produces more isolation, as Susan DiGiacomo learned from experience:

> The day before surgery to biopsy my liver and remove my spleen and several lymph nodes, I met the anesthesiologist. Unsmiling and unwilling to provide much specific information, he told me very briefly what his function would be. My main concern at that point, however, was where I would wake up. I did not want to be alone. I wanted to know where the recovery room was so that my husband could be there when I came to. "That's impossible," he said flatly. When I asked him to explain why, he trotted out a series of hackneyed excuses . . . ending up with "It's not our policy to allow relatives into the recovery room." The surgeon, when approached with the same request, reacted in the same way. (1987:322)

"It's not our policy" seems to be medicalese for "We're not willing to deal with patients on an individual basis." DiGiacomo continues: "Doctors (and nurses) expect to do their work according to established hospital routine. The resulting standardization and depersonalization of patient care are rationalized as necessary for the 'efficient' functioning of the hospital and the benefit of the patient. . . . Patients who take issue with hospital rules incur the wrath of hospital staff, and in consequence are labeled 'bad' patients. . . . I have no doubt that I was so labeled after this encounter" (1987:346).

Should patients have a sudden awakening to the maltreatment that standardization inflicts—a wish, for example, to leave the hospital because of its intrusive procedures or nonnourishing food—they may find punitive tactics in place to stop them: insurance companies often refuse to pay the bills of patients who leave the hospital "AMA"—against medical advice.

Summing up his experience of the third and fourth years of medical school, Melvin Konner, M.D., provides a thoughtful analysis from the practitioner's perspective of the links between the legal, psychological, and social dimensions of the standardization of care:

> Hewing to a standard of behavior toward patients is part of a much larger process of practicing medicine according to the norm. In the norm there is safety. This is true in the ultimate legal sense—a judge will rule on alleged error or negligence contingent on the local standard of practice. If you do what is commonly accepted . . . then you are probably safe. Psychologically, the safety of the norm is even more important and ubiquitous. You *feel* safe, not just legally but morally, to the extent that you do what everyone else is doing. (1987:366)

Konner notes that the standardization of care often takes the form of ritualistic routines so ingrained in the practitioner by constant repetition that they become reflexive, and points out that physicians derive a strong sense of comfort from these routines. In all cultures, people use repetitive rituals to provide themselves with a sense of order, stability, and control. In professions like medicine, where chaos and uncertainty pervade daily practice, cleaving to ritualistic routines in which they can demonstrate clear competence can hold fear at bay and give practitioners a much-valued sense of confidence and control over what are often very uncertain outcomes. While practitioners frequently insist, as DiGiacomo points out above, that standardized routines are necessary for the efficient functioning of the institution, the deeper truth is that many of them would be lost without the confidence-enhancing functions of standardization.

On a wider scale, standardization allows commercial interests such as pharmaceutical and medical technology firms to direct research and ultimately design treatments for application to masses of people. These treatments are presumed to affect each person in the same way, with weight and age the only variables of importance. This belief gives rise to consulting room exchanges in which the patient protests that the medicine, instead of helping, made her feel sicker. It is perfectly correct in this paradigm for the physician to reply, "You must be metabolizing it incorrectly." On rounds during her training as an obstetrical resident, Michelle Harrison "saw a baby with a cut on its face and the mother said, 'My uterus was so thinned that when they cut into it for the section, the baby's face got cut.' The patient is always blamed in medicine. The doctors don't make mistakes. 'Your uterus is too thin,' not 'We cut too deeply.' 'We had to take the baby' (meaning forceps or cesarean), instead of 'The medicine we gave you interfered with your ability to give birth'" (1982:174). In other words, deviations from the standard are presumed to be the patient's fault.

(7) AUTHORITY AND RESPONSIBILITY INHERENT IN PRACTITIONER, NOT PATIENT

In line with its hierarchical structure, the technocratic model invests authority in physicians and in institutions and their personnel. Within this paradigm, a person who consults a doctor is a "patient." This word is surely not casually invoked, since patience is one of the qualities that make a "good patient." Patience is expected when there is a long wait to see the doctor, as well as when doctors insists on pursuing their line of questioning instead of addressing the patient's concerns. Western medicine's value on standardization defines the way patients should behave in order for them to be treated for their complaints.

The doctor is the presumed expert. Physicians are trained to make quick decisions and stand by them. While helpful in emergency situations, speedy decision-making has limited usefulness in a clinical setting. Yet as virtually the only model most doctors learn, it shapes the typical doctor-patient dialogue. Intuitive thinking, brainstorming, creative option generation, and open-ended questions are usually taboo. Obvious cues such as titles and white coats signal the authority of the physician, who can add to his status by withholding information, appearing rushed or annoyed, and using technical jargon the patient cannot understand.

When the doctor is the authority, the patient lacks responsibility, for, in medicine as in other areas of life, authority and responsibility go hand in hand. Many doctors feel that it is incumbent upon them to determine the course of treatment for an individual. They are able to present an option as *the* answer quite easily, by simply refusing to discuss nonparadigm alternatives such as natural healing methods or no treatment at all. In this scenario, a patient's most comfortable role is abdication of personal preference in favor of the doctor's choice.

Technomedicine's investment of both authority and responsibility in physicians and hospitals is a double-edged sword. Although medical personnel do have the power to give orders to patients and establish institutional policies and procedures, they can be and often are held to be accountable for deaths and outcomes that no mortal could prevent. The proliferation of lawsuits against hospitals and doctors over the past two decades is testimony to the way Americans have turned this tenet of the technocratic model against its proponents. As one physician observed, "If you choose to play God, you're going to be held responsible for the natural disasters."

(8) SUPERVALUATION OF SCIENCE AND TECHNOLOGY

Supervaluation of Science. Willis Harman, former president of the Institute of Noetic Sciences, has suggested that Western scientific assumptions constitute the dominant myth of our society. He outlines the three basic assumptions of science as: *objectivism*, the assumption of an objective world that one can hold at a distance and study separately from oneself; *positivism*, the assumption that the real world is what is physically measurable; and *reductionism*, the assumption that we really come to understand a phenomenon through understanding the behavior of its elemental parts (1994:111). Objectivism, reductionism, and positivism characterize the scientific framework within which the techniques used to diagnose and treat human ills are developed, evaluated, and implemented. Thus science makes little room for ambiguity, subjectivity, or individual difference. It focuses on facts and hypotheses that can be proven or disproven through research. As Zerubavel (1991:59) notes, "Science dreads anomalies. . . . Traditionally expected to caulk any crack in the mental wall separating the natural from the 'supernatural,' it likewise excludes whatever transgresses the conventional limits of its discourse or methodology (acupuncture, astrology) as 'non-scientific.'"

The general public tends to assume that doctors are scientists—a questionable assumption. Most medical students receive little or no training in research methodology and analysis; much medical research is criticized by trained quantitative researchers as inconclusive because faultily performed. And physicians themselves tend to uncritically assume a scientific basis for most of what they do—"I'd have to see the study" is a commonly heard phrase from physicians resistant to alternative therapies. Yet doctors routinely use many practices unsupported by science. Ready examples come from obstetrics, where medical tradition and "standards of care" demand numerous interventions in labor and birth that have been proven ineffective and even harmful in randomized controlled trials, including the routine use of the electronic fetal monitor (Enkin, Kierse, and

Chalmers 1989; Goer 1995; Rooks 1997). Further examples include the widespread use of immunization and many high-tech procedures, such as cardiac bypass surgery, never subjected to clinical trials.

The primary measure medical science employs to determine the efficacy of a given intervention or therapy, the randomized clinical trial or RCT, is a valuable tool as far as it goes. It tests new treatments by randomly allocating subjects to a control or to an experimental group, a process intended to eliminate the kind of bias that can occur when patients are aware of the treatment they are receiving. The gold standard in RCTs is the double-blind trial, in which neither patient nor practitioner knows whether the patient is receiving a standard treatment, the experimental treatment, or a placebo.[7]

Perhaps the major problem with RCTs is that, true to the technocratic paradigm, they often do not take into account nonquantifiable phenomena, and they assume that everything that should be controlled for *can* be controlled for, so that outcomes will be meaningfully comparable across large groups. Yet many variables cannot be controlled for; one of these is the impact of the experimenter (doctor) on the subject (patient). Tone of voice, eye contact, and touch have been found to figure so prominently in activating an individual's healing response that one might conclude that any experiment involving contact is open to question. Furthermore, if the wrong questions are being researched, even the most careful randomizing will not make the study meaningful or useful.

As Larry Dossey notes, "Just as behaviorism considers the rat's 'mind' to be a superfluous or silly concept, many research methodologists consider the human mind to be generally inconsequential in double-blind testing" (1995a:10). Dossey discusses three assumptions of the double-blind study, which, though rarely articulated, underlie its methodology and describe its limitations. The first assumption is that researchers can duplicate the initial conditions of an experiment in another time and location. The second assumption is that "the laws governing health and illness are immutable; they apply equally everywhere and at all times, have no 'down time' and do not play favorites." The third assumption is that "healing is a process taking place in a physical universe. Introducing immaterial factors such as 'consciousness,' 'mind,' or 'the spiritual' into medicine is to become bogged down in a metaphysical swamp" (1995:60). Because in many cases these three assumptions do not reflect reality, the limitations of the double-blind RCT are self-evident. Nevertheless, it remains the gold standard in the scientific evaluation of medical treatments, and the fact that this kind of science is supervalued in the United States has to date effectively prevented the fair evaluation of many alternative therapies.

Supervaluation of Technology. As overvalued as science in the medical field are the contributions of technology. If a woodworker uses an elaborate set of tools to construct a piece of furniture, the focus remains on his creation; the tools are in the background, merely means to an end. Sometimes this is also true in medicine—the stethoscope can be merely a means for the doctor to hear the heartbeat—but, especially in the case of "high technologies," the machine is positioned in the foreground. More than a means to an end, the machine itself is often perceived as the definitive element in a diagnosis or treatment. For example, when a doctor uses a stethoscope, she touches the patient, speaks to him, listens with her own ears to his heartbeat or his lungs, interprets the sounds she hears through her own bodily perceptions, and arrives at a diagnosis that depends in large part on her physical senses. When the same doctor uses a CAT (computerized axial tomography) scanner or an MRI (magnetic resonance imaging) device, only the machine touches or interacts with the patient during the procedure; the physician's role is reduced to the interpretation of the mechanically mediated results, which in turn are generally regarded as more objective and therefore more reliable than the physician's subjective perceptions.

In *Megatrends*, John Naisbitt coined the phrase "high tech, low touch" to express the American supervaluation of technology and concomitant devaluation of personal contact. This shift in medicine from a human- to a machine-mediated practice has developed in tandem with the transformation of American society into a machine-mediated culture. In fact, Americans are known by anthropologists to be one of the "lowest touch" societies in the world. Minimizing human contact, Americans have maximized instead their contact with technology, as Jerry Mander's *In the Absence of the Sacred* describes: "From morning to night we walk through a world that is totally manufactured, a creation of human invention. We are surrounded by pavement, machinery, gigantic concrete structures. Automobiles, airplanes, computers, appliances, television, electric lights, artificial air have become the physical universe with which our senses interact" (1991:32).

Such technologies not only pervade our cultural environment, but also form the major trajectory of our cultural evolution, which we define as moving from low- to high-technology systems. Evolutionary "progress" has become an intensifying series of interactions with the artifacts we have created. This human-machine coevolution has had an extraordinary impact on medical care, in which "progress" has come to mean the development of ever more sophisticated machines. Such new technologies are usually introduced by their marketers, who tend to describe them solely in terms of their best-case use and minimize any detrimental effects.

The electronic fetal monitor (EFM) is a case in point. This machine, which counts a baby's heartbeat and estimates the strength of a mother's contractions, was invented by physician Edward Hon in the early 1970s in the hopes that it would prevent unnecessary interventions by providing accurate information about the baby's condition and the progress of labor (Kunisch 1989). Its manufacturers sponsored conferences all over the country to "evaluate" its efficacy, offering expense-paid trips to physicians who, upon arrival, found themselves walking through elaborate EFM displays to get to the meeting rooms (Wagner 1997). Now pervasive in hospital birth, the EFM has resulted not in fewer interventions or better outcomes but in higher costs and higher cesarean rates.[8] Nevertheless, the widely touted best-case scenario prevails, with its false story about the necessity for and efficacy of these machines, and many hospitals routinely employ them in more than 80 percent of labors.

Rapid diffusion and acceptance of a new technology often has more to do with its symbolic value than with its actual efficacy. As anthropologist Brigitte Jordan (1993) points out, technology can be so effective, so dazzling, that it captures our interest and effectively hypnotizes us into not only accepting it, but incorporating it into our lives, with little awareness of the profound changes each new technology can bring. Television of course is a case in point. In the hospital, machines also mesmerize: "The amplified fetal heartbeat sounds like galloping horses . . . both the sound of the galloping and the vision of the needle traveling across the paper, making a blip with each heartbeat, are hypnotic, often giving one the illusion that the machines are keeping the baby's heart beating" (Harrison 1982:90). So powerful is this illusion, as Davis-Floyd found during her research on birth, that nurses often become reluctant to detach the mother from the monitor for fear that the baby's heart will stop. While they know intellectually that this is nonsense, nevertheless they are emotionally affected by these machines, which speak with powerfully symbolic, culturally privileged voices, generating a sense of dependence on them not only for information, but also for the safety, even the life, of the child.

Jordan notes that when medical treatment moves from one level of technology to another, the movement is nearly always one way:

> When different levels of technology are available in the same environment, the solution to problems that arise on one level is almost always sought on the next higher level, hardly ever on the next lower level. For example, if a woman's contractions slow down because she has been moved to a delivery table, she is not allowed to resume the previously effective position, but rather is given pitocin to speed up labor, or perhaps a Cesarean. . . . Referral networks are always set up for a one-way flow of clients, from low-tech to high-tech facilities and practitioners. It may well be that this bias for upscaling rather than downscaling is a property of technological systems in general. (1993:212)

The EFM, along with CAT and PET (positron emission tomography) scanners, kidney dialysis machines, and hundreds of others, "upgrades" medical care in keeping with our notions of evolutionary progress. If medicine were not evolving toward the ever-increasing use of machines, it would appear to be sinking into the Dark Ages while the rest of us race on ahead. Few stop to look at the cumulative results of each individual decision to pursue a new technology. Few want to admit that the hospital has to "encourage" the doctors to use the shiny new machine in order to help pay for it. Once it is there, it must be reckoned with, and any decision *not* to use it begins to look like substandard care—a reality that reflects both the financial and the symbolic supervaluation of technology in the American medical system.

(9) AGGRESSIVE INTERVENTION, WITH EMPHASIS ON SHORT-TERM RESULTS

The logical corollary of a focus on "healing from the outside in" is the employment of aggressive tactics to alter the course of disease. From the outside in, most chronic conditions cannot be cured; rather their symptoms can be managed—but only at the price of the side effects of the powerful drugs used. Holistic physician David Edelberg (1994:23–24) details the plight of the chronically ill patients he often sees:

> Our most typical patient at the center is someone with a chronic illness; conventional medicine does poorly with chronic illnesses. The specialist prescribes harsher and harsher drugs. At some point the patient reads the package insert and says, "Oh, my God, he wants me to take *this*? There must be something better to do." That's the sentence that I hear from patients. They come in with a stack of records and a diagnosis of rheumatoid arthritis and say, "My doctor wants me on methotrexate, prednisone, and gold, and I read the side effects and fainted."

As medical research has progressed, it has produced more and more effective pharmaceuticals and medical technologies. Intensifying the aggressive approach of technomedicine today is an armory of possible interventions exploding exponentially, following the technocratic principle, "If it can be done, it must be done," and resulting in the distinct possibility of the virtual transformation of much of biological life.

Technological Intervention: The One-Two Punch. Since the dawn of the Industrial Revolution, Western society has sought to dominate and control nature. And the more we controlled nature, including our natural bodies, the more we feared the aspects of nature we could not control. This led to the emergence of a phenomenon that anthropologist Peter C. Reynolds (1991) has labeled the "One-Two Punch" of technological intervention. Take a natural process that is working well—say, a river in which salmon annually swim upstream to spawn. Punch One: "Improve" it with technology—build a dam and a power plant, generating the unfortunate by-product that the salmon can no longer swim to their spawning grounds. Punch Two: Fix the problem created with technology with more technology—take the salmon out of the water with machines, let them spawn and grow the eggs in trays, feed the babies through an elaborate system of pipes and tubes, then truck them back to the river and release them downstream.

Reynolds's brilliant insight was that, while most people see Punch Two as an accidental byproduct of Punch One, the deeper truth is that *Punch Two is the point.* We in the West have become convinced that altering natural processes makes them better—more predictable, more controllable, and therefore safer. For example, when the Corps of Engineers lined the banks of large sections of the waterways of the Everglades and installed floodgates, most people considered the change an improvement. No matter that the long-term effect has been to lose huge portions of this natural resource to soil erosion.

Such sacrifice of the long-term for the short-term solution is characteristic of the aggressive intervention of the One-Two Punch in medicine as in other realms of social life. The focus is on the quick fix, "a pill for every ill," while the long-term costs of this approach are too often ignored. Physician David Edelberg describes an experience that reflects this short-term focus:

> One time I was making rounds in a hospital and I had this vast number of charts. . . . And I said, "There are ten people in the hospital. Of these ten, seven are here for diseases of lifestyle. Three are here because of complications of treatment. There is something flawed. And now I'm racing to my office to put out fires that will not prevent those people from filling these beds in ten years. The man with epigastric burning now, in ten years will have a coronary and be in the intensive care unit, and my contact with him has just been putting out fires. If I could help him change his lifestyle and see where the problem is I might be doing something for someone." I was really beginning to question if I was doing anything for anyone at all.

The quick fix Edelberg's patients were expecting, which only leads to more problems later on, reflects the cultural pervasiveness of the One-Two Punch, and describes a powerful motivating force in American society that might be called the *technocratic imperative.* This impetus to improve on nature through technology at the expense of personal responsibility has as its ultimate aim to free us altogether from nature's limitations. Beyond seeking freedom from disease through a pill for every ill, we seek freedom from the limitations of the earth through the development of space technology; from the limitations of our bodies through computers, robotics, and prostheses; from death through cryogenics; and from the limitations of natural reproduction through the new reproductive technologies, from artificial insemination to in vitro fertilization. On a global scale this aggressive, manipulative approach has resulted, over time, in the "taming of the wilderness," the penetration of humans into every corner of the globe, and the pollution of the natural environment from pole to pole. In the realm of American health care, this approach has resulted in the medicalization of the entire human life cycle.

Intervention in the Human Life Cycle: Medicalization from Conception to Death. Medical care in the United States has become a conception-to-death experience. The beginning and end of life, once considered private, family events, today often involve massive medical intervention. Determining who shall be born, who shall live, and who shall die consumes an enormous amount of human and economic resources—a manifestation of the effects of the technocratic imperative.

For example, as recently as two decades ago, it was accepted that some couples had children and others did not. However, during the 1980s, childlessness became a potentially treatable "condition" due to the development of an array of expensive and highly interventionist techniques that offer a chance of artificially induced conception (see Davis-Floyd and Dumit 1998). The existence of these technologies in effect obliges couples who sincerely wish to conceive to pursue an ever-intensifying course of experimental treatments with low odds of success. Since environmental pollution affects sperm, some sperm banks today, in true One-Two Punch form, even go so far as to recommend artifical insemination with sperm that has been "lavaged" (a technique of selecting out the healthiest and most motile sperm) for couples who live in polluted areas (Schmidt and Moore 1998)—a short-term technofix that is far easier to carry out than the long-term solution of cleaning up the environment.

Even if conception occurs "normally," that is without the assistance of a fertility specialist, pregnancy and birth are routinely handled as medical events. So thoroughly are they altered by medical technology that obstetrical residents quickly come to believe they can't take place any other way. During her residency, Christiane Northrup "didn't think it was possible to deliver a baby without an IV, rupturing the membranes, an internal uterine catheter, and a fetal scalp electrode." The normal newborn, in a medical setting, is evaluated, examined, weighed, and treated prophylactically within minutes of birth. Pediatricians take over where the obstetrician leaves off to advise mothers on breastfeeding, diet and nutrition for their baby, handling developmental stages, and discipline—areas of life once the province of elder women. The first years of life are a round of periodic checkups, immunizations, screenings for disease, and medical treatment of minor illness, including colds, influenza, childhood illnesses, and accidents.

Later childhood and adolescence represent the only years typically exempt from medical intervention, unless a youngster falls into the burgeoning diagnostic categories of learning or developmentally disabled, or exhibits a behavior disorder. The onset of the first menstrual period is a ticket for reentry to medical care for young women, while young male and female athletes turn to sports medicine specialists to improve their performance and heal their injuries. Women are expected to use medical advice and treatment for any disturbance with menstruation, fertility, pregnancy, and lactation; men for any impairments in sexual functioning or in the quality of their sperm. Menopause has recently entered the fold as a condition which requires medical diagnosis, treatment, and monitoring, while the diagnosis of "aging" raises the question of hormone treatments and plastic surgery to help the old appear young.

This medicalization of the human life cycle has special implications for women. Anthropologists Emily Martin (1987) and Robbie Davis-Floyd (1992) have documented the bias against women inherent in biomedicine, which defines the prototype of the properly functioning body-machine as male. Where female biology differs from male, medicine tends to view it as inherently dysfunctional. Thus, medical textbooks traditionally use metaphors of decay and degeneration to describe female biological processes such as ovulation, menstruation, and menopause, while reserving to male processes such as sperm production glowing terms of regeneration and abundance (Martin 1987:48). Barbara Ehrenreich and Deirde English (1973a) and others have documented the intense masculinist bias pervasive in medical practice for centuries; in the 1800s in the United States, for example, women were regularly hospitalized for "hysteria"; removal of the uterus, thought to be the seat of "female problems," and excision of the clitoris were routine treatments for this and other "female complaints."

The role of women in the health care system and their participation as patients confirm the alignment of medicine with patriarchal values and a concomitant devaluation of the feminine. Women live in a world where their rights are more circumscribed than men's, despite society's overt commitment to equality. As a result, they are more apt to take direction from an authority—a quality that makes them "good citizens and good patients." Women make the majority of visits to doctors. They have been convinced that almost all of their biological processes and body parts need periodic monitoring and are likely to require treatment.[9] Defining women's bodies as inherently dysfunctional locks them into technomedicine's One-Two Punch and keeps them tied to the authority of the medical care system. They are easily influenced to involve their children in the same system, and are often the driving force behind men's participation.

Midlife brings forth the full panoply of lifestyle and auto immune conditions for both genders, and individuals suffering from these crowd the waiting rooms of every primary care physician in the country. Heart disease, arthritis, diabetes, cancer, chronic fatigue, neuromuscular diseases, as well as digestive and respiratory dysfunction require "workups" to define their characteristics and provide a treatment plan. Although there are many weapons in the arsenal of palliation and relief for these conditions, their recalcitrance causes as much distress for many physicians over time as it does for their patients. Yet all of these diseases respond to improvements in nutrition, lifestyle, psychological well-being, and many alternative therapies. Perhaps the most unfortunate result of the technomedical model's emphasis on aggressive intervention is that the attention it commands, the drama that often surrounds it, and its emphasis on short-term, immediate results have created health care consumers who are impatient with slow-acting treatments, even when they offer the promise of long-term cures.

(10) DEATH AS DEFEAT

Medicine wages its final heroic battle when death appears. If it rears its head in old age, modern medicine is ready! One-third of the $160 billion Medicare budget is spent on individuals with less than one year to live; nearly half of that is spent during the last month of life (Califano 1994:63). Such aggression against death causes many people to seek legal protections against the onslaught of technology. The pressure for life at any cost is so intense that individuals often find that they must battle with family members and medical professionals to refuse disfiguring, painful, and potentially dangerous treatment, to be allowed to succumb to their illness.

In a model where death is the enemy and dying tantamount to failure, mortality is a mighty foe. The death of a human being is a defeat for a medical system that strives for ultimate control over nature. Death is a painful reminder that such striving is illusory—no matter how much we dissect life in order to understand it, no matter how many operations we perform or prostheses we insert, we cannot eliminate death. Medical ethics are attempting to grapple with the conundrum created by a mechanistic approach to dying that is unable to account for qualitative issues. With machines to breathe for us and beat our hearts, drugs to stimulate and simulate major bodily functions, and transplants within and across species to overcome organ failure, the question of death has become highly complicated.

In the arena of the dying, medicine still operates as though its resources were endless. Staving off death costs $62 billion dollars in intensive care each year. Although care given in the last days of life has long been known to be more costly than most medical episodes, doctors have shown little inclination to change except in the most obvious cases, owing to a combination of training, ethical and legal concerns, and deference to patients' families. Medical heroics require that more and more technology and techniques be developed. Again we return to the interventionist guiding principle of medical research: "If it can be done, it must be done," which is, as we have seen, a perfect reflection of our relationship to the natural world. The ecological disasters we are generating on our planet in the name of capitalism and progress result from exactly this approach. Within the medical realm, however, the One-Two Punch takes a more insidious form, pursuing apparently virtuous goals of saving (or producing) life at all costs, preventing death, and aggressive, single-minded intervention. This focus on dramatic and aggressive measures obscures the options of accepting death when appropriate, and otherwise relying on slower, less certain, but more complete methods of remediation, including long-term lifestyle changes and prevention through education and public health.

(11) A PROFIT-DRIVEN SYSTEM

The shaman and druidic priest were supported by the community in exchange for their skills. As society became more complex, all those who worked to benefit others, including healers, came to expect payment in the form of goods or money. However, not until the rise of pharmacology and technology did medical care become completely unaffordable, requiring elaborate financing schemes to ensure its availability. No other essential commodity in life lies beyond the economic grasp of Americans of average means. They can save money and buy a home; they can send their children to public schools and universities. But it has become an accepted fact of American life that medical care is priced outside the reach of most individuals, and will require some form of third-party payment. This option has allowed for the development and proliferation of elaborate and expensive medical technology and pharmacology. The interlocking economics of insurance companies, pharmaceutical and medical device corporations, and medical institutions comprise the single largest element in our gross national product. The momentum of this economic monster is impossible to calculate, but it is readily experienced by any movement or individual who gets in its way.

The social programs initiated in the 1950s and 1960s set the stage for exponentially increasing medical costs by, in effect, allowing government to subsidize health care. Beginning in the 1970s, there have been waves of legislation aimed at containing costs, with the focus shifting from the hospital to the physician to the patient. One might laud the various attempts at cost containment if indeed they had produced a system that sized itself down to something less than double-digit percentages of the

GNP. However, the feeding frenzy continues; today HMOs and insurance and techno-pharmaceutical companies show astronomical profits, while hospitals and doctors cinch in their belts another notch.

One might be tempted to ask how the idea of health got lost in health care. Seldom in the past fifty years has there been any attempt to evaluate the health care system in terms of outcomes or health status. For example, the war on cancer, initiated by Richard Nixon, has cost $32 billion in government-funded research with only a 1 to 2 percent improvement per year in the rate of cancer deaths by 1994, which were still 6 percent higher than in 1970. Since the Flexner Report, every attempt to reform the U.S. medical system in this century has targeted only its financing methods. There is an incredibly strong belief that the proper rearrangement of money will produce a healthy population. Even the Clintons were seduced by this thinking and studiously avoided suggesting that the very foundations of the system—its underlying belief system—may be the cause of all the financial havoc it has produced.

What drives the system? How we spend our health care dollars relates directly to how we spend our research dollars. How pure is research? Many of our interviewees suggested that the directions of even supposedly pure research are not scientific at all. Others feel that potentially beneficial areas of research are overlooked because they are not profitable. One-half of the medical research that takes place in this country is called applied research and is driven by the potential profitability of the products and techniques discovered.[10] Pharmaceutical companies spend $15 billion annually to develop products for treatment and new diagnostic techniques (Califano 1994:41). Much of this research has resulted in techniques that "cure" childlessness, test for and abort defective fetuses, and then ironically provide life support to premature infants, often at a cost of $100,000 per child. Such aggressive therapy frequently saves babies' lives but results in lifelong problems such as retardation and blindness—a prime example of the folly of specialization in pursuit of goals completely unrelated to each other or to the whole of life and society. Many have pointed out that providing adequate nutrition, prenatal care, and social support to poverty-stricken pregnant women to *prevent* prematurity and low birth weight would be far more cost-effective than to concentrate, as we presently do, on salvaging preemies at enormous cost after the fact. But this sort of preventive action would not support or reflect the technomedical paradigm's emphasis on profit or its supervaluation of technology. This particular version of the technocratic One-Two Punch (fail to prevent prematurity, then save the life of the premature baby with incubators, feeding tubes, and respirators) is no cultural accident. It works to fulfill the technocratic myth of transcendence through technology, and thus both expresses and supports the core values of the technocracy far better than prevention ever could.

In the field of drug research alone, the FDA approves between twenty and thirty new drugs for use each year (Fisher 1994:138). This means that a doctor ten years out of training is virtually ignorant of the latest therapeutics—an information gap the pharmaceutical companies rush to fill. Their representatives go door-to-door in doctors' offices, carrying well-stocked sample cases, gifts, and literature promoting their products. These salespersons are often de facto educators, and physicians tend to rely on their information and assistance. It is common for sales reps to scrub in for surgery to teach a physician how to use a new piece of equipment.

If doctors choose to broaden their search for information, where else can they look? To courses that fulfill the requirements for continuing medical education for licensure, to the three leading journals for physicians: The *New England Journal of Medicine*, *The Lancet*, and the *Journal of the American Medical Association* (*JAMA*), and to the hundreds of other publications of the various medical specialties. Unfortunately, both continuing medical education courses and medical publishing are heavily subsidized by the pharmaceutical and medical technology corporations, and medical journals are thick with pharmaceutical ads. A 1992 study published in the *Annals of Internal Medicine* found one-third of these ads to contain misleading information, "particularly in regard to efficacy and the conditions for which that drug should be used" (Fisher 1994:144). Although their ability to influence content has been limited in recent years, pharmaceutical companies still have a major hand in most of the continuing education courses offered to physicians.

Thus, for the physician, the closed feedback loop begun in training, where technomedicine shapes course material, and continued through clinical practice, where physicians learn by example how to prescribe and use the latest "weapons" against disease, is extended indefinitely through reading professional journals and undertaking continuing education courses. "We are brainwashed by the pharmaceutical industry," our interviewee Len Saputo believes, "which is very potent in directing how our education occurs in the first place in the medical centers and in ongoing training. They sponsor all kinds of things we take advantage of because we are compensated in some way for it. But they have ulterior motives, which are very understandable and businesslike. We wind up thinking in those dimensions far more than I think is wise. So we have to be careful about how we are influenced economically by outside groups who determine what we learn."

Pharmaceutical and medical technology companies constitute by far one of the most profitable industries in the United States. The median after-research profit rate in 1993 for the makers of the top-selling prescription drugs was more than five times higher than the median profit rate for all Fortune 500 companies in the same year (Pollack 1995). The subtle grip pharmaceutical companies have on the health care scene is apparent in a scenario Neal Rolde describes in *Your Money or Your Health* (1992). Two drugs used to dissolve blood clots in heart attack patients entered the scene simultaneously. One, TPA, cost $2,200 a dose; the other, streptokinase, cost $76 to $300 a dose. "Although studies had shown them to be equally effective . . . American doctors generally chose the high-priced brand, unlike doctors in other countries" (Rolde 1992:163). Had they chosen more economically, the savings in 1990 alone would have been $200 million. The multipronged marketing effort of Genentech, the company that produced TPA, explains this apparently irrational behavior. Genentech's representatives heralded TPA's benefits so aggressively that doctors feared malpractice suits if they did not use it. The standard of care is set by doctors themselves; all it takes to establish a standard is usage. In this case usage was guaranteed through an elaborate study of thirty-seven thousand patients conducted to establish TPA's "superiority."

A disturbing study revealed that, in 1990, while doctors wrote 240 million prescriptions for antibiotics (close to one for each person), in nearly 1 million of these cases, the only diagnosis given was for a cold, which is known to be unresponsive to antibiotic therapy (Fisher 1994:40). This situation results from the popular belief, reinforced by pharmaceutical companies, that doctors do their job when they give "medicine" to their patients. This belief prevails despite the fact that strains of bacteria totally resistant to antibiotics of any sort are proliferating. Many critics of overprescribing have predicted that nothing short of a plaguelike situation resulting from such overprescribing will change the reliance of doctors on drugs.

The profit motive that drives much of the medical industry corresponds neatly to the profit motive that plays out in other realms of American life. Several of our physician-interviewees noted that the chicken pox vaccine was developed and integrated into the mandatory immunization program not because chicken pox is a serious disorder warranting prevention, but because employers do not want to give time off to parents who need to stay home when their children are isolated with chicken pox. Thus we see how financially motivated cooperation among pharmaceutical research, organized medicine, business, industry, public health, and educational institutions can impact the lives of virtually every child in America.

The profit-driven medical system has become so embedded in and identified with the political economy of American culture that its modification in any substantial way could send that political economy into spasm. Behind the shield of pure science, the same type of moneyed interests that, in other arenas, create bombs or war or dispassionately destroy the environment are now creating "health care." And they do so in direct alignment with the beliefs and values of American culture.

(12) INTOLERANCE OF OTHER MODALITIES: TECHNOMEDICAL HEGEMONY

According to David C. Thomasma, "[A]s Western medicine came to predominate around the world because of its curative powers, alternative therapies, which appeared less substantial based on science and evidence, fell by the wayside. Their elimination from serious consideration engenders a monochromatic view of health and disease, a truncated version of being human, [and] a reduction in the human power to heal" (1995:74).

Like the dominant culture that spawned it, technomedicine until recently saw itself as the only game in town. Obviously there were other systems, but these other modalities were seen as invalid in relation to the dominant system. Technomedicine's proponents did not take seriously the holistic challenge to its claim to exclusive dominance of American health care until a study with startling findings was published in the *New England Journal of Medicine*. Conducted by David Eisenberg and his colleagues (1993), this study revealed that one third of Americans use some form of alternative health care, on which, in 1990, they spent about $14 billion, $10.5 billion of which was cash out-of-pocket—almost as much as the $12 billion spent out-of-pocket on hospitalization in the same year. In addition, the study found that over a twelve-month period, Americans made 425 million visits to offices of alternative medical practitioners (chiropractors, acupuncturists, homeopaths, and so on), exceeding the number of visits made during the same period to all internists, family practitioners, GPs, gynecologists, and pediatricians combined. This groundbreaking study was a tremendous shock to medical doctors, who had previously believed that their system was the only system that counted.

The word "hegemony" refers to an ideology espoused by the dominant group in a given society. One of the essential qualities of hegemonic ideologies is that they are contested by other groups. In a small-scale society, such as that of the Bororo of Brazil, there could be no such thing as a hegemonic religion, or a hegemonic medical system—there was simply Bororo culture, which interpreted the universe in a certain way that was shared by everyone in the culture (Crocker 1985). But in a large-scale, diverse, multicultural society such as that of the United States in the late twentieth century, no one set of ideas about medicine, religion, economics, or anything else is shared by everyone. Nevertheless, there are ideologies that are obviously dominant: in economics, the hegemonic ideology is capitalism, and in health care, it is the technomedical model.

When an ideology is hegemonic, as the technomedical model became after the publication of the Flexner Report, all other competing ideologies become "alternative" to it. Thus healing modalities such as chiropractic, homeopathy, naturopathy, Ayurvedic medicine, acupuncture, Chinese medicine, and so forth have been viewed as alternative to allopathy. While these modalities command increasing respect and usage, allopathic technomedicine still makes the cultural rules, sets the standards for care, and even writes the definitions of all types of disease. Reviewing a book that recounts the brouhaha over attempts to prove the efficacy of homeopathy, physician Rupert Holmes outlines the institutionalized process that silences many attempts to bring forth new information from research:

> Unwanted scientific information is paralyzed by excessive demands for repetitive proofs. The resulting unwanted knowledge is then denounced by "experts." Papers reporting new results are directly censored by anonymous reviewers who operate as the secret police of scientific thought. These individuals determine which papers are published—the direct equivalent in modern times of the *nihil obstat* of the Catholic church. The armory of suppression also includes the perverse use of legitimate technical tools such as statistics, mock attempts at duplication of results, scientific harassment, scientific rumors, and abuse of financial or institutional power. In the final analysis, most scientists operate under an illusion of objectivity, have blind faith that natural phenomena can be reduced to simple known causes, and fail to see the fundamental contradiction between seeking knowledge and seeking power. (Holmes 1996:6)

It is obvious that our presentation of the twelve tenets of the technomedical model in this chapter is also constituted as a critique.[11] Because this paradigm is hegemonic, it needs no more defenders; they are already legion, as are its well-known and thoroughly advertised successes. Thus we have not hesitated to criticize its deficiencies. Any system—medical, economic, religious, or otherwise—that gains sociocultural ascendancy and then rigidifies, shutting out new information and refusing to incorporate contradictory evidence, is in mortal danger both to itself and to the public it serves. Such hegemonic systems can benefit from frontal attacks, which can serve to keep them flexible and responsive to the changing realities of changing times. It is in that spirit that we have presented our analysis.

2 *Medical Training as Technocratic Initiation*

> In most ways medical education is more like high school than a graduate program. The emphasis is on learning mechanical tasks within a rigid structure rather than developing an inquiring mind. It is akin to eight to twelve years of boot camp.
>
> —TERRY TYLER, M.D.

Only a long and complex training process could produce individuals who have the ability to handle life-and-death situations adroitly, to ignore personal needs consistently while continuing to help others, and to suppress emotional response during the most intense situations. Medical training in the United States functions as an initiatory rite of passage, transforming medical students into doctors.[1] It thus carries the burden, not only of transmitting knowledge and skills, but also of imbuing students with the values and beliefs basic to the technocratic paradigm of medicine. Across cultures and throughout history, humans have used similar kinds of rituals to bring about such transition from one social status to another.

Ritual and Rite

A ritual, very simply, is a patterned, repetitive, and symbolic enactment of a cultural belief or value (Davis-Floyd 1992). Rituals often serve simultaneously as symbolic enactments of deep cultural beliefs and as techniques to achieve practical ends. In our analysis of medical training, for example, we will show that teaching techniques and technical routines serve significant ritual purposes above and beyond the communication of information and the "management" of illness.[2]

In all societies, individuals undergoing major culturally recognized life transitions must cross a bridge of rituals commonly known as a rite of passage. Rites of passage consist of three principal stages: separation of the participants from their preceding social status; a "liminal" period of transition in which they have neither one status nor the other; and an integration phase in which they are absorbed into their new social state through various rituals of incorporation. For example, in the rite of passage that constitutes medical training in American society, the separation phase begins as soon as the initiate departs for medical school and gradually merges into the transitional phase, which lasts for seven full years—four years of medical school and at least three years of residency. This transitional or "liminal" phase of being "betwixt and between" is the most salient feature of all rites of passage, especially important in initiation rites. This phase, if the rite of passage is successful, creates a profound interior transformation in the initiate by means of the rituals that make up the rite. According to renowned ritual scholar Victor Turner, "It is the ritual and the esoteric teaching which . . . grows girls and makes men. . . . The arcane knowledge, or gnosis, obtained in the liminal period is felt to change the inmost nature of the neophyte, impressing him, as a seal impresses wax, with the characteristics of his new state. It is not a mere acquisition of knowledge, but a change in being" (1979:238–239).

In rites of initiation, the "gnosis" which so changes the neophytes' inmost nature usually consists of essential elements of the core value and belief system into which they are being initiated. One of the chief characteristics of the liminal or transitional period is the gradual psychological opening of the initiates to such new learning, ideally accompanied by the desired interior change. Many initiation rites involving major transitions into new social roles (for example, Marine Corps basic training) achieve this opening through a combination of physical and mental hardships that break down the initiate's *belief system*—the internal mental structure of concepts and categories through which he perceives and interprets the world and his relationship to it. The breakdown of this belief system leaves the initiate profoundly receptive to new learning and to the construction of new categories. As Turner puts it, "The passivity of neophytes to their instructors, their malleability, which is increased by submission to ordeal, their reduction to a uniform condition, are signs of the process whereby they are ground down to be fashioned anew" (1979:239).

As they convey individuals from one social state to another, simultaneously inculcating them with the core value and belief system of the society, rites of passage also work to renew and revitalize that belief system to assure its perpetuation. The technomedical model is continually renewed and revitalized as it is taught to nascent physicians. Its perpetuation is vital to the perpetuation of the technocratic system as a whole. In all human societies, those in charge of the human body serve as society's representatives: they are responsible for inculcating the values of their culture into the bodies for whom they care. Thus the profound connections between technomedicine and technocratic society are reinforced through the rite of passage of medical training. In what follows, we will see how the above characteristics of ritual and rite are employed during the long and arduous process of medical training to turn fledgling medical students into full-fledged physicians who first internalize, and then perpetuate, the core values of the technocracy.

Psychological Transformation in Medical School and Residency

MEDICAL TRAINING AND COGNITIVE FUNCTIONING

In every rite of passage, the initiates differ from one another in intellectual ability and complexity. Ritual deals with these differences by reducing all participants, at least temporarily, to the same simple cognitive level, which John McManus (1979) describes as "Stage One." A Stage-One paradigm is a closed system whose adherents try to make reality appear to conform to its picture. Stage-One thinking is black-and-white thinking in either/or patterns that do not allow for the consideration of options or alternative views. Such cognitive reduction precedes the conceptual reorganization that accompanies true psychological transformation. In Turner's words, the initiate must be "ground down" in order to be "fashioned anew."

In initiatory rites of passage, the ritual techniques of hazing, strange-making, and symbolic inversion are employed with great effectiveness to achieve this grinding down. *Hazing* techniques, often employed in fraternity and military initiation rites and induction into religious cults, involve wearing down and disorienting the initiate through exhaustingly repetitive activity (in basic training, digging a series of ditches and filling them up; in fraternity pledge rites, frantically running from phone booth to phone booth to receive the next set of instructions). *Strange-making* (Abrahams 1973) involves making the commonplace strange (e.g., shaving the heads of basic trainees or religious initiates so they will lose their sense of identity and familiarity). *Symbolic inversion* means metaphorically turning things upside down and inside out, disrupting the order of everyday life to generate what Roger Abrahams (1973) called "the power attendant upon confusion" (see also Babcock 1978), meaning that this sort of disruption breaks habitual patterns of thinking and leaves initiates open to establishing new ones.

During medical school and again in residency, hazing, strange-making, and symbolic inversion are effectively employed. For example, medical school reduces to lowly status individuals formerly at the top of their classes in college or already successful in another career. As one physician noted: "The first two years of medical school are like backtracking. No fun. Your last two years in college, you tend to do more graduate-level work in smaller classes and you have more freedom about what you learn and how you learn it. Then you are suddenly popped back into an environment like first-year basic science courses in college, where you kind of get what's thrown at you. . . . There's no freedom about what you learn—everybody learns the same thing." First-year residents (formerly known as interns) must begin again at the bottom of the status hierarchy with enormous amounts of "scut work" to perform. Their lowered status is indicated by the language they often use to refer to themselves: "scuzz monkeys," "worms," and "moles" (Stein 1990:210).

The first two years of medical school have traditionally been the same for all medical students, no matter what their eventual specialty: intensive study of the basic sciences—which include biochemistry, neurophysiology, anatomy, histology, and bacteriology—punctuated by countless quizzes and exams. Often taught by research scientists, not physicians, these courses are usually presented as pure science, divorced from any practical function. "Learning" biochemistry, for example, often requires endless rote memorization of chemical formulas, with little or no sense of why or how these might be useful to a physician. In *Gentle Vengeance: An Account of the First Year of Harvard Medical School*, Charles LeBaron recalls:

> Introductory lectures on the "Embden-Myerhof Glycolytic Pathway" . . . What is it? Are we synthesizing something, breaking it down? Does it take place in the ocean, outer space, crayfish, where? Does it start things off, end them? In short, what's it all about? Silly concerns. Just plunge right in and start getting it all down cold:
>
> > Rabbit muscle adolase—Class I, Type A, MW 160,000, four sub-units of MW 40,000; Formula: Alpha-2, Beta-2, but isozymes of varying ratio Alpha/Beta are found. . . . See handout. Consider reaction in direction of synthesis of hexose-P. (1981:62–63)[3]

The apparent irrelevance of much of this material to clinical medical work is a source of great discontent to many medical students, especially to those who entered medical school with ideals of helping humanity. As one physician noted, "Most of us look on the basic sciences as something you put up with until you get to the real heart of the issue. I don't know why they even had a lot of the courses. We took bioengineering and biostatistics. Even a lot of biochemistry is extremely detailed and really has no relevance. The Krebs cycle is a classic example—a biochemical cycle where you have to learn all these enzymes and then when you get through you never use it. My sister in med school now tells me the same thing. She can't understand why she is going through all these detailed analyses of DNA structures and things like that." The enormous quantity of much of this irritatingly irrelevant material adds to its effectiveness as a hazing technique. One physician's assessment is that

> Medical school is not difficult in terms of what you have to learn—there's just so much of it. You go through, in a six-week course, a thousand-page book. The sheer bulk of information is phenomenal. You have pop quizzes in two or three courses every day the first year. We'd get up around

> six, attend classes till five, go home and eat, then head back to school and be in anatomy lab working with a cadaver, or something, until one or two in the morning, and then go home and get a couple of hours sleep and then go out again. And you did that virtually day in and day out for four years, except for vacations.

Alex Cadoux added, "Much of medicine was treating numbers, not people. What counted was your class rank, and where was your internship. All the external parameters. I guess I still harbor anger at myself for buying into this system hook, line, and sinker. There were points of interest, points of joy in learning. But they were fairly rare, because there wasn't enough time to digest the information. We were constantly cramming down the volumes that we were responsible for. . . . It was high-volume learning, not integrated."

One result of such an overload of information—which one physician described as "like trying to drink water from a fire hose"—is the increasing isolation of the student-initiates. It is characteristic of rites of passage that the initiates are separated as a group from the rest of society, in order to ensure their removal from the everyday conceptual world. This social separation is prerequisite to achieving the necessary cognitive retrogression, as Jack Mansberger explained:

> Little do you realize that when you get to the next step, it's going to be just as bad as the one before it, or worse. And then all you want to do is finish that one. So you lose all sight of what you really want, and of what you enjoy. I mean, I used to love to go backpacking, I used to love the woods. And there's no time to do that. You become totally isolated. It's what the system does, is take up all your time. And that indoctrinates you that the system is the only thing in the world that's important. It's not necessarily caring for patients or love or anything like that. It's just the system, that's it. So you're indoctrinated in that, and you lose the entire rest of the world.

In the first two years of medical school, pressures of threat and uncertainty mount. A competitive emphasis on grades and tests, the unpredictability of pop quizzes, the overwhelming bulk of the work at hand, and the increasing isolation—all combine to reduce the initiates' range of cognitive functioning. It is not that medical students become less intelligent; rather, the span of their intellectual capacities and concerns becomes constrained. A kind of tunnel vision develops: the cognitive overload that first- and second-year medical students experience forces them to focus only on what is immediately in front of them. They become progressively less capable of self-reflection and of the psychological distance from the socialization process that such self-awareness might have helped them to achieve. The positive side of this, as Bethany Hays pointed out, is that "you become able to focus on a problem with many variables, under intense pressure, and to solve it without becoming mired down in personal issues—a great skill at three in the morning when someone is bleeding to death." The downside, Hays continues, "is that you learn to problem-solve under pressure in purely technomedical terms. If a solution coming out of some other model might have been better, you're not going to find it." When one is totally immersed in one model of reality to the exclusion of everything else, one can easily lose sight of the importance, even the existence, of other ways of thinking and being. As Karin Montero put it, "I worked so hard, I was so busy, that I didn't think very much."

REDUNDANCY AND EMOTIONAL NUMBING AS TRANSFORMATIVE TECHNIQUES IN MEDICAL TRAINING

For maximum effectiveness, a ritual will focus on sending one basic set of symbolic messages, which it repeats over and over again in different forms. Symbols work through the right hemisphere of the brain; we thus receive their messages as a gestalt that is physically felt through the body and the emotions, often bypassing the intellect.[4] Repetition and the hazing process of physical exhaustion, begun during medical school and intensified during residency, work together to ensure that the resident will internalize the set, established routines of standard medical practice—and the separation-based core value system that underlies them—so thoroughly that she can perform them on automatic pilot. Obstetrician Bethany Hays explained, "As senior residents at Baylor, we knew that we had done more twins, more breech deliveries, more C-sections, more complicated forceps than anybody out in practice. We were the experts by the time we finished that residency. The price we paid for that was that we were exhausted, we didn't have time to think about what we were doing; it was just do it, and do it, and do it some more."

Many hospitals require their residents to perform repetitive and redundant daily chores that have little to do with training to be a physician. These include delivering lab specimens, carting patients around, changing sheets on hospital beds, starting IV lines, drawing blood, and doing secretarial record keeping. This "scut work" occupies a quarter to a third of residents' time, the equivalent of six months out of a four-year residency, or about eight hours out of a thirty-six-hour shift (Duncan 1993:64). In addition to its effectiveness as a hazing technique, the tradition of using residents to perform this scut work saves hospitals and attending physicians millions of dollars a year. Residents, typically paid well below minimum wage, often make less per hour than nurses, physician's assistants, and orderlies. Not only does this system provide financial benefits to the hospitals, it also works to ensure that when residents, drastically underpaid and exploited for years, finally enter private practice, they will feel entitled to the same high fees as their former exploiters, and thus will help to perpetuate the profit orientation of the technomedical system (Duncan 1993:65).

In the haze of cognitive overload and physical exhaustion that characterizes medical school and residency, most students gradually lose sight of the idealistic goals they may have had on entering medical school. If the rite of passage is successful, the new goals medical students eventually develop will be structured in accordance with the values of the dominant medical system. This process is aptly summarized by a resident:

> Most of us went into medical school with pretty humanitarian ideals. I know I did. But the whole process of medical education makes you inhuman. . . . I've seen people devastated when they didn't know *an* answer. . . . The whole thing can get you pretty warped. I think that's where the feelings begin that somebody owes you something, 'cause you really, you know, you've blocked out a good part of your life. People lost boyfriends and girlfriends, fiancees and marriages. There were a couple of attempted suicides. . . . So you forget about the rest of life. By the time you get to residency, you end up not caring about anything beyond the latest techniques you can master and how sophisticated the tests are that you can perform.

For many physicians-in-training, an emotional numbing accompanies the psychological transformation this resident describes. Emotions can be inconvenient in medical school: they can interfere with one's ability to dispassionately dissect a cadaver, grasp the beating heart of a dog minutes before its death, absorb enormous amounts of decontextualized information, and treat the many tragic figures who present themselves for care. Gradually, many medical students and residents begin to learn to cut themselves off from their feelings. Jack Mansberger explained:

> After a while, you don't even feel, because you put such a tremendous emotional box around yourself. Particularly in my field, surgery, you know, the long hard hours, the whole bit. You're not supposed to be emotional. Trauma cases come in—there's no room for emotion and all that. So you build this tremendous wall around yourself to protect yourself and keep yourself going. You actually lost sight of where you really were, and the box becomes so thick and heavy. It's what you carry around. It's not until later on, when the weight of that box is so tremendous that it about does you in, that you realize what you've been doing the whole time. And of course your family suffers and everybody else around you suffers.
>
> Q: What were you boxing yourself in from? What would the emotions have been if you had stopped to feel them?

A: I think there would have been a lot of fear, a lot of pain, all that kind of stuff. I mean, you're dealing with people who are dying left and right. Awful scenarios. I mean, just really difficult things to deal with and nobody ever talks about it at all. You just keep going. Just don't stop. It's like if you ever stop you'll get done in. If you stop and reflect on what you're doing, that'll be the end of it—you'll fall back down the hill. The only way to keep going is to keep going up the hill. Because everybody else is going with blinders on, but that's the only thing you can do. If you take them off, you might just quit. You might just say, "I'm going to go and do something else—this is ridiculous!"

Bethany Hays echoes his commentary. When we asked her, "How did you feel about residency while you were experiencing it?" she replied,

I was brain dead, so I really didn't have a feeling about it. I just wanted to be done because they kept telling me that next year would be better—you know, "Don't worry, because next year will be better!" It took me a long time to figure it out, but by the time I was a senior resident, I knew that was a lie, that it was never going to be better. And it took me another fifteen years to figure out why.

Q: Why?

A: Because what they were teaching was incomplete. It had no connections. . . . Like in college, the philosophy majors took pure philosophy—Descartes, Locke, Kant, et cetera—but I was interested in the philosophy of art, of music, of science. . . . I was interested in where philosophy interfaced with other disciplines, because any subject in the center of that subject gets detached from other disciplines. Higher mathematics could exist in a vacuum; it's *applied* mathematics that gets things done. And the same is true of medicine. If medicine is being practiced in a vacuum, without regard to what we are doing, why heal people? Why bother? There's no point in pretending we can keep people from dying. So why bother? If you bother, it must have to do with the fact that those people are in relationships with other people, or are not done learning what they are here to learn. It's all connected. And it's those connections that my medical training just completely ignored.

Ignoring such connections by presenting enormous quantities of information out of meaningful context enhances the left-brained, linear focus of medical training and works to shut down the gestalt-oriented right hemisphere, which is also the processor of the emotions. Such disconnected teaching, in combination with physical exhaustion, information overload, and the repetitive redundancy of many medical tasks, can emotionally numb initiates and regress them away from higher-level, integrative thought. They will develop a kind of narrow tunnel vision in which the gnosis of medicine, separate from all other realities, becomes all-important.

COGNITIVE TRANSFORMATION: LEARNING "THE WAY"

Cognitive transformation occurs in ritual when "symbol and object seem to fuse and are experienced as a perfectly undifferentiated whole . . . and insight, belief and emotion are called into play, altering our conceptions . . . at a stroke" (Moore and Myerhoff 1977:13). A sixty-three-year-old obstetrician presents the outcome of such transformative learning: "I think my training was valuable. The people who trained us, and their philosophy, were unbeatable. Dr. Pritchard—he was *the* man in obstetrics [when I trained with him]. And his philosophy was one of teaching one way to do it, and that was *his* way. And it was basically the right way. . . . I like the set hard way. I like the riverbanks that confine you in a direction. Later on . . . you can incorporate a little bit of this or that as things change, but you learn one thing real well, and that's *the* way."

In medical schools and hospital units, this cognitive transformation of the initiates—this perceptual fusion with "*the* way"—occurs when reality as presented by the technocratic model gradually becomes one with reality as the initiate perceives it. Training programs in other fields may also be focused on "*the* way" to repair an engine, try a case, or polish a gem. But in medical education, the student, like the marine in boot camp or the religious novice, is "decontextualized"—removed from the normal life context and outside interests that could leaven the initiation process. Thus the projection of "*the* way" to practice medicine tends to merge in the initiate's psyche with the exclusion of other ways. Chris Northrup illustrates the extent of this exclusion when she describes her OB training: "I would say we're taught that this baby is basically just a tumor to be cut out. I was so steeped in the training that I didn't begin to see or appreciate the miracle that the body is, particularly in birth."

As we have seen, the intellectual overload of the first two years plays a significant role in this transformational process, despite the fact that most of the content of the courses is quickly forgotten; said one physician, "I was thinking yesterday that I must be a lot dumber than I was when I went to medical school, because I don't remember any of the stuff that we learned. You remember the things that you use clinically, that's all." In contrast, physicians-to-be spend most of the last two years of medical school, and all four years of residency, in just the sort of embodied hands-on experiential learning that *is* remembered (Jordan 1993:ch. 7). A practicing obstetrician recalls,

> I had delivered maybe thirty babies as a medical student. When I was a first-year resident . . . on my first day I was thrown in as the Chief of Labor and Delivery. I had an intern and six medical students under me. A lady came in off the elevator abrupting, we had to do an emergency cesarean

> on her. I had never even seen one, much less done one! And I had to go in there, scared. Well, the second-year resident comes in and walks me through it. It's a "see one, do one, teach one" program, and that's how medical schools are generally run. Somebody shows you how, they walk you through it once or twice. And the next few times, you do it, with them still watching you and guiding you. You do that a few times, and then you start teaching others. And that's the basic philosophy of how you learn. It's not a bad system. I don't know of anything that can replace it. And you learn pretty quick!

Given the effectiveness for learning of this sort of emotional and physical involvement, we might well ask why the first two years of medical school consist primarily of intellectual overload? A rite-of-passage perspective reveals a function, if not a purpose, underlying this educational method. Two years of nothing but science, besides serving to separate the nascent physician from the person that she was, also serve very effectively to separate her from the people whom she will treat. Before she begins to deal with real people as patients, she learns conceptual distance from them.

For example, to study the basic sciences is to be taught to think of the body as a machine. During anatomy lab, medical students dissect the body's muscle groups, organs, and vasculature in finer and finer detail. Discussing the effects of this process, one student noted, "I've had some real perception changes of people. We all have this sort of thing—I'm good at tennis, say, or something else, and therefore, I'm good. I started realizing more and more, I can't help but think of us as machines. And there's none of this individuality and goodness; it's just whether or not you synapse quickly" (quoted in Good and Good 1993:96). As Howard Stein puts it, "In biomedical training, the body is a lifeless machine before 'it' is a person. Death and deconstruction precede, and set the tone for, life" (1993:186). LeBaron elaborates:

> I held the slide up against the light again. Yes, that had once been someone's finger. It had felt coffee cups and pieces of paper and buttons, scalded itself, shook hands, gestured in excitement, caressed faces. Now it lived between pieces of glass in a box. A small chill ran through me. "Strange," I said. "Yeah, isn't it? Here's a piece of penis. A little later, you'll get to a salivary gland from someone's tongue." I looked at him, my eyes widening. Phil shrugged. "After a while, you just don't think about it anymore." I started again, a little more slowly. If this was human flesh, however sliced, dried, or stained, I should at least show it the courtesy of adequate attention. Soon people began to leave for lunch. It was almost one, I was hungry, and another class started at one-thirty. I sped up: esophagus, testicle, intestine. . . . Where are those crazy ter-

> minal bars they said I should see? The heck with them . . . I'm getting something to eat. You get used to things fast around here, I thought as I locked up the microscope. (LeBaron 1981:40)

Growing detachment from both the diseases studied and the people who have them leads fairly rapidly, in the first year of medical school, to the development of cynicism and intellectual arrogance. LeBaron documents this process, describing one of his first-year Harvard class's rare contacts with an actual patient, a multiple sclerosis victim. The class's first reaction was dismay at the actual physical presence of a "CPC—clinical-pathological correlation," as disease victims were named, but soon:

> "Shit, I'd love to do a coronal section on his frontal lobe," said someone behind me. "You'd see demyelinated plaques the size of golfballs." Some knowing snickers. People hadn't started off talking that way; initially everyone had approached our occasional CPC sessions with an almost reverential awe—the word actually made flesh. But now after a year of dog labs, corpses, continual memorization, and no patients, that kind of conversation was part of the background noise. And those expressions of flippancy, cynicism, the sarcastic smiles that had been so conspicuous by their absence back at orientation were already starting to spread through the class like some sinister psychological tide. (LeBaron 1981:213)

The objectification of the patient and the alienation of practitioner from patient so evident in the above quotation are the philosophical correlates of the Cartesian separation of mind and body. This belief in mind-body separation, inherent in the scientific medical view, does not permit the interaction of individual consciousness with the molecules and atoms that comprise the stuff of "scientific" inquiry; thus, as physician Cynthia Carver notes, it is easy to leave people out of the medicoscientific equation: "The first two years of medical school . . . are not taught in a framework of how *people* function. The students are taught about bodies as though the minds, emotions, and lives associated with those bodies were irrelevant. They are also taught about hundreds of pathological conditions and processes as though they were all equal: equal in importance, equal in outcome, equal in incidence" (1981:132).

Teaching about pathological conditions as if all were equal in importance and incidence presents medical students with the very false impression that learning about rare pathologies is just as important in patient care as studying more common conditions is. Most medical schools withhold actual clinical experience, which could teach students very differently, until after the initiates have internalized the basic attitudes and values underlying this scientific worldview. As resident Paulanne Balch explained:

> Medical school is so sterile and abstracted from the person. It's a process that really begins the first day of medical school. You begin by learning about a disassembled set of organ systems. That's about the most integrated it gets. You learn about the digestive system, the circulatory system, the nervous system. You learn about the different body parts and processes, and how they work together, and how to break down information a patient might give you as to which system is involved. Then you develop a treatment program based on the results of your diagnosis. Notice I have not spoken a word about the person. And the crisis, if it occurs for you, is when you sit down with a person to solve a problem they have, and you don't have any tools from your training to recognize the fullness of what a human being is.

Although clinical experience early in medical training has the potential to bring students and patients closer together, in many medical schools it begins in the second semester of the second year, and seems designed to intensify psychological distance. Because this clinical work consists primarily of the highly routinized tasks of doing physicals and taking medical histories, it tends to widen the gap between medical students and the people they are going to school to learn to heal, encouraging them to regard these individuals as "cases"—"the gallbladder in 133" or "the section in 214." This objectification of the patient is further intensified in residency, as this second-year resident suggests: "As interns, we lose why we went into medicine—whatever humanistic interest we had. It's very hard to sit there and listen to someone tell his life story when you've got six other admissions, bloods to draw, you've got to be up all night. Every second you spend being compassionate means that much less time to sleep. So you become very efficient at not really listening to people—just getting the information you need, and shutting them off" (quoted in Harwood 1984:70).

With this internalization of "scientific objectivity," initiates have the opportunity to find a sense of individual identity within the medical paradigm through clinical rotations that expose them to the practice and procedures of various medical specialties, where the highest value tends to be placed on the acquisition of technological and surgical skills. The second two years of medical school allow the overwhelmed student to associate with and seek approval from the masters of the craft. Whisked through the various departments of the hospital—itself the cathedral of technology—students are understandably hungry for the excitement and adrenaline rush provided by the drama of the ER, the intensity of the ICU, and the theater of the OR. With just a few weeks in every department, it is no wonder that the slow pace of, say, an outpatient department fails to capture their imaginations. Applying cream to an eczema, prescribing an antibiotic for a strep throat infection—these mundane treatments just don't measure up to the thrill of bringing life back from the brink, whether in birth or near-death. The value of taking a thorough and time-consuming patient history pales in comparison to the frenzy of caring for accident victims or the drama of participating in organ transplants.

Psychologically medical students are seeking approval and nurturing with the only receptors available—the brain and adrenals. Is it fascinating, high-tech, new? Is it exciting? Will it give me an edge, a high? The process of rotation does far more than expose doctors-to-be to techniques, patients, and the wonders of technology; it exposes them to doctors from whom they will learn the finer points of conduct, ethics, and behavior on which to model their future selves. The cathedral is full of priests. The clergy conducted the ceremonies of the first two years; now the high priests move in for the final preparation for ordination.

Residency permits the new doctor, while still bottom-feeding, to mediate with respect to the new crop of students. What was mental overload in the first two years becomes physical exhaustion in the last four. Rarely, in the course of seven long years, is there an opportunity to reflect, to integrate, to assimilate, or to contextualize the information which has been force-fed through intellectual, physical, social, and cultural channels. As one doctor summed up the cognitive transformation that occurs, "It doesn't seem to matter—male or female, young or old, wealthy or poor—it is only the most unusual individual who comes through a residency program as anything less than a technological clone. This rite of passage that you are talking about is an assembly line to the adoration of technology."

Gender and Medical Training

Before the Industrial Revolution, healing in the Western world was primarily women's work. The technomedical system was created by men; its creation encompassed four centuries of active repression of female healers in the West and the deliberate stamping out of their knowledge and traditions. This repression continued on into twentieth-century America. The Flexner Report resulted not only in the closing of homeopathic and naturopathic schools of medicine, but also in the closing of the separate medical schools for women, which had been established in the 1800s. It took fifty more years for women to be able to enter male medical schools in any significant numbers; when they got in, they found themselves confronting a medical system based on intensely patriarchal principles and values.

In the early 1960s, the population of physician-trainees was 90 percent white and male; by 1993, it had changed to 30 percent women and 18 percent minorities (Duncan 1993:63). The American Medical Association predicts that by 2010, 30 percent of U.S. doctors will be women, compared to 19 percent in 1995. In many of the leading medical schools, over 50 percent of the students in the class of 1998 are women. As more women enter medicine, the question arises, Is it changing them, or are they changing it?

Modern medical education is conducted within a realm where masculinist beliefs predominate. Its rituals of hazing, emotional deadening, and physical suffering are typical of male initiation rituals around the world, from the Spartans to the marines. The feeling here is that in order to leave one way of being and enter a new one (as in leaving the world of childhood to become a man), the initiates must sever all connections with their prior life. This kind of left-brained, separation-based thinking is not found in female rites of initiation, which tend across cultures to be connection-based, to celebrate a woman's ability to grow and change while still remaining connected to her kith and kin (Farrer 1980, Lincoln 1981).[5] Psychologist and writer Carol Gilligan (1993) has shown that this kind of connection still characterizes the upbringing of American women.

Thus it is to be expected that women would have an especially difficult time accepting their medical training and its underlying values and worldview, which fail to recognize the personal, an area where women often excel. The medical system's unwillingness to acknowledge feeling and value relationships, the realm of "the feminine," was the underlying cause of the suffering that the women physicians we interviewed particularly expressed. Ann McCombs said that she "found medical training offensive intellectually and . . . in the area of relationships—being a female in a predominantly male system." The devaluation of the personal that often typifies medical training can be devastating to women students. "The interaction I had with my patients," reports one female physician, "the appreciation they had for me and the fun and enjoyment of being a helping, caring person carried me through years of frustration with the profession. I felt I was in a hostile environment and didn't know where I fit, but at least there was something positive and right happening with my patients. When this was no longer happening, there was little to make it seem worthwhile" (Julia Hall, *MetaPhysicians' Tales*).

A coping strategy Christiane Northrup found useful was to consciously defer gratification—for years. She could accept her "average" academic performance, knowing she excelled in intuitive and relational skills: "I just knew that my ability to find out what was going on with a patient was not average. But I also knew this ability was completely invisible in that world. It wasn't seen or honored. I would do no harm, I would do no harm. I would learn my skills, and then when the time came, when it mattered, I would add this other stuff I was doing—when it was my turn."

Although women have achieved parity in the profession as students and as practicing physicians, many are scarred by the stress and lack of self-expression they endured as women—on top of all the other pressures the system imposes. Many of them told of eagerly awaiting the day they could bring their total being to bear in their work, but fearing the loss of their feminine abilities along the way as the unrelenting pressure of the system forced more and more conformity to the masculine norm. Several of our women interviewees expressed their anger and outrage at a system of training that barely recognized and in no way accommodated their roles as mothers. Bethany Hays recounts "marching into the office of the chairman" of her OB/GYN department at Baylor prior to applying for internship, and asking,

> "What concessions are you willing to make for women in your program?" And he said, "Um, concessions?" And I said, "Well, you know, like the pediatricians have shared and part-time residencies. They can take time off if they have kids, they get leaves of absence if they want to have babies. You know, I'm married now, and I don't intend to wait until I'm forty to have my first baby, and if you want real women in your program, some of them are going to want to have children. And so I want to know, What is your plan for that?" And he was dumbfounded. It had never occurred to him—it didn't have to because they had never had any women in the program. So he said, "Well, uh, uh, I guess if you want to have a baby the third year, you could be on pathology the last three months." And that was it, and I thought "Oh, my God."

The women medical students and physicians we interviewed seemed more troubled than many of their male colleagues by the high degree of personal imbalance required by their profession. Although some of the men we interviewed commented on the grueling conditions of medical school, none touched on the sense of being personally out of balance the way several women did:

> I found medical training extremely difficult. When I finished training I was in a very vulnerable state. It was a real soul-destroying experience. One of the things I found difficult was how little respect there was for the need to balance. I need balance. My life was one-sided and unhealthy. It really bothered me. I went to faculty members and asked for advice on this situation. They advised me to be unhealthy for three years and then become healthy. Get balanced later. This was totally unacceptable to me. (Marilyn Levinson, *MetaPhysicians' Tales*)

Several women described themselves as "ill" during and after medical training. This was often not the type of illness that could be diagnosed and treated, but rather a kinesthetic sense of the effects of unrelenting stress, sleep deprivation, adrenaline states, and social deprivation. Rebecca

Lawrence found herself "becoming more physically and emotionally spent. I felt ill most of the time, not with any one symptom, but just sick. I'd wake up in the morning with a damn-it-all attitude, feeling too sick to eat." Marilyn Levinson was "sick continuously for two years. It started with some type of pneumonia and then bronchitis, bronchitis, bronchitis." A fourth-year female medical student told us in a letter she sent:

> By the third year of medical school, I found myself in a severe depression and sleeping for ten hours a day. Everything I knew about life and living, everything I believed in, was being trampled and pissed on every single day of my medical school experience. Love, joy, deep caring, touch, relationship, individualized care—these had no place. It made me sick, physically and emotionally. I could handle the assault on my body, but the continuous assault on my spirit was too painful to bear. So I took a year off, hoping that by the time I came back I would have found the inner strength to continue while protecting my soul.

Like this student, Rebecca Lawrence took a year off to recover some balance, but lost it almost immediately upon returning to training. "It sure was difficult. I didn't feel my approach was recognized, validated or supported. I started to get real tired again, and when that happened, my desire to be creative with my patients decreased. I started doing the bare essentials again. I fulfilled the requirements to make my supervisors happy, but it wasn't making *me* happy."

Our women interviewees tended to be acutely aware of the moral ambivalence of their position in a system that forces them to cause pain to their patients, often for no apparent benefit. Their attempts to mitigate that pain through emotional nurturance were apt to incur the wrath of the system, so they had to cultivate deviousness in order to be able to practice the kind of medicine they cared about. Rebecca Lawrence said, "I did provide good eye contact with my patients, and did a little caring touch, so my personality did some good. Patients seemed to like the personal interaction, though it was real basic. I would cross out appointments in my book or put in fake names so I would have more time for people, manipulating the system as best I could. But I was basically in a survival mode most of the time."

Some women, like Rebecca Lawrence, risked their careers in subtle and invisible ways to make situations more comfortable for their patients. Others, like Chris Northrup, sometimes confronted the system head-on:

> I had the idea that when I'd be alone with the patient, I'd try to learn what was really going on. I knew many times that the treatment wouldn't be successful because the person didn't want to live. There isn't any receptor site for that information in allopathic medicine. I'd go to tumor confer-

ences every Wednesday, and the guys would present the patient: Forty-eight-year-old multipara, tumor in the pelvis, diagnosed by local M.D., stage-two Pap. . . . Then they'd talk about what kind of cancer she had, what stage it was in, and the specialists would talk about the treatment they were going to give her. You never, ever heard about who this person was. And I'd bring it up. That was stupid—like taking the Star of David into a fundamentalist Christian church. But I knew in myself that I had something to offer and something to say that wasn't being recognized.

One of Northrup's anecdotes illustrates how patriarchal values cross gender lines, in this case being invoked by women. She describes her OB residency as characterized by technologically assisted births. After finally gaining permission from her supervisor to attend some women without the use of electronic fetal monitors, she found that the nursing staff was often unwilling to cooperate, fearing that the outcomes would be bad.

Many women in touch with their capacities for intuition, sensitivity, and empathy were acutely aware that these were neither acknowledged nor valued in their training. Some, like Northrup, had the confidence and self-esteem to know that, one day, they would be able to create a situation where these were valued. Others went forward with agonizing doubt about their ability to find fulfillment. Although male students and doctors also suffer in high-pressure and impersonal situations, the women seemed to suffer doubly because they doubted that they would ever be valued for who they were. One woman physician particularly warns against the idea that women can change medicine or medical training: "I see a lot of women making the mistake of thinking that, when they are in the belly of the beast, they are going to change the beast. It does not work." Bethany Hays, who calls technomedicine "the prototype addictive organization," described to Davis-Floyd the pain of finding out that she could not change the beast:

I tried for fifteen years to change the way OB was done at Baylor, to make birth more humane for women. I felt like I was beating my head against the wall and I couldn't figure out why I couldn't seem to make a difference. I thought there was something wrong with *me*. Then Polly Perez handed me a manuscript one day. It was your dissertation, before it even got published. You were talking about birth as a rite of passage that indoctrinates women with the core values of American culture, and I suddenly realized that it wasn't me, it was the *culture*! I was trying to change an entire culture, and of course it was so much bigger than me that I couldn't make a dent!

Some women coped by choosing a specialty that allowed for a more holistic treatment of the patient. For example, Sandra Kamiak spurned a specialty in internal medicine in favor of psychiatry to avoid the impersonal handling of patients. "People are broken down into parts," she noted in her interview. "It's mechanical. I felt at first that I was going to go into internal medicine, but thought that I would not have enough time with a patient. With ten minutes for an exam, you just don't have time to deal with all the stuff that's going on emotionally. You could do an X-ray or throw a pill at a person, but it didn't seem to be adequate."

The first generations of women to graduate from medical schools as a distinct minority often coped by becoming overachievers. As Bethany Hays put it, "In medical school I just wanted to prove that I could do as good as the guys. I wanted to be the best man for the job, and so, when things happened to me because I was a woman, I always assumed it was because I wasn't doing a good enough job. And so I worked very hard. Like most women, I did twice as much work to get half as much credit. I knew that to actually be given concessions because I was pregnant would be like being given second-class citizenship. I would not have been able to have any power in the program. And so I worked very hard all through my pregnancy up until the day I delivered."

Some women, fearing they would be labeled "soft," not "tough enough," overcompensated by becoming not only better, but also more technocratic—more aggressive, more interventionist, more mechanistic—than their male counterparts. During her research on obstetrics during the 1980s and early 1990s, Davis-Floyd often heard labor and delivery nurses voice the complaint that the new women physicians were "worse than the men" when it came to ordering unnecessary interventions. Now that the numbers are evening, female students do not necessarily feel the same compulsions to beat the men at their own game. Nevertheless, many still feel that their educational process is a continual trade-off of their inner reality for outer rewards.

It is unfair to imply that men make medical school bad and difficult and that all women suffer. The individual men or women involved are not the problem: they are simply participants in a system that is closed, dominant, and derived from a larger system where the same patriarchal/technocratic values prevail. Patriarchal values characterize Western civilization, and the concomitant devaluation of the feminine has produced many social ills (Eisler 1995). Achieving inner and outer balance—the challenge and opportunity of the times—means balancing one's character and practice between aggressive intervention and patience, objectivity and relationship, analysis and intuition. Both men and women physicians face a great deal of confusion as they begin to value the feminine principle in life as well as in medicine. Many of them initially despair of finding any relational way to practice medicine as they have been trained. The gift of such despair is an ability to shift perspective and activate the feminine principle—regardless of the gender of the doctor. The "feminine" qualities of trust, patience, relationship, and surrender then become allies in the search for a new way.

Maintaining Psychological Distance

Human beings are not automatons; rites of passage can fail to transmit the core value and belief system of a given society to the initiate. While most of the forty physicians in our primary study did buy into the medical system during their training "hook, line, and sinker," as one of them put it, some managed to maintain a high degree of distance between their psyches and beliefs and the intensive initiation process to which they were exposed.

An example of the hook, line, and sinker school was a physician whom we asked, "Why do medical students not see patients until late in the second year?" She responded, "I don't know. Mostly it's because you have to have some of the other background before you start playing like you're a doctor. You have to have some basics to work on, and you really have to go back to basic sciences and learn principles about why things work a certain way before you can build clinical medicine onto that." This physician demonstrates the effectiveness of her socialization through her acceptance of the science-before-patients structure of her medical school training. In contrast, a holistic physician demonstrates the difference that psychological distance can make: "As it is now, the basic sciences really get you off the track of what you're there for. Most of us went in with pretty high humanitarian ideals, but by the time you got through the basic science years, most of the people in my class had developed a pretty cynical attitude. If we could have taken clinical rotations and seen patients early on in medical school, we would have come out with a lot better attitude and a better idea of the purpose of the basic sciences."

How did this physician manage to maintain enough psychological distance from his socialization process to be able to analyze it in this highly reflexive way? Realizing early on that his family would suffer considerably if he did not spend *some* time with them, he made a commitment to take off one night a week for that purpose, accepting in advance that it would mean being "a few answers short" on the next day's test: "It was a trade-off, but I think worthwhile in the long run, because I knew that my family would be with me a lot longer than medical school. That difference, whether it's a maturity level or not, was missing in a lot of people. I was older, about twenty-seven; most start at twenty-one or twenty-two." The cognitive separation achieved by this conscious decision not to participate in the competitive values inherent in medical education was intensified by his first child's birth—an overly medicalized and very unhappy event that occurred during medical school. "When [my wife and I] kind of figured out that things didn't have to be that way, I guess it made us both into crusaders."

As physician Cynthia Carver points out, the medical school selection process ensures the admission of students with highly competitive instincts and a strong scientific bent, who "generally went straight through, from high school to college to medical school, [managing] to reach the age of 21 without having experienced anything much other than academic life" (1981:129; see also Stein 1990:180). Students selected *out* by this process include those who, "despite being as bright as the high mark getters, allow themselves to be 'distracted' by. . . . volunteer work, music, art, literature" and other careers (1981:129).

Our interviewees who resisted their technomedical socialization during training were able to do so for a variety of reasons. Those who entered medical school later in life discovered that their life experience gave them a distinct advantage in this endeavor. Paulanne Balch began medical training after a long and successful business career. In response to the question, "Did you feel part of the group while you were in medical school?" she answered, "No, because I'm old enough to be the mother of some of them. There was a group of us who were over forty. We were united by our awareness of a lot of the crap that we were being fed . . . and of the hazing aspects." Others found maintaining a range of outside interests to be essential, as was the case with Dubravka Milas: "As a second-year medical student, I have found that it's so important to get involved in other things besides school—work in a clinic, volunteer for a program that needs your help. If you don't do it now in medical school, you won't do it later either. I'm really finding that to be true. The people who are willing to reach out, they start doing it in their first year. And those that don't, they never do reach out, and so they are the ones who get tunnel vision and get eaten up by the system" (personal communication).

Finding himself unable to maintain outside interests, Peter Grote took a radical step:

> While I was in medical school, I felt that my focus was getting too narrow because I wasn't taking the time to do any other sorts of things. I looked at the people I was surrounded with and saw that most everybody was in the same boat—very narrow in their life experiences and their focus. I saw that those people who did other things for a number of years before going on to medical school were bringing a greater wealth of knowledge and a better attitude and approach to things. So I decided, in the middle of medical school, to take a year off. . . . I got myself involved in a program that summer called Crossroads to Africa. I went to Africa with a small group of other people who were also in medical school or nursing school. We went to a town where there was no medical care at all. We set up a little clinic and spent two months there treating people and trying to teach two

native nurses from the area some things they could keep doing after we left.

Q: What effects did that experience have on you?

A: It had a lot of effects. One was opening my eyes to other cultures. Another was opening my eyes to the benefits of a broader, public health approach to medical care over and above a narrow high-tech approach. I was also very impressed by how happy people were with what in our view was so little. And how willing they were to share everything they had.

Exposure to other ways of healing is a common catalyst for the paradigm shift made by holistic physicians, usually after they complete their medical training. In this case, such exposure gave Peter Grote a cognitive distance from his medical socialization that broadened his vision beyond technomedicine's narrow bounds.

The distancing factors for Barry Elson included yoga training and vegetarianism. Here is how Elson discovered that the emperor had no clothes:

> One unsettling thing about my medical school was that here we had this huge faculty, multimillion-dollar buildings, et cetera, and not a single course on nutrition. I wanted to learn some nutrition so I went to the director of basic sciences education and asked, and he said I'd have to get other students interested in taking it. So I passed a petition around and got a whole bunch of people to sign it, and he said, "Well, it's great that everybody wants to take it, but we don't have anybody to teach it." So I went around to the faculty and I found a gastroenterologist here, a biochemist there, an anatomist there, and we set up an elective. And the first session, here was the gastroenterologist teaching that white bread was better for you than whole wheat bread because it had more vitamins injected in it, and that this whole "health food" thing was completely wrong. And that was in the early seventies. Now, of course, even the federal government recognizes that whole grains are good for you. And I realized that I was dealing with incredible ignorance at a very basic level by narrowly specialized people who didn't know anything about other fields at all. So in a sense I had created a monster, because it reinforced the delivery of all kinds of misinformation. At that point I just threw up my hands.
>
> Q: Why did *you* know about nutrition?
>
> A: I had been studying yoga for awhile, and was a vegetarian as a result of that. Over the years I learned about nutrition from other vegetarians, and then started reading voraciously.

Elson's commitment to the holistic philosophy he expressed through yoga and vegetarianism was so deep that it almost ended his medical training. Ultimately he found that a clear vision of his purpose for being there was essential to his ability to stay the course:

> I went into medical school firmly committed to holistic medicine—I actually thought I had coined the word. I found myself using it in college. Now I realize I must have seen it before that—it was just coming into use in the late sixties. That was definitely my orientation . . . nutrition, stress management, and working with the *whole* person in a collaborative relationship. So the third and fourth years of medical school were particularly ironic and bizarre for me because I'd find myself in a hospital, supposedly a place for helping people get better, and a diabetic, for example, would be getting white bread with caffeinated coffee and sugar—which cause an immediate increase in blood sugar, which puts added stress on the patient's metabolism of glucose, which was already impaired! Basic principles of nutrition were being ignored. The person as a whole, of course, was also being ignored.
>
> And the hospital is a dreary, drabby place with dark-green paint and you get poked and prodded by eighteen medical students, sixteen residents by the time you get out of there. I couldn't image a hospital as being anyplace to heal from anything and of course, we know that's often true. We know an overwhelming percentage of hospital days are spent from misprescribed medicines and many surgeries are done to correct previous surgeries. We know that there's an enormous iatrogenic realm that hospitals are palaces to . . .
>
> So during my training I was a stranger in a strange land. . . . Partway through medical school I seriously considered dropping out. . . . For a while I thought about becoming a naturopath so I'd only be doing things I really believed in.
>
> Q: So why did you decide to stay?
>
> A: I had a vision about what I was doing on the planet. . . . I confronted something very basic about where I was going and what I was doing, and I realized that what I needed to do was go back and play the game some more and become a doctor. . . . I came to understand that my purpose on the planet is . . . to be a "healer" and by that I don't mean someone who does something to someone else, but someone who helps other people heal themselves. I had a very clear vision that that's why I am here, and that vision sustained me during the rest of my training.

Such clarity of vision is a tremendous boon to those who manage to achieve it during or prior to their medical training. In an interesting twist, Elson discovered that some of the medical education he was resisting as abstract and irrelevant turned out to be essential to the kind of holistic healing he later came to practice. Many physicians have used the Krebs cycle as an example of how boring, abstruse, and archaic medical education can be. Yet as Barry Elson explains, he and Alan Gaby have "rediscovered" it in their practice of medical nutrition:

> In the kind of medicine that Alan and I practice, the Krebs cycle and the biochemical intricacies of human metabolism are absolutely essential. They

give us a key to nutritionally unlock the door to healing a wide range of chronic illnesses. It's particularly ironic for me, because here I was this philosophy/psychology holistic kind of guy in the first two years and I was one of those people who said, "I don't need to know this biochemistry . . . I need to relate to my patients."

But where I was completely wrong, was that I was making the assumption that the doctors I was going to be learning from knew what they were talking about when it came to treating metabolic disorders appropriately. Their solutions were to throw drugs at them. My solution now is to find a way to nutritionally speed up those enzyme processes that are lagging, so the body can function more efficiently and heal itself. And the Krebs cycle is an essential part of that. It's a completely different paradigm. . . . I think that's an analogy for what we try to do interpersonally in holistic medicine—it's a whole synergistic model, rather than an analytic one.

The reason Elson originally missed the importance of the Krebs cycle no doubt had much to do with how it was taught. As noted earlier, much of the information in the basic science courses is taught as if it had no connection to anything beyond itself. In a conversation with a fellow student, Charles LeBaron elaborated:

> You know, I spent three years working in a institution for the retarded . . . and there was never a time there that was as intellectually deadening as now. . . . Look at biochem—I counted seven separate stages in that pyrimidine synthesis. What's it all mean? Why are we memorizing it? . . . When I was studying physics back in night school, we calculated the mass of the Milky Way, did all sorts of problems with harmonic motion, nodes and antinodes, blackbody radiation, quantum energy levels . . . I can't see how it has any practical value. But it seemed to me that measuring the mass of a galaxy was fun, revealed some principles about natural phenomena, and showed how accessible immense and faraway objects could be to mathematical analysis. So I know why I was there. . . . Memorizing the seven steps of the pyrimidine synthesis just to memorize them doesn't give me any sense that I'm doing anything but wasting my time and developing a contempt for the subject matter and the people who are teaching me. (1981:107–109)

To this tirade, LeBaron's classmate responded, "Maybe there's a theoretic significance that you don't see?" LeBaron answered, "So why don't they point it out?" and she replied, "Perhaps they assume we see it." LeBaron replied,

> Fine, let's say it's of tremendous significance. . . . Let me give you an analogy. The rose window in the north face of Chartres Cathedral is extraordinarily complex and beautiful. When I visited Chartres, the guide turned

> his back to the rose window, faced us, and proceeded to describe in exact detail each image on each shard of glass, the symbolism of the colors, the mosaic pattern of the panes. . . . He had dedicated his life to studying it. If, instead of explaining the rose window to us, he'd forced us to try and memorize all those images and recite them back by rote, the whole thing would have been worthless and unpleasant. At the very best, we could only have parroted what he'd said himself. Now, let's say one of these cycles is a rose window of biochemistry. Should we just memorize it, recite it, and forget it? Or should we be taught how to understand its meaning and roles and interaction in life? (1981:109–110)

After the final lecture in LeBaron's first-year biochemistry class, the instructor put down his pointer, shut off the slides, and summed up his impression of the science that he had made his lifework:

> "The extraordinary fact about living creatures, living processes, is the structure, the order they manifest in the face of disorder. Each process is interlocked, each life depends on another, the prey upon the predator, the predator upon the prey, cycle upon cycle, pathway branching upon pathway in a web of inconceivable beauty. We don't exist as units alone in an inanimate world but as part of that intricate web. It is this sense of location in the midst of loneliness, repose in the midst of chaos, that constitutes the aesthetic and the real reason for the study of the chemistry of living things."
>
> [I] sat there stricken as people filed out, hurrying off to the library. I thought again about the rose window at Chartres. . . . You son of a bitch, I thought. . . . I can understand being so immersed in the day-to-day world of test tube research that nothing larger ever invades the mind. But if you *know,* if you see that beauty, how could you defile it by teaching it to us in this way? (1982:136–137)

As we hope the above analysis of medical school as an initiatory rite of passage has made clear, the sort of disconnected teaching that so wounded LeBaron's soul is an accurate reflection of the separation-based worldview that, since the early 1900s, medical training has been designed to perpetuate. Those who resist internalizing this worldview during medical training form a ready pool of candidates for expansion into holistic practice.

Trends in Medical Education

Although all of our interviewees took issue with the attitudes and values that underlay their medical training, most were unequivocal in their appreciation of the knowledge, skills, and experience they gained. In particular, those students who had ferreted out more progressive medical training situations found much to appreciate. Deborah Malka found that "the University of New Mexico had one of the finest programs in the state. Students learned in tutorial style in small groups of six instead of large lecture classes. We learned by case study approach"—a patient-oriented teaching tool. Anu de Monterice discovered Case Western Reserve to be "a very progressive school. Dr. Spock was there. They tried to integrate the curriculum, using clinical experience earlier, which is unusual. Then they tied the systems together. Quite a good education." What Ann McCombs loved about McMasters, an experimental medical training program in Canada, was that "it was set up to teach you to think, the way law school teaches you to think. It's not about how much factual information you've got, it's about what you can do with it. Because when that factual information becomes obsolete, you need to be able to bring in another set of facts and use them. What you have to learn is problem-solving, and that's a lifelong skill."

A second reason for valuing medical education was the feeling that it lent a credibility to physicians' future work within the holistic realm. Christiane Northrup found that she "liked the grounding of it. I like the tradition of medicine, the whole of learning those skills, learning how to get someone out of trouble. It gave me the underpinnings and the tradition to say what I am now saying with more authority than if I had not gone through that. I know what I'm talking about, and I believe people listen in a different way than they would if I had not had that training." Bethany Hays said that her medical training gave her "the technical skill and knowledge to be able to sort of walk between the worlds. I managed to do medicine differently because I did it so well. They couldn't criticize; they couldn't question my outcomes. Believe me, they watched; they scrutinized. If I had had bad outcomes, I'd have been buried long ago."

Ed Neal also noted the benefits of having "the 'Good Housekeeping stamp of approval.' I don't have to fight with someone if I want to do acupuncture or something. Power comes from my medical training. Power is not a bad thing. . . . It's good to be able to stand up and say to my colleagues that people have souls. And they listen." Neal appreciated the rigors of his medical training, recognizing the character-forging worth of the long hours and difficult work: "I'm proud to be an M.D. The best thing about the training is not the treatments you learn, which are not very effective in primary care. I'm really proud of having done the work. It's hard work. What was really of value was being in the fire. It was very grounding that way. When I work with alternative practitioners, sometimes it seems a little fluffy because they haven't seen people puke blood at three in the morning, when things aren't pretty, or spiritual—when you connect with life and death and pain and suffering."

Our interviewees agreed that the challenge in medical training is to keep what is worthwhile in the current system while reshaping its underlying core values. Cadavers can be dissected with respect or with disdain; patients can be appreciated as individuals or treated perfunctorily. The physicians we interviewed, most of whom completed their medical education in the 1970s and 1980s, were reporting on their socialization into a paradigm of medical education that is currently undergoing some modification in response to sociocultural influences. In the prime of their life careers, they and their cohorts wield powerful influence over current developments in medicine. Fortunately, the medical care system is responding to pressures from patients to place a higher value on qualities such as equality, communication, and noninvasive techniques.

Terry Tyler asks, "Is the pain of medical education a necessary initiation? For most doctors there is no transcendence of the pain, or of the ego. A deliberate initiation needs to be carried out with a great deal of love. Then there is the possibility of transcendence. My hope is that there will be an upswelling of protest from people going through the medical training process. Perhaps they will say, 'We need to be whole. We need to be healed in order to be healers.'"

A look at developing trends shows some important shifts in that direction. First is a recognition that physicians may benefit from earlier exposure to clinical experience. We have suggested a strong correlation between delaying actual contact with patients and the unconscious adoption of technocratic values. Some medical schools have begun to incorporate patient care into the first-year curriculum, beginning on day one. One impact of a curriculum that integrates clinical experience with basic science is a renewal of interest in primary care. During the 1980s the number of doctors entering primary care dropped 14 percent as the trend toward specialization gained ground. However, this trend seems to be reversing in the 1990s as more medical students become aware of the need for primary care physicians. A surprising finding in our interviews with holistic doctors was how many of them had considered choosing surgery as their specialty, yet a serendipitous event like the location of the residency, a family obligation, or the Vietnam War intervened and pushed them into primary care. Of our forty interviewees, twenty are board-certified as primary care physicians.

Primary care is defined as first-line care and is provided by the physician who is first consulted when a problem is suspected or develops. Many times warm and long-term relationships develop between primary care doctors and their patients, in contrast to the impersonal interactions often characteristic of patient-specialist relationships. "The time is ripe for change because all parties—students, faculty, and the public—agree the system isn't working," says former surgeon general C. Everett Koop, who has introduced a new approach to medical training at Dartmouth Medical School. Dartmouth requires first-year medical students to do a seven-week primary care rotation with a doctor in the community and to assume responsibility for the care of a family during that time. They experience the humanistic rewards of primary care firsthand at an impressionable stage, before the seduction of technology has swayed them. "Most people feel there is a tremendous information overload during the first two years of medical school," says Dr. Jonas Schulman, associate dean of education at Emory University's School of Medicine in Atlanta, as reported in the *San Francisco Examiner*, October 4, 1992. "What all of us are trying to do is get students involved with patients early, before they are able to visualize them as diseases."

A related benefit of this trend is a conscious attempt in some schools to model communication skills to medical students in the hope that they will develop more effective styles as practitioners. The strategy involves acceptance of students' emotions, rather than repression, and a conscious rejection of the emotional deadening that accompanies traditional medical education, as the same issue of the *Examiner* reveals in a report on a Dartmouth anatomy class: "Nervous students in surgical gloves and aprons filed into a fluorescent-lit laboratory and lined up alongside steel tables where cadavers lay ready for dissection. Instead of feeling pressured to maintain a stoic composure, these first-year medical students were encouraged to cry, laugh, faint, or leave the room if they wanted to. None did, but many said they appreciated the 'permission' to do so."

In contrast, here is Terry Tyler's experience of his medical anatomy class during the 1970s:

> The first week of medical school, we were required to dissect a fetus. We were arranged in teams of four around a dissecting table with the cadaver on it, all mummified in gauze bandages and stinking of formaldehyde. On that first day we were faced with a fetus, which had been placed on top of the cadaver. Our group had a full-term baby, which had been stillborn. The very first thing we were to do was to take a meat cleaver and do a saggital section through the head of this fetus. That is, we were to cut its head in half from front to back. Out of that class of eighty-five students, six did not return the next day. I think they might have made the best doctors.

With that suggestion, Tyler acknowledges the importance of feeling and compassion in medical practice. Dr. Koop echoes this sentiment, as the July 3, 1994, *San Francisco Examiner* reports, suggesting that technology, which in many ways has undermined the interpersonal aspects of healing, can also be part of its reestablishment: "Suppose you're a third-year student working in the clinic. You see a patient who had a major convulsion yesterday—the first one of his life. He asks you: 'What's wrong with me? Will it happen again? Is it curable?' Well, a third-year student knows nothing about that. But, with software that connects us to the National Library of Medicine, he can punch 'grand mal seizure' into the computer and get facts on the prognosis, therapy, and likely recurrence. He'll learn a little bit, retain some of the specific knowledge; but he'll get experience in problem-solving and listening to patients that will be more important than memorization."

The scenario in which technology frees a doctor to focus on the interpersonal aspects of a medical interview fulfills a prediction John Naisbitt made in *Megatrends* (1980) that at the turn of the century the blending of "high tech and high touch" would reintroduce the personal element into a culture he foresaw as increasingly alienated by technology.

Growing public awareness of the abuses of residency and the danger posed to patients by exhausted residents who fall asleep during surgery, prescribe the wrong medication, or write down the wrong information in the chart has sparked calls for more humane hours and more time off for residents. Many are on call every other night, while working thirty-six-hour shifts every other day. A study compared a group of postcall residents who had slept approximately thirty minutes in the preceding thirty-six hours with a non–postcall group of residents who were not fatigued. While manual dexterity, reaction time, and short-term memory were relatively unchanged by sleep loss, the study found, creative thinking suffered appreciably, as did originality, verbal fluency, motivation, and the ability to maintain constant vigilance (Nelson et al. 1995). The director of the residency program of the neurology department at Baylor Medical Center in Houston, Dr. Cliff Gooch, notes that

> in order to make residency less intensive, it is necessary to hire more people to do the work that residents have done. Some places have done that, and I think it's a positive step in the right direction. What's working against that, though, are the HMOs, which are really causing the financial crunch that medicine finds itself in now. . . . In an ideal world, residents would have exactly the right balance of supervised experience and autonomy [and] would be freed from doing a lot of the more mundane tasks that are not really necessary to their training. [Scut work is] part and parcel of residency training now in public hospitals, because they don't have enough money to pay enough people to do those things. . . . You really want to give the resident what they need without taking undue advantage of them. (quoted in Flint 1996:12)

Another trend in medical education is increasing willingness both to conduct research in and to offer courses in alternative medicine. Harvard Medical School, for example, has endowed a Mind/Body Medical Institute Chair, the first in the field of behavioral medicine; Dr. Herbert Benson, who conducted the research behind the "relaxation response," currently holds it. Harvard professor David Eisenberg, who teaches a course in alternative medicine, strongly advocated the rigorous evaluation of alternative therapies in testimony before a Senate subcommittee in 1993, and stated that "research centers should be built in the midst of our most respected medical institutions to insure credibility and fair-mindedness" (1996:22). By 1997, the NIH's new Office of Alternative Medicine had funded ten such centers across the country in well-respected universities from Stanford in California to Columbia in New York.[6]

In 1995, of this country's 125 medical schools, 26 offered a total of 42 courses in alternative or complementary medicine, which translates to 21 percent of medical schools offering at least one course in alternative medicine. In 1996, that number increased to 51 courses offered in 31 medical schools, including Harvard, Stanford, Yale, and Johns Hopkins. In 1997 the numbers rose to 60 courses offered in 37 medical schools. In other words, by summer 1997, more than 30 percent of the nation's medical schools were offering at least one such course.[7] Offering a course is not the same as requiring one; nevertheless, the increase in the number and availability of these courses certainly points to the expansion of medical education beyond the boundaries of the technocratic paradigm. Many of these classes are introductory or survey, clearly not designed to provide medical students with skills in alternative techniques. But their existence indicates a new level of responsiveness, not just to students, but to the overall health care environment.

In this chapter, we have shown how initiation into the technomedical model is accomplished through rituals that effect a psychological transformation of student to physician, a transformation that generally takes place in alignment with the core value system of technomedicine. At the end of their seven-year-long rite of passage, the student-initiate is admitted into the ranks of the most prestigious and powerful professional group in our society. The new doctor goes forward, fully imbued with the values and capable of using the arsenal of techniques available in the technomedical paradigm.

That paradigm has resulted in many dramatic improvements in diagnosis and treatment of illness and disease; it has also left many patients angry and alienated by its cold and impersonal treatment and has been unable to help them with many of their illnesses. Its emphasis on aggressive intervention has done a great deal of harm, and its high costs have become a major problem in the American economy. Many physicians themselves remain far from satisfied with the limitations and Stage-One nature of their technomedical training. And general agreement exists in the health care field that the hard edges of techomedicine must be softened.

PART II

The Humanistic and Holistic Paradigms

3 *The Humanistic Model of Medicine*

> Now patients are more involved with their care, and the therapeutic relationship has shifted from paternalistic to patients being partners in their own care. . . . On the whole, I think that's the new paradigm of what we would call, in America, traditional medicine. I by no means think that holistic physicians have a lock on that.
> —CLIFF GOOCH, M.D.

While the majority of the physicians who comprise our primary research base are holistic, a small number are not. This was not intentional on our part—we were seeking to interview only holistic physicians. But the boundaries between holistic and humanistic practice are blurry, and it is often not possible to tell one from the other in an introductory conversation. Looking for holistic practitioners, we sometimes found instead physicians who seemed very different from traditional technocratic M.D.'s, but who also seemed different from the holistic M.D.'s whose worldview we were increasingly coming to understand.[1] Occasionally we were surprised when a physician we had thought of as holistic emphatically rejected the label and its accompanying paradigm of care. For example, one of them said, "I never thought that I was holistic; it was humanism to me. I always thought of holistic medicine as people who don't know anything about orthodox medicine, but who were naturopaths or learned herbs. They didn't know much about drugs and surgery. Holism did not equate to what I was doing. Humanism felt right for me. Humanism means putting the human element into medical education. It is psychological, sociological, humanistic."

Over time we came to realize that these physicians, who deviated significantly from the technomedical model in the way they relate to patients and in their personal attention to the human side of the medical consultation, also deviated from the holistic model in their allegiance to technomedicine and in their resistance to many of the alternative modalities that holism embraces. Expanding beyond the narrow confines of technomedicine into a more caring and relational approach to patients, they traveled no further. Some may have found humanism a comfortable resting place, a halfway point on a journey they will later resume. But others clearly found in humanism an approach to healing and a set of beliefs that could both satisfy and challenge them for a lifetime.

This chapter discusses this humanistic approach, one that speaks of reform rather than revolution. Without overthrowing the dominance of allopathy or undermining popular belief in its efficacy, the proponents of this approach seek to soften the hard edges of technomedicine. Humanists try to treat patients with compassion and respect, to add the interpersonal dimensions of healing to the allopath's technical expertise. Humanists, in theory and in practice, pose a far lesser threat to the allopathic system than holistic physicians, who present a more radical challenge. Humanists wish simply to humanize technomedicine—that is, to make it relational, partnership-oriented, individually responsive, and compassionate. Theirs is an approach based on common sense and good interpersonal skills, one that values and seeks to revitalize the Marcus Welby–type physician—the family doc, the community pediatrician. This caring, commonsensical approach, which reflects the availability of these M.D.'s as individuals, their communication skills, and their deep concern for their patients is garnering wide national appreciation and support. Clearly less radical than holism, clearly more loving than technomedicine, this humanistic paradigm has the most potential to open the technocratic system, from the inside, to the possibility of widespread reform.

As much an attitude as a paradigm, the humanistic model can be characterized as follows:

(1) Mind-body connection
(2) The body as an organism
(3) The patient as relational subject
(4) Connection and caring between practitioner and patient
(5) Diagnosis and healing from the outside in *and* from the inside out
(6) Balance between the needs of the institution and the individual
(7) Information, decision making, and responsibility shared between patient and practitioner
(8) Science and technology counterbalanced with humanism
(9) Focus on disease prevention
(10) Death as an acceptable outcome
(11) Compassion-driven care
(12) Open-mindedness toward other modalities

Underlying Principle and Type of Thinking: Balance and Connection

Whereas the technomedical paradigm is based on the principle of separation, and the holistic model on its opposite, the principle of integration, the principle underlying the humanistic approach is connection: the connection of the patient to the multiple aspects of herself, her family, her society, and her health care practitioners. Humanism requires treating the patient in a connected, relational way as any human being would want to be treated—with consideration, kindness, and respect. This paradigm insists on the deep humanity of the individuals involved and stresses the importance of the patient-practitioner relationship to the healing process. Characterized by a balance between left- and right-brain hemispheric functions, a humanistic approach to healing requires no fundamental change in the left-brained allopathic approach beyond talking to a patient while she undergoes a painful procedure, or reaching down to take her hand while conveying a diagnosis she may be afraid to hear. Right-brained skills of empathy, relationship, and emotional connection can simply be incorporated into allopathic treatment. Thus the boundaries between the technomedical and the humanistic approaches are also very blurred; many technomedical practitioners regularly take the trouble to be caring and to that extent can be considered humanistic.

The best analogue for the term "humanism" in the medical literature is the term "biopsychosocial," which suggests a willingness to see the patient as multidimensional, to understand the human being as far more complex than the reductionism of the biotechnical model allows. As a corollary, this term acknowledges that the roots of illness can be emotional and mental, and recognizes that healing must occur on those levels also. Although a significant amount of research has appeared in medical journals attesting to the connection between the mind and body, the allopathic paradigm fails to acknowledge this connection when it looks at causes and cures for illness, an omission that the proponents of this approach seek to rectify. Yet they generally do not go so far as to insist, as holists do, that mind and body are one.

History of the Humanistic Model of Medicine

The origins of the humanistic model lie in the era of the general practitioner, when personality, intuition, and the desire to serve one's community played a major role in patient care. In that era, the personality of the doctor was significant in part because it was one of his most important instruments. Peter Nunn, an interviewee, trained in England when healing was an art that depended heavily on the physical and intuitive skills and experience of the practitioner. He recalls, "We still had the old-guard doctors who were preantibiotics. I remember the Queen's physician, Lord Evans, going around and just picking up the patient's hand, giving a complete diagnosis from the hand, from the texture, the pulse, the temperature, obviously looking at the patient. I saw him diagnose thyroid disease that way in a woman who had been in for weeks and no one knew what was wrong with her."

During the 1960s Americans were mesmerized by the prime-time saga of Marcus Welby M.D., whose dedication and compassion fulfilled their longing for a doctor whose work was truly a vocation. Contrast that with the 1990s show *ER*, in which high-tech emergency care is given to patients whose eventual outcomes and personal situations are minimally known to the doctors, whose primary job is to "stitch 'em and ditch 'em."

Even as the friendly family doc was vanishing from the American medical scene, a number of prominent physicians and researchers began to call for a new model that strongly resembled his approach. They gave it a name: the biopsychosocial model (Engels 1977), to indicate that equal attention should be paid to a patient's biology, individual psychology, and social environment. George L. Engels, M.D., who originated the term "biopsychosocial," describes the impact of seeing his mentor John Romano in 1941 "sit down with a patient on medical rounds and engage him as though in the privacy of his office"—an experience that eventually culminated in Engels's move "beyond the biomedical to the biopsychosocial" (1995:xix). In a series of publications, Engels (1977, 1980, 1988) described the benefits of this model, which center on reincorporating the social and psychological domains into the medical treatment of illness.

An early interpreter of Engels's theory was psychiatrist Arthur Kleinman. In *The Illness Narratives* (1988), Kleinman describes an experience during his medical training in the 1960s that fixed his interest on the human dimensions of illness. As a neophyte clinical student, he was charged with attempting to soothe a badly burned seven-year-old girl as, struggling and screaming, she was placed in a whirlpool bath and the burned flesh was tweezed from her raw, open wounds. Nothing he tried soothed her in the least until he hit on the strategy of asking her to tell him what it felt like to be so badly burned and to have to endure such pain every day. Surprised, she stopped screaming and told him. Every day thereafter, she continued to narrate her experience to him, and she ceased to struggle and resist her treatment. They both learned an important lesson: talking about the experience of illness can help to order it and make it more bearable.

Later Kleinman treated an elderly woman who had syphilis, which she had acquired from a serviceman in World War I and which had inexorably shaped the trajectory of her life. She taught Kleinman the difference between the doctor's focus on disease and the patient's experience of illness. Through these and many other such experiences, Kleinman came to believe that, although not taught in medical training, the interpretation of narratives of illness—which he defines as "the innately human experience of symptoms and suffering"—is "a core task in the work of doctoring" (1988:xiii).

Another pioneer in the humanistic arena was Herbert Benson, famous for his discovery and naming of "the relaxation response." Proving as he did that change in mental and emotional states could have an impact on physical states was revolutionary—and came from the belly of orthodoxy. Fundamentally, research like that of Kleinman and Benson simply documents for the record what thoughtful individuals discover in the course of living, whether they are doctors or not. As Albert Einstein noted, "The whole of science is nothing more than a refinement of everyday thinking" (1950:59). Certainly this is true of the scientific research underpinning the humanistic model. Bill Moyers expressed it this way:

> In science class we studied the material world, which we expected would someday be understood and predicted down to the last molecule. In philosophy we studied models of reality, based on the rational mind, that took no notice of conditions male and female, sick and well, rich and poor. . . . Yet every day in this divided world of mind and body, our language betrayed the limitations of our categories. "Widow Brown must have died of a broken heart—she never got sick until after her husband was gone." My parents talked about our friend the grocer, who "worried himself sick," and my Uncle Carl believed that laughter could ease what ailed you. (1993:xi)

In 1993 Moyers produced a four-part public television series on *Healing and the Mind* that awakened the nation to the possibilities of a health care approach that incorporated the mind in the healing of the body; the series gave visibility to many of the studies we describe in this chapter. Eager to inform American viewers about the healing powers of the mind, and wanting to be a bridge-builder rather than an iconoclast, Moyers stuck very close to what we describe here as the humanistic approach, avoiding some of the more radical and revolutionary claims of holism.[2] His series and its accompanying book, *Healing and the Mind*, sparked the formation of discussion and self-help groups across the nation, and greatly increased public awareness of the value of humanistic and holistic alternatives to conventional care.

Of course, there is far more to the history of the humanistic model than we can describe here. Suffice it to say that in the wider cultural arena, the social transformations of the 1960s and 1970s made the American public aware of the importance of interpersonal and intrapersonal communication. Psychology became a popular subject, as individuals strove to understand themselves and others on a deeper level. Concomitantly, social reform led to a great interest in the humanistic treatment of disenfranchised groups. The demands of women, blacks, Hispanics, and others for equality and respect influenced medicine along with every other social realm. Twin prongs within medicine have both sparked and sustained the development of this model. Many physicians practiced humanistically all along, or began to do so out of their own desire for more meaningful and relational contact with their patients. Others came to humanism through medical research, devoting great portions of their academic careers to demonstrating the value of the humanistic approach. It is somewhat ironic that their efforts were rendered necessary by the stubborn insistence of the dominant technomedical paradigm on the mechanicity of the body and the fundamental separation of the patient from both the practitioner and the disease. Although this insistence is counterintuitive, it has taken two decades of research in the humanistic and holistic fields to prove. And although the mind-body connection has been proven, its implications are still not generally accepted or acted upon.

Whereas many of the developments in the holistic revolution have been driven by groups outside mainstream medicine such as naturopaths and chiropractors, the impetus for the humanistic reformation has largely arisen from inside the ranks of the medical profession. Nurses were the first to call for the system's humanistic reform (Benner and Rubel 1989; Peplau 1952); later on they were joined by an ever-increasing number of mainstream physicians, including, among many others, George Engels, Herbert Benson, Arthur Kleinman, Robert Smith, Dean Ornish, David Spiegel, David Eisenberg, and Candace Pert. The fact that some on this list might also be cited as fundamental to the recognition of holistic medicine shows how closely these two paradigms are linked. As we will see in chapter 4, holism does not exclude humanism, but rather incorporates it.

Today humanistic reforms have been or are being implemented in a growing number of medical schools and residency training programs; we will describe some of these in the following sections. But at the same time as we acknowledge that medical humanism has been largely developed from within the cultural and medical mainstream, we must also note the influence that those outside the mainstream have exerted. Hegemonic paradigms like the technomedical model are extremely difficult to crack open from the inside without strong accompanying external pressure. The burgeoning field of holistic medicine and its increasingly widespread utilization by the American public have given fair warning to the medical mainstream that change is long overdue. The coming of age of medical humanism in many ways is a response from within the system to this strong external pressure from the proponents of holism. This fact helps us see the complexity of the interactions among the three paradigms of care we discuss in this book.

The Twelve Tenets of the Humanistic Model

(1) MIND-BODY CONNECTION

The humanistic approach neither demarcates a total separation between mind and body, as does technomedicine, nor claims oneness for mind and body, as does the holistic model. While conceptualizing mind and body as separate, the humanistic model recognizes the influence of the mind on the body and advocates forms of healing that address both. Proponents of this paradigm see body and mind as being in constant communication. Thus the humanistic paradigm insists on the importance of the "mind-body connection" in illness and healing.

During the 1960s, Herbert Benson began research that eventually demonstrated this connection. After his experiments with monkeys showed that they could lower their blood pressure in response to certain stimuli, a group of meditators asked him to do the same sort of research on them. Benson and some colleagues designed an experiment (Benson, Beary, and Carol 1974) to measure various physiological responses of the meditators during three twenty-minute periods: a quiet period, a meditation period, and another quiet period following the meditation. The results were striking. Compared to the simple resting state, the volunteers consumed 17 percent less oxygen while meditating and produced less carbon dioxide. Their breathing slowed from a normal rate of fourteen or fifteen breaths per minute to ten or eleven, and the lactate in their bodies dropped precipitously (high levels of lactate are associated with anxiety, low levels with tranquillity). In addition, brain wave patterns changed during meditation, producing more of the low-frequency alpha, theta, and delta waves associated with rest and relaxation and fewer of the high-frequency beta waves associated with normal waking activity. Benson later found that this relaxation response can be stimulated by a wide variety of methods (including hatha yoga, hypnosis, and progressive muscle relaxation) and can help in the treatment of many medical problems, including high blood pressure, heart disease, cancer, infertility, and chronic pain (Benson and Klipper 1976; Benson 1984, 1987; Benson et al. 1992). Unlike many holistic physicians, Benson does not claim that this relaxation response itself can heal. Rather, he states, "To the extent that any disorder is caused or made worse by stress, the relaxation response is useful. It is never a substitute for regular medical care" (1993:236).

Further understanding of the physiology of the mind/body connection comes from the field of psychoneuroimmunology (PNI). PNI researchers seek to document the actual physical and chemical communication between the central nervous system and the immune system, and the mediating roles that hormones play. Nerve fibers extending from the hypothalamus, where the pituitary is located in the brain, reach deep into the thymus and bone marrow. Because the pituitary is both gland and nerve fiber, it mediates between signals from the endocrine and nervous systems. When a physical invader, such as a bacterium or a virus, triggers the immune system to respond, the gland action of the pituitary stimulates the production of hormones. Similarly, if emotional stress causes excess hormonal secretion, nerve endings that detect the presence of homones in the body alert the immune system. In short, mental, emotional, and physical processes do not take place separately; because of the mediating functions of hormones, every mental function has an emotional and physiological component and vice versa.

PNI research represents one of the many areas of crossover between the humanistic and holistic paradigms of medicine. Humanists draw obvious conclusions about the existence and importance of the mind-body connection, but they fail to take PNI findings as far as they might; holists take a further step toward the concept of mind-body unity. In *Healing and the Mind*, Candace Pert, a well-known researcher in the field of PNI, describes the transition that has been taking place in scientific thinking about the relationship between brain and body:

> In real life the brain and the immune system use so many of the same molecules to communicate with each other that we're beginning to see that perhaps the brain is not simply "up here," connected by nerves to the rest of the body. It's a much more dynamic process . . . the old emphasis on the brain is breaking down now that we're discovering, for example, that cells of the immune system are constantly filtering through the brain and can actually lodge there. When people discovered there were endorphins in the brain that caused euphoria and pain relief, everybody could handle that. But when they discovered they were in your immune system, too, it just didn't fit, so it was denied for years. The original scientists had to repeat their studies many, many times to be believed. It was just very upsetting to our paradigm to find mood-altering chemicals in the immune system—and not just the chemicals, but the receptors as well. (1993:180)

Conventional scientists had difficulty accepting the existence of mood-altering chemicals and receptors in the immune system because it implies that changes in mood and attitude can directly affect changes in immune response. Pert struggles with finding the right metaphors to express the philosophical implications of this research on the mind-body connection:

> I used to say that neuropeptides and the receptors are the physical substrate of emotions. Then someone yelled at me and said, "What do you mean, 'physical substrate'? That makes it sound as if they're the foundation of emotions. How do you know the foundation isn't in another

> energy realm? Why don't you say neuropeptides are the biochemical correlate?" It's tricky. I don't have the right language because I'm not sure. I can say that what it looks like to me is that the currency with which mind and matter interconvert might be emotions. Emotions might actually be the link between mind and body—although I hate the word "link," because it's mechanical and Newtonian, and it suggests fences. (1993:186–187)

Pert's work and thought are fundamental to the development of the scientific underpinnings of both the humanistic and the holistic paradigms. Her search for the right language reflects her struggle over whether to replace the technocratic model's insistence on mind-body separation by "going all the way" to the holistic model's stress on the oneness of body and mind, or by stopping at the uneasy middle ground of the humanistic emphasis on their connection, which keeps them separate even as it brings them closer together.

(2) THE BODY AS AN ORGANISM

Although in some ways the human body is *like* a machine, it is a fact of biological life that the body is not a machine but an organism. Such a conclusion for most people represents simple common sense. Yet it has powerful repercussions for treatment, as the way the body is defined will shape the way it is treated by a culture's health care system. Much of the techno-medical style of treatment stems from its definition of the body as a machine, including the notion that mind and body are separate. Yet, as a group of humanistically oriented researchers has pointed out, "Even medical therapies that are the most machine-like would be ineffective without the innate healing powers of the organism," which has "properties that no machine has: those of growth, regeneration, healing, learning, and self-transcendence" (Tresolini et al. 1994:20).

Defining the body as an organism charters the development of an array of treatments that may be irrelevant to a machine but matter a great deal to an organism. Unlike machines, mammalian organisms feel pain and respond emotionally to interactions with others and to changes in their environment. Most mammals seek privacy and protection when they are ill; most mammals respond positively to the comfort of a loving touch and shrink from contact that is harsh or punitive. Thus a paradigm of healing based on a definition of the human body as an organism would logically stress the importance of kindness, of touch, and of caring.

As we will see in the following chapter, the holistic model defines the human body as an energy field. In spite of the strong scientific basis for this definition, to many practitioners such a definition seems equally as fantastical as the technomedical model's definition of the body as a machine. The middle ground provided by the humanistic model's definition of the body as an organism thus has great appeal for those who wish to expand beyond the narrow parameters of the mechanistic approach but who balk at the holistic expansion from matter to energy, which they see as extreme.

(3) THE PATIENT AS RELATIONAL SUBJECT

In chapter 1, we described "the patient as object" as the third tenet of technomedicine, an approach that involves treating the patient's body and ignoring her mind. In chapter 4 we will describe the holistic model's third tenet as "healing the whole person in whole life context," an approach that addresses the multiple components and relationships of the individual in her environment, and acknowledges that full healing may be well beyond the abilities of any one practitioner, but may require multiple healers practicing a diversity of modalities. The humanistic model generally eschews holism's wide range, focusing instead on remediating technomedicine's objectification by treating the patient as a person instead of as a machine to be fixed.

In *Love, Medicine, and Miracles*, Bernie Siegel recounts his joy at the simple discovery that his patients were people. Burned out on his surgical cancer practice, he considered other careers: "I couldn't decide what I wanted, but I realized that most of my choices had to do with people. Even in the painting I did as a hobby my only interest was portraits. Then it finally dawned on me. Here I was, seeing a score of patients every day, as well as their families, dozens of doctors and nurses, and still I was looking for people. I'd thought of my patients merely as machines I had to repair" (1986:14).

In addition to seeing the patient as a person, this biopsychosocial approach acknowledges the profound effects of the social environment on the individual and seeks to incorporate this awareness into treatment. Perhaps the most often cited study in humanistic medical care is that conducted by David Spiegel, M.D., and his colleagues on "The Effect of Psychosocial Treatment on Survival of Patients with Metastatic Breast Cancer" (1989). In the early 1980s, Spiegel began organizing support groups for women with advanced breast cancer because he "wanted to learn how to help the dying. . . . As a psychiatrist leading weekly 90–minute sessions, I watched the women cry together over the deaths of group members, cheer small victories, and plot strategies for coping with recalcitrant husbands, stubborn children, and difficult friends. I was struck then, and continue to be impressed, by the almost instant rapport these women shared, the often unspoken sense of understanding that grew out of their similar circumstances" (Spiegel 1993:331).

These groups, part of a study Spiegel and his colleagues were conducting at Stanford University on the health benefits of social support (Spiegel et al. 1989), yielded the expected finding that participation helped the women emotionally. Spiegel's original motivation for following up on the women in his groups was to disprove the notion, popular in the mid-1980s, that psychological factors could actually affect the course of cancer. Thus he was shocked and amazed to find, when he sat down to analyze the numbers, that the women in his groups not only felt better emotionally, but ultimately lived an average of eighteen months longer than did women with comparable breast cancer and medical care who did not attend such groups—which meant that the women lived twice as long from the time he and his colleagues first saw them. This added survival time was, according to Spiegel, "longer than any medication or other known medical treatment could be expected to provide for women with breast cancer so far advanced" (1993:331–332). This study, which received widespread attention, awakened many physicians to the beneficial effects of good relationships and social support on both the psychological and the physiological aspects of illness and disease.

Other studies have shown that stress can reduce immune system functioning, and that this reduction can be mitigated by social support. For example, research on medical students by psychologist Janice Kiecolt-Glaser and immunologist Ronald Glaser at Ohio State University College of Medicine (1991, 1992) showed that certain cells in the students' immune systems became less effective during the stress of exams. But medical students who felt connected to family and friends showed a much less pronounced immunological change than those who described themselves as lonely.

Spiegel's study has been followed by a number of large-scale studies that show a lower risk of dying at any age to be associated with having close social relationships. The classic example is a study conducted by epidemiologists Lisa Berkman and Leonard Syme (1979) on residents of Alameda County, California, which examined the relationship between the death rate and four types of social support: marital status, contact with extended family and friends, church membership, and other group affiliations. Berkman and Syme found that those individuals who were least socially connected were twice as likely to die as those with the strongest social ties, even when health habits such as smoking, alcohol use, physical activity, obesity, and use of preventive health programs were taken into account. Likewise, sociologist James House of the University of Michigan studied the social connections of 2,754 adults, and found that the most socially active men were two to three times less likely to die within nine to twelve years as those of a similar age who were relatively isolated. The risk for socially isolated women was one and a half to two times as great (House, Landis, and Umberson 1988).

Research like Spiegel's that has looked specifically at people who are already sick shows that once serious illness strikes, social support continues to affect one's chances of staying alive. For example, internist James Goodwin and his colleagues (1987) found that married cancer patients did better medically and had lower mortality rates than the unmarried; Redford Williams and his colleagues at Duke University (1980, 1992) found that having a spouse or other close confidant tripled the chances that patients with coronary artery disease would be alive five years later, and epidemiologists Peggy Reynolds and George Kaplan (1990) at the University of California at Berkeley found that women with the least amount of social contact were 2.2 times more likely to die of cancer over a seventeen-year period than were the most socially connected. All of these researchers have been careful to eliminate the obvious confounding variables such as smoking and alcohol abuse, differences in socioeconomic status, and access to health care.

These studies and many others like them consistently show that more and better social support from family and friends is associated with lower odds of dying and better odds of healing at any given age. The increasing number of these studies and the consistency of their findings has given tremendous impetus to the call for the humanistic reform of the medical system, which had previously ignored the variable of social support and the importance of treating the patient as a person in relationship with others.

In 1992 the Pew Health Foundation Commission and the Fetzer Institute (see note 1) established a Task Force on Psychosocial Health Education to develop an agenda for "encouraging the development or expansion of educational programs that reflect an integrated biomedical-psychosocial perspective" (Tresolini et al. 1994:8). Despite nursing's long history of emphasizing caring relationships, the task force noted, this practice has not become a defining force in health care. To affirm the centrality of relationships in the healing arts, the task force asserted the need for a new phrase, "relationship-centered care." They felt that this focus could help to overcome the reductionism implicit even in the "biopsychosocial" approach, as well as the lack of focus on relationship in the term "patient-centered," which was also being used to describe the humanistic approach: "The phrase 'relationship-centered care' captures the importance of the interaction among people as the foundation of any therapeutic or healing activity. Further, relationships are critical to the care provided by nearly all practitioners (regardless of discipline or subspecialty) and a source of satisfaction and positive outcomes for patients and practitioners" (Tresolini et al. 1994:11).

The concept of relationship-centered care is making significant inroads into the reform of the technomedical system. For example, one offshoot of Bill Moyers's series *Healing and the Mind* was a round table on self-help groups sponsored in May of 1997 by the Kansas Health Foundation and several major hospitals in Kansas, and attended by representatives from fourteen managed-care providers in the state. Open dialogue and collaborative work resulted in the creation of systems of referral, quality assurance, and funding for meeting space, telephone systems, printing, and so on for thousands of self-help groups that offer relational support to people with a wide variety of illnesses, from alchoholism and arthritis to cancer and cystic fibrosis. Funding was also allocated for training Kansas health care providers—physicians, nurses, social workers, and so on—to understand the value to patients of self-help groups and relationship-centered care (Janis Claflin, personal communication).

(4) CONNECTION AND CARING BETWEEN PRACTITIONER AND PATIENT

The studies described above carry the further implication that close contact and good relationships between patient and physician can also improve the patient's chances of recovery. The implication for clinical practice is that not only should physicians do all they can to encourage patients to reach out to others, but also they should use the healing power of the doctor-patient relationship. Although most humanists are found in traditional medical settings and conventional practices, they are not afraid to establish a real human connection with their patients, to open to them in wonder and interest, and to come to know them not just as patients but as individuals. Oncologist Dawn LeManne expresses this perspective: "I have profound respect for every patient who comes to me. Inside myself, every encounter with a patients is a sacred encounter. When I'm standing in front of the exam room, with my hand on the door, I have the sense that this is a special event. It could take three minutes; it could take an hour, but this is a special encounter. This is a feeling that I bring to my work. It's not something that I decided to do one day. In essence I do that with each encounter."

Like LeManne, Amy Saltzmann identifies the heart of humanism as the focus on the individual rather than the condition: "It's a subtle difference. It's looking at someone as the MI [myocardial infarction, or heart attack] who just came in as opposed to looking at the woman with three kids who works for an electrical engineering company who just had a heart attack. The difference is where your focus is. Is your focus on the person or on the disease and the tests and the medicine?"

The physicians we identified as humanistic instinctively knew that their very presence and attention to their patients were healing influences. Glenn Masterson describes his delight as well as his patients' satisfaction with the style he has cultivated:

> I've got a large geriatric practice—somehow my name went around the mobile home park. I love these older people. They're wonderful. One thing I like is they're not in a hurry. You take a middle-class mom with two or three kids, and she's got a schedule, she's in a hurry. But these old people, they've got a book, and they've got a wealth of experience, great stories to tell. They read the paper and tell me what's new in medicine. I spend a lot of time talking to them.
>
> Q: How do you see yourself as different from other physicians?
>
> A: I listen to patients. I think my patients appreciate that I care about them. I've had so many patients tell me that just listening to them is therapeutic.

Masterson has tapped into the central task of the doctor, described by John Berger as providing "an individual and closely intimate recognition of the patient. If the man can begin to feel recognized . . . the hopeless nature of his unhappiness will have been changed" (1967:68–69).

The humanistic ability to connect is often put to the test. Interviewee Ed Neal describes working with someone "you can't stand" as a challenge he is sometimes required to meet as a physician. One of the MetaPhysicians describes how he dealt with this sort of challenge: "I spent so many years disliking my patients. It seems a lot of doctors don't like patients—they are somewhere between neutral and negative. Now I am aware that there is someone beyond the patient's face, beyond the institutionalized being, beyond the 'chronic low back pain.' The veils that separate me from others are losing their power. This love I am feeling is something I want to explore more" (Gene Ross, *MetaPhysicians' Tales*).

Bernie Siegel talks about the struggle to balance professional distance and personal relationship, defining "rational concern" as a way for physicians and caregivers of all types to connect without losing themselves in the process:

> I became aware that . . . I had adopted this standard defense against pain and failure. Because I was hurting, I withdrew when patients needed me most. This became especially apparent when I returned from a long vacation . . . for a few days, I reacted only as a human being. Then I could feel the emotions slipping away and the professional veneer taking over. Yet I wanted to hang on to this sensitivity, because the coldness doesn't really save anyone from the pain. It just buries the hurt on a deeper level. I used to think a certain amount of this distancing was essential, but for most doctors I think it goes too far. Too often the pressure squeezes out our native compassion. The so-called detached concern we're taught is

> an absurdity. Instead we need to be taught a rational concern, which allows the expression of feelings without impairing the ability to make decisions. (1986:14)[3]

Humanistic physicians tend to derive a great deal of satisfaction from their work. The great majority of doctors who practice in this style may not even be aware of the increasing amount of research proving the benefits of humanism; they practice that way out of the force of their own personalities, as a response to their vocation as healers. For them the relational components of their work, whether with their staff, colleagues, or patients, are the most rewarding. They actually feel better as a result of their relational approach, seeing it not only as good for their patients but also as good for themselves, as Ed Neal relates:

> A farming family came to the intensive care unit. The husband was dying. He was in a coma, on a ventilator . . . and it was my job to turn the ventilator off. What happens when you do that is that the heartbeat gets slower and slower. So I did it and started to walk out of the room. The wife said, "Don't go, stay here." So I did, and we all held hands. I'm starting to cry now because I cry whenever I remember this. Each person said, "This is what this man meant to me and this is how much I love him." Afterward, I felt great all day—warmed up like I was sitting in front of a fire. And it dawned on me that whenever there is healing, it's like a fire that touches everyone involved.

In "'Learning Medicine': The Constructing of Medical Education at Harvard Medical School," Byron and Mary Jo Good suggest that the juxtaposed "central symbols" of *competence* and *caring* represent a cultural tension developed throughout medical education that is linked to a dualistic discourse characteristic of contemporary American medicine:

> Physicians must be competent; they should also embody caring qualities. Competence is associated with the language of the basic sciences, with "value-free" facts and knowledge, skills, techniques, and "doing" or action. . . . "Caring" for these students is expressed in the language of values, of relationships, attitudes, compassion, and empathy, the nontechnical or as one student called it the "personal" aspects of medicine. It is also conveyed in terms such as "the laying on of hands." Competence is closely associated with the natural sciences, caring with the humanities. Competence is a quality of knowledge and skills, caring a quality of persons. (1993:91)

The Goods go on to note that this juxtaposition of competence and caring, present throughout the history of Western medicine, reflects the larger struggle in American society between science and culture, technology and humanism, which in the West are often seen as opposing forces.

> Medicine . . . accepts this dichotomy as fundamental, then defines as essential to the role of the physician qualities of both of these cultures. . . . Competence is given primacy, as is bioscience as the presumed basis for medical practice, and the language of competence has come to be increasingly powerful in expressing the self-worth of the physician, in negotiating boundaries among specialties, and in providing the sole grounds for compensation for failures of medicine to provide benefit. Central to medical education is the demand to educate competent physicians while maintaining the qualities of caring. Contradictions, both socially and culturally constituted, necessarily result. (1993:93–94)

It is precisely these contradictions that the humanistic approach to medicine seeks to resolve. In chapter 1 we heard Bill Manahan's impassioned description of the inner turmoil that witnessing human suffering can produce in the compassionate physician. From what we have learned about medical education, it is apparent that the traditionally trained physician has received little guidance in how to cope with, let alone express, such feelings. Doctors faced with suffering, whether in an emergency or routine situation, are expected to process information quickly, arrive at, and often implement a course of treatment. In technomedical circles, emotions are thought to interfere with such abilities. In both humanistic and holistic settings, feelings are accepted as part of the healing response.

For example, physician Robert Smith offers a course on patient-centered interviewing for residents. He specifically teaches them to talk about their own feelings in peer support groups and then offers them techniques for staying open to empathize with the feelings of others instead of shutting down. Rachel Naomi Remen, M.D., author of *Kitchen Table Wisdom* (1996) and founder of the Commonweal Institute, offers a course at the University of San Francisco School of Medicine specifically designed to teach medical students "how to maintain one's integrity, how to deal with grief, to recognize and be open to the sacred" (Remen 1995). In the class on grief, students are taught to recognize dysfunctional ways of coping with grief, to identify their personal strategies for dealing with loss and disappointment, and to learn supportive strategies for helping others deal with grief. Such re-formation of medical training works to resolve the tension the Goods identify between competence and caring by balancing students' technomedical competence with specific caring and relational skills.

(5) DIAGNOSIS AND HEALING FROM THE OUTSIDE IN *AND* FROM THE INSIDE OUT

Where the technomedical model emphasizes diagnosis and healing from the outside in, and the holistic model from the inside out, the humanistic model calls for a moderate application of both approaches. It does not ask for reliance on inner knowing, as does the holistic model, nor does it confine itself to valuing external diagnosis, as does the technocratic model. The physician-patient communication it emphasizes allows physicians to elicit information from deep within the patient and combine it with objective findings.

Accordingly, humanists find that knowing how to listen is as important as knowing what to say. The complexity of this task lies in allowing the patient enough freedom to express whatever is important while continually seeking the thread that will lead to a clinical grasp of the problem, whether its roots lie in the emotional, social, or physical realms. Thus, listening skills are crucial for obtaining the correct mix of data required for diagnosis.

Biotechnically oriented physicians rely on objective findings, not only in the sense of laboratory and physical examination results, but also in the way patients describe their condition. They follow generally the differential diagnostic method—an approach aimed at ruling out possibilities and ultimately revealing the cause of the complaint. So, for example, a patient describing a pain will be asked to specify whether it is sharp or dull, what time of day it occurs, and whether it radiates. These are not inquiries into the patient's subjective state, but attempts to diagnose. A humanistic physician, on the other hand, may ask many of the same questions, but in addition will also be interested in patients' sensitivity or tolerance for pain, their resourcefulness in applying home remedies, the nature of their social support network, and the meaning of this illness in their current life.

In *The Nature of Suffering and the Gods of Meaning* Eric J. Cassell notes, "Being responsive to the face of suffering remains the attribute of individual physicians who have come to this mastery alone or gained it from a few inspirational teachers." Our interviewee Bill Manahan had just such an inspirational teacher: "Carl Rogers was extremely important to me in becoming a humanistic M.D. in the 1970s. He taught me about active and passive listening, and it was a huge step—to actually *listen*, really listen, to my patients." In an effort to make this mastery more available, proponents of the humanistic approach are actively promulgating programs designed to teach residents skills that facilitate open communication with their patients, including the "active listening" Manahan describes.

George Engels has found that "the answers you get from a patient depend on the questions you pose and how you pose them" (1996:xi). With this statement, he introduces *The Patient's Story: Integrated Patient-Doctor Interviewing*, a manual physician Robert C. Smith has written to provide just the sort of basic methodology for patient interviewing that has been lacking in medical training. Smith emphasizes the idiosyncrasy and confusion of past methods of teaching interviewing to students, noting that this methodological vacuum may itself have encouraged students to acquire "human data" erratically and unsystematically: "By *human data*, I mean information that the patient communicates in words or through nonverbal but uniquely human modes of expression, for example, a frown. . . . I offer a challenge to the student: Keep human data foremost and do not rely primarily on the physical examination or the laboratory tests. Interviewing is the key skill of the physician. . . . Not only does it provide most diagnostic and therapeutic information about the patient, but it also is the major determinant of the doctor-patient relationship and outcome of care" (1996:1).

Noting that a clinician will perform from 120,000 to 160,000 interviews during a career, Smith points out that the biomedical model teaches students to elicit symptoms of disease using a "doctor-centered" interviewing process. The physician elicits many bits of nonpersonal data, then synthesizes them into a description of the patient's disease. The typical doctor-centered interview begins with the doctor eliciting the patient's chief complaint. From there, the doctor attempts through diagnosis to define it, though treatment to remediate it, or through referral to further clarify it. But humanistic doctors know that the presenting complaint often masks an underlying problem. A person complaining of fatigue, depression, and body aches may actually have lupus or may be despondent over a failed marriage. Practitioners must adopt an open-ended learning approach in order to create the space and time necessary to bring forth the underlying dynamic. Once this appears, the action required may be far different than that prompted by objective symptoms only.

This open-ended learning approach forms an important part of what Smith (1996:4) calls the "patient-centered interview." Instead of asking a series of closed, rapid-fire questions, the physician simply encourages patients to express what is most important to them, which will usually come out as a combination of personal data and data about symptoms. Allowing patients to lead keeps their ideas and concerns paramount. Smith recommends a judicious combination of both doctor- and patient-centered interviewing, as initially the physician must scrutinize for any symptoms that might require immediate action. If urgency is not an issue, the interviewer should "meet the patient's needs not by taking control but by allowing the patient to lead the conversation and to discuss the symptoms or personal issues she prefers. Ideas in the initial dialogue originate in the patient's mind rather than in the doctor's; later, the doctor will insert her ideas into the exchange" (1996:6). Smith stresses the "powerful humanistic rationale" for integrating patient-centered principles and addressing patients' needs first, so that patients can be heard and understood "in a way that validates them as human beings rather than as objects of study" (1996:6). Such an approach in an ultimate sense involves power sharing between doctor and patient and an enhanced sense of autonomy on the part of the patient, who, atypically, is not rendered dependent on the doctor by this approach. Clearly, the patient-centered interview can form an invaluable part of the humanistic physician's ability to be both competent and caring, both of which these interview skills facilitate.[4]

As we will see in the following chapter, holistic physicians give credence to intuition as a diagnostic skill. Likewise, many humanists have found that as they learn to be more in touch with and responsive to their own emotions and those of their patients, concomitantly they begin to access their own intuition. In her interview, Deborah Malka explained that most physicians, increasingly trained to be dependent on tests, "have to work hard at trusting their intuitive part, because it's trained out of you. If you can't prove it, you can't say it's there." The humanists who do work hard at getting to know and trust both their own intuition and that of their patients can add to technomedicine's emphasis on diagnosis from the outside in a dawning respect for the possibilities inherent in diagnosing from the inside out.

(6) BALANCE BETWEEN THE NEEDS OF THE INSTITUTION AND THE INDIVIDUAL

Most American medical institutions, such as hospitals, clinics, health maintenance organizations, and nursing homes, are designed to support and implement technocratic principles. These institutions are so highly regulated with respect to infection control, medical/surgical and nursing procedures, security, and liability that it is rarely within the ability of an individual to effect significant change, especially when it comes out of another paradigm. Doctors, however well intentioned, are expected to function within the institution's rules and regulations and are virtually powerless to modify procedures.

Nevertheless, humanists can soften the hard edges of technomedical institutions in several ways. For example, they can use technomedical interventions judiciously. Conservative management of conditions at the primary care level can mean fewer referrals to specialists, sparing the patient the alienation within the medical system that such a referral may entail. Combining intuition with rational modes, humanistic physicians are likely to trust themselves more and to defer hospitalizing a patient whenever possible. They are also more likely to make their daily rounds feel meaningful to the patient.

One nationally recognized attempt to design a more humane hospital is the Planetree experimental unit within the California Pacific Medical

Center in San Francisco, opened in 1978. Among Planetree's innovations in patient services were: allowing patients to wear their own clothes and taking their meals in a dining room if possible; offering bed and board to the patient's support person; educating patients about their condition; and providing them with unrestricted access to their medical charts. Although the original unit has been discontinued, Planetree now has sixteen affiliate institutions, each offering some innovations in hospital care, from facility design to massage and closed-circuit educational television. A few affiliates even try to make emergency rooms and intensive care units more user-friendly, in an effort to strike a more viable balance between institutional and individual needs.

(7) INFORMATION, DECISION MAKING, AND RESPONSIBILITY SHARED BETWEEN PATIENT AND PRACTITIONER

The poles between empowerment and dependence form the framework within which doctors and patients make decisions. Clearly, health professionals are trained to bring linear information to bear in their decision making. In addition, the humanistic paradigm allows nonlinear, subjective processing to play a significant role, resulting in a balanced or empathic style of thinking. "Empathic" refers to the ability of one person to understand another's reality even if that reality is beyond their direct experience. Even when straightforward evidence of disease is present, doctors still have considerable latitude regarding how mutual they are willing to allow decision making to be. In the technomedical model, each situation has a matching action. The humanistic model opens situations to multiple options, as indicated by this humanistic obstetrician: "If you . . . don't want a sonogram, or a hospital test for some reason, and you know that there's a 1/10,000 chance that that test may actually prevent death or some other complication, and you're willing to take that chance, I think it's your right to make the decisions, up to a point. Now where is that point? . . . We can't really prove that a hospital birth with a certain structure in which every kind of test is done is the very best. So I think women *need* to have a choice in their experience" (quoted in Davis-Floyd 1987:307).

The doctrine of informed consent theoretically establishes the guideline for information sharing between patient and doctor. What it says, in essence, is that patients have a right to understand their diagnosis and prognosis, their proposed treatment and its risks and benefits, and their treatment options. In the technocratic model the discussion of options outside of conventional medicine is generally impossible due to the doctor's allegiance to technocratic approaches and ignorance of alternatives. Discussing no treatment as an option is equally unlikely. Within the humanistic model, a discussion of treatment choices leads naturally to an exploration and sharing of values. Here doctors are more likely to respond favorably or at least neutrally to a patient's wish to try alternative methods. Non-treatment as an option may also be more acceptable, particularly in the face of painful or disfiguring treatments. Although the humanist may not be any more informed regarding these options than the technocratic doctor, the shift results from the physician's regard for the individual's right to control her fate and to make reasonable decisions about it.

In *The Illness Narratives* (1988), psychiatrist Arthur Kleinman expands the notions of the patient's right to information and the "patient-centered interview" to a more dialogic approach. He describes the value of engaging patients in a conversation about their experience of illness instead of simply trying to diagnose their disease. He suggests that the goal of the practitioner should be to enter into the experience of illness as patients perceive it by listening carefully to their illness narratives. To understand more deeply a patient's story, the physician can employ anthropological techniques of ethnographic analysis to interpret the patient's symptoms as symbols of deeper life issues and to grasp the influence of the patient's cultural, personal, and family explanatory models. Kleinman feels that understanding the "personal and interpersonal significance of the illness" is essential to finding the key to a cure (1988:233).

Kleinman goes on to suggest that "the real challenge for the physician is to engage in negotiation with the patient as colleagues involved in care as collaboration"—an empowering process in which the physician translates between the patient's "lay model" of his illness and the "professional biomedical model," encouraging the patient and his family to express their disagreements and criticisms, and negotiating with them about these areas of conflict. As part of that negotiation, the physician must "expose his uncertainty and the limits of his understanding, as well as his critical reactions." Kleinman notes that "the negotiation may end up in a compromise closer to the patient's position, a compromise closer to the doctor's position, or a joint lesson in demystifying professional and public discourse. . . . Most of the time, in my experience, the negotiation will result in a compromise acceptable to all parties" (1988:243)—one that fosters mutual respect, open communication, and the process of healing. Like other humanistic and holistic physicians, Kleinman stresses the value and importance of the placebo effect, which can be activated purely through the strength of the physician-patient relationship and thus should be tapped in every healing encounter.

Medical sociologist Eliot Freidson (1988:322) asserts that the need for information is apt to result in conflict simply because a lay culture is encountering a professional culture at a moment of crisis. To balance this, the doctor needs to communicate a trustworthiness to the patient so that the patient can accept or reject recommendations without feeling either bullied or negated. A sense of freedom pervades the atmosphere when a physician has mastered the art of shared exploration. Although some physicians might fear liability with this level of information-sharing, the Consensus Conference on Doctor-Patient Communication held in Toronto in 1992 found that most lawsuits against doctors are the result of communication faults rather than errors in medical judgment. In other words, the open sharing of information, decision making, and responsibility between patient and practitioner works both to minimize the risk of lawsuit and to enhance healing.

(8) SCIENCE AND TECHNOLOGY COUNTERBALANCED WITH HUMANISM

Humanistic physicians take science as their standard and use virtually the same tools and techniques as technomedical doctors. The difference lies in timing and selection. Humanists may be more willing to wait, more apt to be conservative, more open to mind-body approaches. Humanists who are primary care doctors (family physicians, internists, pediatricians, gynecologists) may delay referring to a specialist and attempt to resolve a problem using more conservative methods, provided they have the consent of the patient to do so. Humanistic specialists will naturally be inclined to use the technology at their disposal, but like oncologist Dawn LeManne quoted above, will emphasize caring and relationship alongside it, a combination John Naisbitt (1980) captured in the phrase "high tech, high touch."

(9) FOCUS ON DISEASE PREVENTION

Almost all the physicians in our study expressed awe and admiration for the high technology available to treat trauma and serious infectious diseases. Yet they also noted that these costly technofixes could never do as much for as many as preventive care. Len Saputo allowed that "after the horse is out of the barn, there's nothing better than Western medicine. We can do some amazing surgical things, some amazing biochemical things, that are to be absolutely viewed with respect, true achievements. But their adherents don't look at other aspects of health care—prevention and wellness—nearly to the degree that they could. These are just as scientific, and infinitely more cost-effective." The humanistic approach seeks a balance between these approaches; many humanists, while adherents of biomedicine, are also strong proponents of science-based public health initiatives that stress keeping the horse in the barn—prevention for the many more than high-tech cures for the few.

Most doctors in practice for any length of time will share their frustration about "mopping up" after careless lifestyles. Yet this is what constitutes a great deal of medical care. The oxymoron "preventive medicine" describes a contrasting approach that attempts to stop disease and accidents from occurring in the first place. This strategy lies in the arena of public health and deals primarily with the public environment. Its proponents advocate clean air and water, good nutrition, and health care for the indigent and most vulnerable members of society. Programs to prevent teenage pregnancies, to provide nutritious food for low-income mothers and infants, and to ensure basic medical care to Head Start youngsters reflect a societal nod at protecting vulnerable populations against the obvious forms of disease. Interviewee Joel Fort feels that prevention needs to be incorporated into every specialty so that it becomes a "societal consensus": "For at least thirty-five years, I have been a very active proponent in all kinds of forums for preventive medicine. Most people are unwilling or unable or too uncomprehending to practice it. We need a societal consensus that prevention in all areas—accidents, health, diet—should be a massive campaign. We should enlist, if necessary, the profiteering advertising agencies to run ads in prime time to get us to buy prevention as they get us to buy destructive products."

A deeper look at prevention would focus on personal motivation. Patients from all social strata might be motivated to care for themselves better if they believed that their doctor cared enough about them to design a plan for self-improvement and monitor its implementation. Trust and concern must be present before individuals will undertake change. While this may not be the best use of the most expensive medical personnel, the personal power of the medical doctor can have profound influence and impact.

Prevention has been limited to the public health arena presumably because it does not turn a profit, unlike the sale of high-tech medical equipment and pharmaceuticals. No one benefits in any immediate sense when people stop smoking, and tobacco companies in particular tend to lose. But a model in which compassion, not profit, is the driving force, has room for prevention and for broad-stroke social programs that reflect political agendas that protect the disenfranchised. Thus the public health paradigm, which stresses long-term, large-scale disease prevention and health promotion, corresponds closely to the humanistic paradigm, which stresses long-term individual and family (biopsychosocial) disease prevention and health promotion. In fact, humanists often leave private medical practice for work in the wider arena of public health, as anthropologist Melvin Konner discovered. Early in his medical school career, Konner found himself in conversation with two such physicians, who had given up both successful research careers and powerful administrative positions to take leadership roles in the field of public health. One had designed and implemented a program to screen newborns for hypothyroidism, which if undetected can cause profound mental retardation. They both insisted that

> public health measures, not medical care, were responsible for all the important reductions of morbidity and mortality in modern times [and that] medicine had accomplished nothing significant at all. I protested. Coronary artery bypass surgery? Appendectomy? Antibiotics? Nothing I mentioned impressed them in the least. The treatments were overrated, the numbers of people saved were trivial compared with the numbers, past and future, saved by preventive medicine. I felt like an idiot. Here I was, taking my first steps in clinical work, defending the whole enterprise of clinical medicine in an argument with two men who had spend decades practicing medicine at its best and who had abandoned it and insisted it was useless. (Konner 1987:40)

Arnold Rosenberg, a physician and research scientist, noted his own increasing dissatisfaction with his research career:

> Here I was, working in the laboratory on a cellular level to get a better understanding of cancer and heart disease, the big things. . . . But the more I learned and studied, the more I realized that both heart disease and cancer were unnecessary diseases. They were diseases that our civilization created . . . almost totally preventable diseases of our lifestyle. It seemed wasteful to me to continue to devote my life to trying to find a pill to help people continue wrong lifestyles while we got rid of their symptoms of these big diseases. . . . I felt very unhappy about that—it was so very unfulfilling. (*MetaPhysicians' Tales*)

Another physician who was practicing humanistically and left the practice of medicine for the public health arena is Marsden Wagner, who for fifteen years served as director of the Maternal-Child Health Division of the World Health Organization. After many years of an active pediatric and neonatology practice that left him "dissatisfied and restless, feeling that I was just practicing rescue medicine, not solving the child health problems of the community," he returned to UCLA for two years of postgraduate study in the science of medicine and public health: "The single most important thing that happened to me during those two years," he reports, "was being exposed to a different paradigm. While the medical paradigm focuses on the individual who comes for help, on sickness, on curing, and for the most part uses the biological approach, the public health paradigm focuses on populations, on health, on prevention, and uses a bio-psycho-social approach. Once that paradigm shift happens, there is no turning back" (1997:367).

The field of public health is vast and cannot be discussed in any detail here. Here we simply seek to point out the correspondences between the public health paradigm and the humanistic model. Both seem to be compassion-driven; both focus on disease prevention, health promotion, and public education. The public health paradigm takes a broad-scale, populationwide approach, while the humanistic model focuses more specifically on the individual relationships among family, patient, and provider and the effects of these relationships on illness prevention, diagnosis, and treatment.

(10) DEATH AS AN ACCEPTABLE OUTCOME

In technomedicine, where death is the enemy and all resources are recruited to stave it off, the death of a patient usually signals failure. Lifesaving procedures for low-birth-weight infants, often implemented without respect for their eventual quality of life, high-tech intervention for the terminally ill, and life support for otherwise unconscious individuals all represent attempts at sustaining the fragile thread of life against all odds. But the public has signaled its interest in a more moderate approach to sustaining life. Individuals can sign living wills in advance, requesting that life-prolonging measures be limited. The durable power of attorney allows individuals to name family members who can carry out their wishes in the event of their incapacitation. The Hemlock Society, which focuses on the needs and rights of the terminally ill, asserts in its brochure that among the rights of U.S. residents is the ability to determine their own course of treatment, to refuse or stop treatment once it has begun, and to refuse CPR in their own homes. The hospice movement has brought death back into the home by supporting the dying individual and the family, not with major medical intervention but with the comfort of pain relief. These highly humanistic interventions stem from a philosophy, as we have seen, that profoundly honors a patient's individuality and freedom of choice.

One of our interviewees, Dawn LeManne, is an oncologist who deals intimately with death and views it as part of the process of being human:

> I don't look at death as the ultimate defeat or illness and suffering as the exception. One thing that working with oncology patients has taught me is that one day each of us will encounter a situation where things didn't go as we planned. And to approach it as "Why me"?—as a terrible calamity that had never happened to anybody else on earth before—is counterproductive. I think that it also helps me stay in the here and now. Every day is a blessing, every encounter is a blessing. We just have to make the best of what we have. This is very different from nihilism. Please don't think that I just go in there and give up. But there's a certain way of approaching it that helps me stay right with the moment and get with the program. Do what needs to be done, and make the most of our human encounter as well as our medical encounter—whatever that might be.

Elizabeth Kubler-Ross first popularized the notion that death might be approached consciously. The techniques she employed in her large workshops included emotional release and a focus on completions—what needed to be done before a peaceful death might be enjoyed. These sessions and her writings (1969, 1975) positioned death as "the final stage of growth." Further evolutions of her pioneering work have defined the death process as something of great significance within an individual's biography—an event to be planned, approached, and lived with as much intention and grace as possible. The meaning of "healing" deepens and broadens as death approaches: so much besides the physical illness can be healed. The process of dying under both the humanistic and holistic paradigms becomes an opportunity to heal one's relationships with spouses, lovers, children, friends, oneself, and God. Grievances can be forgiven, old wounds mended, unmet needs and wishes fulfilled. In such cases, the death of an individual can provide tremendous opportunities for healing for families and entire communities.

For the humanistic or holistic practitioner, facilitating this process can mean developing a rich relationship with the dying, and coming to a deep understanding of their psychology and their past. It may also mean attending them at their final hours, as many are choosing a "home death" rather than an institutionalized one. On the personal level, this often requires the practitioner to develop the ability not only to welcome death instead of feeling any sense of failure in its presence, but also to work to find and express its meaning. Several beliefs assist practitioners in this endeavor. First is belief in the vitality of the spirit and its ability to live separately and beyond the body. Rudolf Steiner, founder of the Anthroposophical Movement, put it this way: "The moment of death seen from the other side is the most beautiful experience . . . a glorious picture of the eternal victory of the spirit over matter." Doctors who wish to live this belief usually must overturn the materialism that underpinned their long years of training and indoctrination. Second is the ability to face the idea of one's own death with equanimity and to avoid projecting personal fears into others' situations. Third is surrender to a will and universe whose purpose is essentially a mystery and whose ways cannot be fathomed. Every doctor has experiences of the unlikely recovery as well as the unwarranted death. When death comes, it must be greeted as a friend bringing a gift—the opportunity to experience one's birth into the world of spirit. Many humanists are deeply religious, often with a Christian orientation that contrasts with the more Eastern orientation of many holistic physicians who tend to see death neither as an end nor a permanent shift to a spiritual level of being, but as a turning of the great wheel of life.

(11) COMPASSION-DRIVEN CARE

> We are so busy chasing after money that we've forgotten we are brothers and sisters.
>
> —MICHAEL GREENBERG

Humanistic physicians are travelers on the road from the left-brained, linear thinking characteristic of Western society since the Industrial Revolution to the right-brained, intuitive, empathetic style of thinking that characterizes what Rianne Eisler (1987, 1995) calls "partnership" cultures (in contrast to the "dominator" cultures characterized by patriarchal values). When they hold the hand of a patient undergoing a painful testing procedure, when they sit down by a patient's bed and look that patient in the eyes, when they listen for a long time to a patient's story, then share a story of their own, humanistic physicians are working to re-create a place in medicine for the human values of partnership, relationship, compassion, and caring. Nurses have provided these to patients for over a century. But nurses have been both female and structurally subordinate—a double whammy in the hierarchical and patriarchal medical system, and a situation that has made technocratic physicians (including women) all the more anxious to distance themselves from nursing by acting like doctors—a role that at least in the hospital has been defined in part by its structural opposition to the role of the nurse. Only after three decades of scientific research documenting the benefits of this humanistic approach are technocratically trained physicians allowing themselves to be human, letting go of the fear that others will think them weak and incompetent if they open themselves to their own feelings and learn skills for processing their patients' feelings without becoming emotionally overwhelmed.

Although most humanists practice within the for-profit medical system and are bound by its constraints, in many cases their motivation is not profit but compassion. For example, interviewee David Gershan, who is studying anthroposophical medicine, works in a county medical clinic that serves low-income patients who are often blamed both for their poverty and for their poor health status. His compassionate nature sees it differently:

> The cases are difficult and you have this frustrating bureaucracy behind you as you try to find resources for the patient. No one should have to worry about medical care. Period. No one should have to work to be financially entitled. Whether one receives welfare or not represents two sides to one malady. We have a history in the world of inhuman treatment of people. In this country we are faced with the psychological fruits of slavery, classism, and racism. There is no way that the whole population can compete in this laissez-faire economy. Those who can compete confront the same illness as those who are not making it. Like grades, there's no "A" if there's no "F." Our system depends on the subjugation of people

> financially and culturally. Welfare shows one sick system trying to fix another sick system.

Another humanistic physician, Joel Fort, who has devoted his life to reforming the social aspects of medicine through teaching and innovation in clinical practice, suggests that the members of the medical profession extend themselves financially in order to serve those who otherwise cannot afford good care: "I think every doctor should be asked to donate at least 10 percent of their care to the poor. If organized medicine would recognize that so many people are suffering, they might recognize that we have an implicit ethical obligation. Also, I think we should pay more taxes. I'm not advocating socialized medicine because of my concern about the abuse of bureaucracy. But we should provide for people who have nothing."

Many humanistic physicians spend time every year providing medical services to the poor, often in Third World countries. One such physician from San Antonio, Texas, travels once a year to Guatemala to spend two weeks performing cataract surgery on dozens of indigenous Guatemalan Indians, many of whom walk for days over the mountains to arrive at his clinic for their only chance to see again. Karin Montero, a nascent holist who has practiced plastic surgery humanistically for many years, goes to El Salvador once a year for three weeks to operate on children with cleft palates and give them perhaps their only chance at a normal appearance. Bill Manahan, who for years practiced as a humanistic physician before moving to holism, has spent many months volunteering in clinics that serve the poor in inner-city and rural areas in the United States and Africa.

For these reasons we have identified the driving ethos of the humanist as compassion—the ability to sense and feel the needs of others even if they are outside of one's own experience. The compassion for their fellow humans that drives humanistic physicians to do such work in other countries drives them as well to provide patient- and relationship-centered care when they come home.

(12) OPEN-MINDEDNESS TOWARD OTHER MODALITIES

The humanists we interviewed accepted the notion of the scientific and normative basis of Western medicine. Most had no intention of learning alternative healing techniques, although in general they were open-minded and would support patients who chose to use alternatives—as long as the overall treatment program included conventional care. Their attitudes toward alternative therapies ranged from dismissive to intrigued. This physician expresses a typical view:

> We don't have all the answers, and sometimes it's reasonable to pursue other forms of care. And I'm not opposed to that but I can't recommend or advocate it. I would see it as reasonable for a person to which nothing else can be offered but comfort and supportive care. I mean, we're all going to die, and nobody wants to face their own mortality. If there is a condition that won't respond to technocratic medicine . . . if something can't be offered for their physical health, at least provide them with psychological health. (Cynthia Hernandez, M.D., quoted in Garza 1996)

The range of humanistic practice extends from a simple softening of the hard edges of technomedicine at one end to the beginnings of holistic practice at the other. While many humanists adopt Hernandez's attitude—a sort of bemused tolerance—others, not content to stop at relating to their patients, advocate dietary and lifestyle changes that border on the holistic, and take a more proactive stance toward other healing alternatives. Many patients, in addition to caring and connection, want their physicians to respect their desire to experiment with treatment outside of allopathic medicine, and place high value on the humanist's open-mindedness toward such experimentation.

Physicians in transition to humanism need not undergo any noticeable change in beliefs about what causes or cures disease. Simply being more considerate, more caring, more willing to touch and communicate positions physicians within the humanistic model. They can still order "every test in the book," ignore the role of nutrition, express skepticism about the efficacy of alternative healing modalities. Humanistic doctors are not necessarily on the road to holism. Their compassionate stance offers many physicians a lifetime of satisfaction. Most will not undergo the radical shift in values that permits them to go beyond compassion to employ the healing power of that mysterious thing called energy in overcoming disease. This is the realm of the holistic physician.

4 *The Holistic Model of Medicine*

> Holistic medicine uses those modalities which are least harmful first. It works with people in their context and creates other kinds of healing contexts. It sees each person as unique and it understands the spiritual dimension of health care as well as of each person's life unfolding.
> —JIM GORDON, M.D.

If the technocratic model of medicine is the ruling hegemony, the holistic model of medicine is the ultimate heresy, moving far beyond all of the premises and assumptions upon which technomedicine is based. Of the three paradigms we discuss, the holistic model encompasses the richest variety of approaches, ranging from nutritional therapy to traditional healing modalities such as Chinese medicine to various methods of directly affecting personal energy. Some holistic practitioners study a particular modality while others employ an eclectic approach, often of their own design. Holism often calls on individuals to be active, asking them to make major modifications in their lifestyles. It may also ask them to be passive, to simply receive prayer or a transfer of healing energy.

Given the fluid nature of holism, no one description may fully do it justice. Nevertheless, we venture an attempt, and identify its tenets as follows:

(1) Oneness of body-mind-spirit
(2) The body as an energy system interlinked with other energy systems
(3) Healing the whole person in whole-life context
(4) Essential unity of practitioner and client
(5) Diagnosis and healing from the inside out
(6) Networking organizational structure that facilitates individualization of care
(7) Authority and responsibility inherent in each individual
(8) Science and technology placed at the service of the individual
(9) A long-term focus on creating and maintaining health and well-being
(10) Death as a step in a process
(11) Healing as the focus
(12) Embrace of multiple healing modalities

Underlying Principles and Type of Thinking: Integration and Fluidity

The principles of connection and integration that underlie the holistic paradigm arise from the fluid, multimodal, right-brained thinking that, after centuries of devaluation in the West, is finally beginning to regain lost ground (Eisler 1995). While the whole brain is involved in all brain functions, it is possible to say that the right hemisphere is predominantly involved in perceiving the gestalt, the whole. In contrast to the classifying and segmenting unimodal approach of left-brained, linear systems of thought, fluid thinkers use multimodal means of perception to apprehend the whole and to intuit the ever-shifting relationships of its parts:

> While the language of words, of abstracts, of concepts, is shaped by culture and tends to move in the thought-forms of culture, the language of things, of images, can, if we open to it, take us deeper. The contexts of the images, the stories, have been twisted to tell the stories of the patriarchy, but if we let the *things* themselves, in all the richness and complexity of their existence, speak to us, we reverse the reversals, or more—we dive below the cement-banked channels of consciousness and reach the underground rivers that are its source. Take for example . . . the tree. I see the leafless winter sticks of its branches sprout green buds, leaves, blossoms; I see them swell into this fruit that is itself a seed. And so for me this constellation becomes an experience of renewal, and I feel it in the flesh of my own woman's body, which seems so vulnerable, so mortal; yet I can know, with a sense deeper than words, how it renews itself. (Starhawk 1988:26–27)

Precisely because this type of thinking does not take place in a linear fashion and cannot be logically explained and replicated, it has been systematically discredited in Western thought. It is thinking of, with, and through the body and the spirit—holistic thinking, fluid thinking that transcends logical reasoning and rigid classifications in favor of what Starhawk (1989), one of its principal spokespersons, calls the "spiral dance." She means the spiral of the vortex, the tornado, the creative matrix in which all things are tossed around and mixed up beyond any making sense. From the deep integrative chaos of this energy vortex arises the surprise—the unpredictable relationship, the unexpected connection, the revealing intuition—that so often constitutes a prime element of holistic healing.

History of the Holistic Model

The consciousness revolution that began in the 1970s eventually touched on all aspects of public and private life. The theme, whether in civil rights, feminism, or educational reform, was to remove impediments to individual freedom. Legislation laid the foundation for the psychological, cultural, and political reformation that has been required to take the impulse for freedom to an experiential level in most individuals. But it has taken a long time for this freedom of choice to extend to health care, which has been almost singularly spared from reform. Instead, parallel systems of healing, most culled from other cultures or from the "underground" realm to which they were consigned at the beginning of this century in the United States, developed in the shadow of orthodox medicine.

The term "holism," from *holos*, the Greek word for "whole," was adopted by some of the pioneers of this movement to express their inclusion of the mind, body, emotions, spirit, and environment of the patient in the healing process.[1] The development of holistic medicine is equivalent to what Grossinger (1982) calls "the new medicine revival" of the 1960s and 1970s. He traces a convergence of native traditions from the East and West with the concept of the mind/body as an energy unit, as postulated by Sigmund Freud and elaborated by Carl Jung and Wilhelm Reich. These ideas found fertile ground in the counterculture movement, which demanded that an equally radical and self-empowered medicine support it, and the ecological movement, which insisted that the debris "out there" only mirrors the toxins within. In the short space of a decade, it became acceptable to "work on" oneself psychologically and physically, and desirable to do so within a framework that incorporated the values of self-reliance, freedom, and innovation.

At the populist level, the Boston Women's Health Collective offered liberation to a whole generation of women through the 1969 publication of the original *Our Bodies, Our Selves*—a virtual owner's manual for the female body. The growing feminist critique of male medical techniques, procedures, and ideologies led hundreds of women from Massachusetts to California to volunteer to examine and treat each other. Some of these lay clinicians became midwives offering women alternatives in birth; a good many went on to medical school, where they challenged the gender imbalance and patriarchal value system.

On the West Coast, a group of homeopaths led by Bill Gray, M.D., from Stanford invited the esteemed George Vithoulkas, a world-renowned Greek homeopath, to give lectures on homeopathy in the hopes of infusing its underground practice with a new enthusiasm and professionalism. In the early 1970s chiropractors, long marginalized and persecuted by the medical profession, organized to launch an unrelenting and ultimately successful campaign for legitimacy. Naturopathy quietly came back with the establishment of the first training programs in the United States in twenty years. Somatic therapies became popular through the inspiration of Wilhelm Reich as interpreted through the work of various innovators. Psychotherapy got off the couch and into the living room through the popularization of Transactional Analysis by Thomas Harris (1967), gestalt therapy as interpreted by Fritz Perls (1969), and the encounter movement. Seekers went East and teachers came West, bringing new instructions in the art of living in peace and health.

Macrobiotics introduced the idea of food as medicine, and organic farming forged a link between nutrition and ecology. Growing awareness of the importance of nutrition spawned a generation of vegetarians and a new kind of nutritional science given early impetus through the work of Roger Williams (1956, 1959, 1971) and Linus Pauling (1971). Shoestring-budget health food stores, living room–based Edgar Cayce study groups, and small-scale sectarian yoga instructors now became the focus of the endless seeking of flower children and political radicals alike. And midwives, nearly eliminated by physicians by the 1950s, staged their own nationwide renaissance, developing new skills and creating their own local and national professional organizations (Gaskin 1977; Litoff 1978; Rooks 1997).

Out of all this cultural ferment emerged doctors who, having experimented as individuals, gradually assumed leadership within the medical professional arm of the holistic health movement. Many volunteered in the free clinics that served the needs of the hippies and poor. Pediatrician Mike Holt recalls: "I volunteered to be the doctor when the Rainbow Gathering came to California because some of my friends from the Grateful Dead days urged me to have this experience" (*MetaPhysicians' Tales*). Others learned the value of multidisciplinary cooperation in government-funded clinics. One of us (St. John) administered such a clinic in Chicago in the early 1970s that required each new patient to see not only a doctor or a nurse-practitioner, but also the optometrist, dentist, nutritionist, mental health professional, and social worker—all of whom were employed within the health center. The Peace Corps provided an avenue for some medical doctors to develop their skills in conjunction with native healers in other cultures.

Some of the seminal publishing in this era provided theoretical models for the evolving understanding of the mind-body connection. Examples are Hans Selye's *Stress Without Distress* (1974) and Kenneth Pelletier's *Mind as Healer, Mind as Slayer* (1977). The earliest holistic centers grew out of community support for alternatives in treatment. Early pioneers with national visibility included Bill and Gladys McGarey, an M.D.-husband-and-wife team in Arizona who began using the many nature-based treatments recommended by the late psychic Edgar Cayce; Evarts Loomis, who founded perhaps the first holistic healing center in the country, Meadowlark, in northern California in 1959; the Hahnemann Medical Clinic doctors who resurrected homeopathy in Berkeley; Norman Shealy, M.D., whose pain clinic in Wisconsin became recognized for its integrative methods; and the physicians in Pennsylvania and Chicago who learned to use the Indian teacher Swami Rama's eclectic techniques.

While our study focuses on holistic M.D.'s, it is clear that they are, in a sense, the last of many waves to wash over and transform the way we regard and practice healing in America. Yet their leadership has helped to bring what might have remained a marginalized movement into the mainstream. In chapter 5 we will explore more specifically how personal and cultural influences caused the physicians in our study to make the shift in values that aligned them with the holistic model we describe here.

The Twelve Tenets of the Holistic Model

(1) ONENESS OF BODY-MIND-SPIRIT

Mind and body, rent asunder by Cartesian rationalism, and reconnected in medical humanism, are re*united* in holistic medical care. The worst problem here is language: we are so used to speaking in terms of mind-body separation that even holistic healers find themselves still using the words "mind" and "body"; when they are careful, they will refer to the "bodymind" to indicate that it is all one thing, or write footnotes insisting that, although they may still use the words "body" and "mind," the body is incorporated in the mind and vice versa. A large part of the initial impetus for the reuniting of mind and body in holistic healing was the dawning realization that the brain, which even the most devoted Cartesians would admit is the physical seat of the mind, is not located only in the head—above, and therefore superior to, the body—but in fact extends throughout the central nervous system. Understanding that the brain is distributed throughout the body makes it much harder to talk or think about body and mind as separate entities.

Applying the principle of mind-body unity in practice means that it is impossible to treat physical symptoms without addressing their psychological components. Psychoneuroimmunologist Candace Pert explains:

> Viruses use [the same receptors as the neuropeptides that carry emotions] to enter into a cell, and depending on how much of the natural juice, or the natural peptide for that receptor is around, the virus will have an easier or a harder time getting into the cell. So our emotional state will affect whether we'll get sick from the same loading dose of a virus. You know the data about how people have more heart attacks on Monday mornings, how death peaks in Christians the day after Christmas, and in Chinese people the day after the Chinese New Year. . . . Another example: the AIDS virus uses a receptor that is normally used by a neuropeptide. So whether an AIDS virus will be able to enter a cell or not

> depends on how much of this natural peptide is around, which, according to this theory, would be a function of what state of emotional expression the organism is in. Emotional fluctuations and emotional status directly influence the probability that the organism will get sick or be well. (1993:190)

If the mind is the body, and the body is the mind, then how one responds to the treatment of even so mechanical a thing as a broken arm will have as much to do with how one thinks and feels about that broken arm as about what kind of cast is put on it. This premise is intensely threatening to conventional physicians, who have felt perfectly justified in cramming their days with a series of five-minute encounters, writing prescriptions, and moving on. The insufficiencies of this approach, in light of the findings of the psychoneuroimmunology (PNI) researchers, become salient. Like humanists, holistic physicians are finding that they need much more engagement with the patient—more interaction, more dialogue—to get at those intangibles of mind and emotion now seen to be as much a part of the illness or trauma as its physical manifestation. Against this complex backdrop of the flux and flow of neuropeptides and their accompanying emotions and physical symptoms—what Pert describes as "a fluid, dynamic system"—the relative simplicity of "a pill for every ill" can seem very appealing.

To further complicate matters, the holistic paradigm does not stop with mind-body oneness but insists on the participation of the *spirit* in this newly rediscovered human whole. What exactly the spirit is, few can say, yet there is a general consensus among holistic healers that the spirit, or soul, is very much a part of each human being, and continues in some form after the physical body dies. Asked by interviewer Bill Moyers, "Then are you saying we're just a circuit of chemicals?" Candace Pert responded, "Well, that gets to be a philosophical question. One way to phrase it would be, can we account for all human phenomena in terms of chemicals? . . . As a scientist, I believe we're going to understand everything one day, but that this understanding will require bringing in a realm we don't understand at all yet . . . that extra-energy realm, the realm of spirit and soul that Descartes kicked out of Western scientific thought" (1993:180).

For millennia, most of the world's major religions have insisted on the existence of a universal spirit and individual souls. In not only accepting the soul's existence, but also consciously incorporating it into the healing process, holistic healers bring medicine back into the world of the spiritual and the metaphysical from which it was separated during the Industrial Revolution. In short, holistic healers reintegrate not only body, mind, and spirit, but also medicine and religion. As Bethany Hays expressed it in her interview, "Only recently did I realize that since healing occurs in the spirit, not in the body, my calling is more in the line of mysticism than medicine. The only problem is that I have no idea of how to do this work. I guess I will have to do on-the-job training!"

Many of the holistic physicians we interviewed are spiritually conscious people who incorporate that spirituality into their practices as well as their daily lives; many of their patients see no separation between their spiritual lives and the medical treatments they undertake. A few of our interviewees expressed a perspective that extended far enough to encompass medicine itself as a spiritual path, among them Larry Dossey:

> One of the reasons I think kids ought to continue to go into medicine, as screwed up as the profession happens to be currently, is that it is a fabulous spiritual path. Where else do you get put into situations where you have the opportunity to learn something you can learn nowhere else in such a short period of time—except, for instance, during war? Medicine is an opportunity to walk through a doorway of personal transformation . . . it's a fabulous opportunity, let me just put it right there. Sort of thing that's never played out in medical school, but if you're willing to really enter into [the experiences you are offered] . . . you can embark on a great spiritual path, you can!

With the understanding that mind and body are one comes awareness that one must take responsibility for one's thoughts and the values that direct them. Edward Bach, a British physician known for the flower essences named after him, maintained in his book, *Heal Thyself*, that the "real primary diseases of man are such defects as pride, cruelty, hate, self-love, ignorance, instability, and greed." He felt that these states of mind generated all physical disease. Carolyn Myss, a medical intuitive who worked with Norman Shealy, M.D., for many years and achieved 93 percent accuracy in intuitively diagnosing his patients, makes some penetrating observations about how the mind affects the body. She became puzzled when she realized that

> the promise of health does not motivate a person either to heal or to change the habits which almost certainly guarantee the creation of an illness. . . . After years of being perplexed by this phenomenon and frustrated with people who could be healthy but choose otherwise, I have concluded that the promise of being a healthy person is . . . not the motivator for change that one might think it is. Health is the result of a commitment to live a more conscious life—to become more responsible for one's health and emotional well-being—and that is the overwhelming challenge to many people. (Shealy and Myss 1988:147–148)

In a later work, Myss (1996:71) refers to "woundology"—the compulsion to cling to wounds out of fear of upsetting the balance of power with a significant other, or simply out of the wounds' contribution to personal identity.

As Myss and Dossey imply, the spirituality of holistic healers tends to be fluid, and to take the form of a loose identification with Eastern or New Age philosophies more often than with Judaism, Christianity, or Islam. This phenomenon is very much in keeping with the fluidity of the holistic paradigm itself. Where the technomedical model is rigid and separatist, the holistic model, like the energy it acknowledges and honors, recognizes no sharp divisions or distinct boundaries. This is another reason that holism is so threatening: in many people's minds, to trifle with boundaries is to invoke chaos. And indeed, chaos theory and systems theory both inform and underpin the holistic paradigm and its insistence on the oneness of body, mind, and spirit.

(2) THE BODY AS AN ENERGY SYSTEM INTERLINKED WITH OTHER ENERGY SYSTEMS

About this principle most of our interviewees were very definite and very specific. When we asked them, "What is the human body?" they replied:

> An energy field . . . It's the description that fits the data the best!. . . . Because if it's an energy field, then the mind-body connection is not an issue. If it's an energy field, the ability to influence it with subtle energy becomes very easy to understand. If it's just a collection of chemicals, then there are a lot of pieces you can't understand. You can break it down into the smaller and smaller pieces, and basically what you're going to end up with is energy fields. (Bethany Hays)

> Energy, energy, energy! It's just different forms of energy. The physical part is the most dense form and it's the part we can see and touch and feel. It has sensors but we're multidimensional beings. No question in my mind about it. I can feel it. I've always been able to feel it, I just didn't know what I was feeling. I work with what I can see and touch and feel, because that's what I know best, but I'm very clear that it's all energy and that it's about transmuting it from one plane into another plane. (Ann McCombs)

> I think the human body is a variety of energy that is vibrating more slowly than light. It's trapped light and it is the vehicle through which God has a body to experience Her creation. . . . And I think it's fraught with sacred meaning that we haven't even begun to realize yet. (Christiane Northrup)

> It's an energetic system. It's a blessed receptacle for the soul. It's a joy, it's a trip, it's fun. It's meant for celebration. (Jim Gordon)

As these healers attest, the holistic paradigm moves far beyond the narrow view of the body-as-machine, past the humanistic view of the body as an organism, all the way to a limitless view of the body as energy. Defining the body as an energy field or an energy system provides a powerful charter for the development and use of forms of medicine and treatment that work energetically such as acupuncture, homeopathy, intuitive diagnosis, Reiki, hands-on healing, magnetic field therapy, and therapeutic touch. "Energy medicine" acknowledges the possibilities that an individual's health can be influenced by such subtleties as the vibrations of anger or hostility or the electromagnetic fields created by power plants and microwaves. It may employ strictly energetic healing modalities such as light therapy, magnetic field therapy, and polarity therapy. All of these presuppose nonphysical reality. Practitioners of energy medicine work with the invisible subtleties of energy flow, blockage, and release, and pay attention to the energetic rhythms of their own body wisdom as they go. As Larry Dossey explained in our interview:

> The body is part of the hierarchy of consciousness. My working belief is that the hierarchy of consciousness extends though the bottom levels of what we call matter, even down to the level of the atoms and electrons and subatomic particles, so I would want to say that my body has a certain wisdom. It is conscious to a certain degree. My body can inform me in certain ways that maybe a change is needed or maybe . . . it has tired of being abused or stupidly treated by my habitual thought processes and crazy behaviors. I think my body does contain consciousness and can be wise in certain ways. So why shouldn't it talk to me? I think it does.

While most of our interviewees were quite clear in their commitment to defining the body as energy and accepting all that definition implies, it is important to note that some physicians who describe themselves as holistic, and who incorporate many of the elements of holism into their practices, do not fully accept this definition, as its implications might take them farther out onto a conceptual limb than they are willing to go. In other words, while they feel quite comfortable advocating dietary changes, nutritional supplements, meditation, psychotherapy, exercise, and nontoxic pharmacological products (all of which are well grounded in science that is continuous with contemporary immunology and nutritional research), they are uncomfortable with forms of healing that involve the manipulation of subtle energies, such as Reiki healing and homeopathy. A given physician's transitional journey into the wide-open meadows of holistic medicine may or may not lead all the way to the realm of energy discourse, where the unsettling implications of the new physics and systems and chaos theory hold sway.

The technomedical view leaves little room for any nonphysical reality. Yet today's physicists relish documenting the vanishing frontier between matter and energy. Medical research would require complete restructuring if it accepted such conclusions from other disciplines. For example, while medicine hotly refutes the impact of the investigator on research, physics recognizes the Heisenberg Principle, which acknowledges the inevitable influence of the observer on the observed. New research is demonstrating that even the intentionality of the experimenter can profoundly affect the outcome of an experiment (Wiseman and Schlitz 1996). Without this second tenet of the holistic paradigm, this influence is inexplicable. How can an observer totally separate from the observed phenomenon affect its behavior? Acceptance of this second tenet answers this question: the observer and the observed are not separate, but are energy fields in constant interaction with each other.

(3) HEALING THE WHOLE PERSON IN WHOLE-LIFE CONTEXT

This tenet of the holistic model of medicine, a logical corollary of the first two, acknowledges that no single explanation of a diagnosis, no single drug or therapeutic approach, will sufficiently address an individual's health problems; rather, such problems must be addressed in terms of the whole persons and the whole environments in which they live. It is no accident that the most commonly asked question in holistic health is "What's going on in your life?" This question, which has become almost a cliché, expresses the holistic view that illness is a manifestation of imbalance in the bodymindspirit whole.

Like many humanists, proponents of the holistic approach do not stop at the simplistic explanation that the sore throat you just developed, the cough you can't shake, are the straightforward results of bacteria invading your body. Bacteria permeate us constantly; most of the time, our immune system protects us. If it is too weak to do so, we must ask what has weakened it. Here holism accepts to the fullest findings from psychoneuroimmunology and other fields that the immune system can be depleted by exhaustion, depression, emotional stress, a negative attitude, anxiety and fear, the cruelty of a colleague, the alcoholism of a family member, the loss of a loved one, toxins in the air and the water, the stresses of technocratic life. (One of our interviewees, for example, had injured his right arm twice in one year, and was finally willing to accept the injuries as a message from his body to slow down and reevaluate his Type A approach to life.) The corollary of this view, of course, is that the immune system can be restored by multiple means, from dialogue to dream analysis, from exercise to organic food.

An illustrative example comes from the treatment Jim Gordon (1996:92–115) prescribed for his patient Leslie Newman (a pseudonym), a "perfectionist and workaholic" who came to him for help with a worsening case of multiple sclerosis. Gordon's initial treatment plan included a diet of only raw food for three weeks to cleanse her system, Chinese herbs to balance her immune system, yoga lessons, and a half-hour of walking every day. As their relationship deepened and trust grew, he began to draw her out about the pressures and miseries of her life as a successful attorney in an extremely lucrative practice, and to tell her about the effects of those kinds of stresses on illness. He advised her to keep a journal and do twenty minutes of wild and fast dancing every morning as a form of meditation, a powerful and immediate way of breaking her old patterns of rushing off to work and living only in her intellect. As her condition improved, Gordon advised Leslie to employ the power of her mind to let go of the notion that she "had MS," a chronic, incurable condition. He told her to "drop MS before it drops you." He also asked her to begin to follow her dancing with a period of quiet awareness meditation, during which she would focus on what was going on in her body and her mind—what she was feeling, what she longed for, who she was. After a year and a half of such work, during which time her condition steadily improved, Leslie gave up the high-powered job she hated in favor of working with the rural poor in Colorado, and moved there with her lover. Six months later she sent Gordon a Christmas card; it read: "Merry Christmas. I'm well. Love, Leslie, your former MS patient."

Obviously, healing whole people in their life contexts is light years away from the technocratic model's treatment of the patient as object, and even from the humanistic treatment of the patient as relational subject. This holistic approach recognizes, as Jim Gordon did with Leslie Newman, that total healing involves attention to the individual-in-multiple-relationships: body-mind-spirit-emotions-family-friends-community-environment—a very tall order! This approach also acknowledges that total healing for a given individual or family may be well beyond the abilities and scope of practice of any single holistic healer. In keeping with this belief, holistic physicians do not practice compulsively and addictively, trying to heal everyone and everything. Instead they learn one or two new modalities well, acknowledge their limitations, and find out enough about other healing systems to know when to refer.

For example, interviewee David Edelberg has designed a clinical model for holistic practice that involves him or a fellow M.D. in the initial interview with each patient, but relies on other professionals for treatment: "I know what all the practitioners [in my wellness center] do. I know the difference between the Feldenkreis and Alexander techniques. I can do a little acupuncture and a little homeopathy, but I do not regard myself as an alternative practitioner. When it comes to selecting which modality to use for a specific problem, most of the time the patient knows what to choose. In fact, if the patient has an idea of what will work and I have a different idea, I go with hers, because most of the time patients know what will work for them."

In envisioning an ideal "countersystem" to technomedicine, sociologist Stephen Lyng suggested that in such a system, "the practitioner's primary role would be educational, while the patient would assume primary responsibility for selecting a diagnosis and treatment regimen from among the various alternatives presented" (1990:61). Edelberg and many of his holistic colleagues have created just such a countersystem. Honoring the wisdom of whole individuals in the context of their environments and all their relationships, holistic physicians sees themselves as advisors, and know that the patient must be the one who makes the choice. On a deeper level still, holistic physicians sense, and sometimes experience, themselves and their patients not as separate, but as united in the healing realm.

(4) ESSENTIAL UNITY OF PRACTITIONER AND CLIENT

Many holistic practitioners try to drop the word "patient" in favor of "client," as this term implies a mutually cooperative, egalitarian relationship, in contrast to the relationship of subordination, of patiently waiting on the practitioner's convenience. Where the humanistic model emphasizes the value of a mutually respectful connection between practitioner and client, still essentially separate and distinct beings, the holistic model offers the possibility that they are not separate but are fundamentally one. If the body is an energy field, then as they interact the energy fields of client and practitioner can merge.

Thus, when Leslie Newman entered Jim Gordon's office for the first time—hostile, demanding, and a half-hour late—Gordon resisted the temptation to refer her to someone else. Instead he dealt with the increasing tension between them by suggesting a ten-minute breathing exercise. As they counted their breaths, they synchronized their rhythms, getting more in touch with themselves and "on the same wavelength" with each other; the rapport they developed as a result proved essential to the success of their healing relationship. Indeed, Deepak Chopra (1991), a physician, author, and primary spokesperson for the holistic health movement, suggests that the best way to diagnose is to "become one" with the client—a far cry from the clinical detachment still taught in most medical schools:

> More and more, I . . . have come to feel, when I am face to face with patients, that I *am* them. I lose the sense that we are separate. We are not. I can feel their pain as they describe it. I can understand them without blame and want them to get well because I will be getting well myself. This intimacy . . . does not embarrass either me or them. It is a very

> simple equation, really, one that is part of natural medicine. It only requires me to feel that I am a doctor, not just someone who has put on the mask of doctor. . . . Before the art of medicine comes the art of belief, but before either comes the art of Being. (1991:160)

In acknowledging and "being" in that oneness, Chopra finds that an answer to the riddle of the illness or disease often spontaneously arises. Likewise, Carolyn Myss, whose work we described earlier, diagnoses people's illnesses through a process of intuitively entering their bodies and moving systematically through their energy system (*chakras*) and the associated glands and organs. From this journey, she states, she can also determine emotional states and personal history.

The concept of essential unity, however, is less a matter of "entering into" than of recognizing no separation. This recognition can extend from something as simple as acknowledging that "there but for the grace of God go I," to the type of transcendent experience related to us by Larry Dossey, a well-known writer and spokesperson for holistic healing. One of us (Davis-Floyd) interviewed Dossey in Austin, Texas, at a scientific meeting. The day before the interview, a man sitting in the audience listening to a paper being presented had suddenly collapsed, with blood and vomit gushing out of his mouth. It was determined later that he had suffered a massive heart attack. Dossey, the only physician in the room, had rushed to his side and immediately administered mouth-to-mouth resuscitation. During the interview, Davis-Floyd asked Dossey how he was able to overcome the repugnance one might be expected to feel over ingesting blood and vomit. He replied that most physicians overcome that repugnance by doing the resuscitation in a mechanical way, putting their consciousness somewhere else. But over the years he had come to understand the value of doing the act with the whole of himself. He found that when he brought his total consciousness to bear, the blood and vomit transmuted into sacred substances that bound him to the other man, with whom, through attempting resuscitation, he could become completely one. He called this transmutation "spiritual alchemy."

(5) DIAGNOSIS AND HEALING FROM THE INSIDE OUT

As we mentioned previously, the two major theoretical and clinical approaches within the history of Western healing have been those of the empiricists and the rationalists. The empiricists relied on experience; they tended to see illness as a whole, albeit with many symptoms, and "believed that pure observation of the patient is the root of knowledge in medicine" (Coulter 1982:473). Their goal in treatment was to stimulate the self-healing mechanism, the "vital force" within the patient, which would lead to the resolution of symptoms.[2] For the rationalists, who tended to rely on science and the objective world for information and verification, "logic and pathological theory always played a major role" (Coulter 1982:474). As we have seen, the rational approach of allopathic medicine targets symptoms directly and works toward their elimination. If the symptoms disappear, the person is considered cured. Healing is directed from the outside in—the magic bullet approach.

Proponents of the holistic model point to the limitations of this outside-in type of medicine. Examples include the inability of antibiotics to keep pace with bacterial mutations and the iatrogenic results of many pharmaceutical, diagnostic, and surgical procedures. The holistic approach begins instead with the body's own immune system—a proxy for the vital force. When strong, this immune system successfully keeps us healthy in spite of our constant exposure to the germs that permeate our environment. When we get sick, instead of focusing on the outside invader as the cause, the holistic model looks to the failure of the immune system to perform its functions, and asks why it is weak.

To find the answers, holistic practitioners often rely on approaches that are both rational and empirical, including nutritional science, immunology, and psychology. Understanding that the body, mind, and spirit are one, and that individuals as full participants in their environment are fully influenced by it, holistic practitioners know that the causes of immune system failure, or that of any other bodily system, may lie in many places—in the psyche of sick individuals, in their family relationships, in the fact that they live in a heavily polluted zone, or in a combination of all three plus many more. No test or diagnostic procedure can tease out all of the interrelated stresses on any one individual, but, as Chopra and others point out, in deep and open communication with the healer, given plenty of time and the development of trust, the individual can usually communicate to the healer enough information "from the inside" to provide the keys to a successful, usually multimodal, approach to treatment. Even serious and supposedly chronic disease may respond to this approach, as Jim Gordon's treatment of Leslie Newman showed.

Like Leslie Newman, many patients seek the services of a holistic practitioner out of desperation, after conventional treatments have failed. Thus the patient often arrives with diagnosis in hand, one obtained by the outside-in methods of technomedicine. It is then incumbent on the physician to probe more deeply into the roots of the illness. In reaching a more holistic diagnosis and formulating a treatment plan, the holistic healers will apply this fifth tenet to themselves as well. While they may, if appropriate, order further "outside-in" diagnostic tests, they will primarily diagnose and treat from the inside out—in other words, they will rely to a significant extent on the knowledge that arises from their own intuition, just as they will trust the inner knowing of their clients.

Intuition is defined by the third edition of the *American Heritage Dictionary* as "the act or faculty of knowing or sensing without the use of rational processes; immediate cognition." Brigitte Jordan (1993) defines authoritative knowledge in a given community of practice as the knowledge on the basis of which decisions are made and actions taken. While technomedical practitioners tend to regard textbooks, diagnostic tests, and the experience-based advice of experts as authoritative, and to devalue and often dismiss the still, small voice of intuition, holistic practitioners (like some humanists) tend to regard intuition as a primary source of authoritative knowledge, along with the books and the machines, and actively work to cultivate their intuitive abilities as a way to tap into what they perceive as the deepest healing powers available.[3] Thus, in holistic practice, "diagnosis and healing from the inside out" can refer to the information that arises from deep inside both patient and physician—a phenomenon explained at its core by their essential unity.

(6) NETWORKING ORGANIZATIONAL STRUCTURE THAT FACILITATES INDIVIDUALIZATION OF CARE

As in the wider society, individualization of medical care is inevitably accompanied by change in the overall structure of the organization. In the business world, corporations are shifting from vertical management hierarchies to "flat corporations" (in which, in theory, employees are personally empowered to act autonomously, consult with managers when useful, and dialogue with the CEO by e-mail)—a transformation paralleled by holistic transformations in medicine. The holistic model of healing values relationship, communication, and interconnection more than status, prestige, or conformity to the system. Thus a diagram of the relationships among a given set of holistic practitioners and their clients would show not a vertical hierarchy but a web.

Such mutuality and interconnectedness often characterize relationships among holistic practitioners themselves. Holistic M.D.'s network with chiropractors, acupuncturists, homeopaths, midwives, and others without expecting the deference that is traditionally their due within the medical hierarchy. In wellness centers and other enterprises that bring various types of practitioners together under one roof, holistic physicians are as likely to be employees as owners. For example, Women-to-Women Clinic, where Bethany Hays and Chris Northrup are based, is not owned by these two obstetricians but rather by one of them jointly with a nurse-practitioner, who thereby became the employer of the other M.D.

Holistic physicians, trained in technomedicine, have seen the damage standardized hospital policies and hierarchies can do to the individual spirit—their own and their patients'. They do what they can within the hospital system—prohibit two A.M. weighings, encourage patients to call if a problem arises with hospital staff, allow family members to stay all night and to bring the patient healthy food—to treat people as individuals and not as members of a disease category. In general, they do their best to respond to the individuality and unique needs of each patient within the constraints imposed on them by hospital and legal regulations. A key concept here is the notion of patient autonomy, described in (7) below.

Those who practice outside the hospital often go to great lengths to make their care responsive to the uniqueness of each client. Our favorite example is provided by Patch Adams, founder of the Gesundheit Institute, a holistic healing community in northern Virginia. Confronted one day with a schizophrenic who suddenly stripped naked and began to roll in the mud, Patch contemplated him for a moment, then also ripped off his clothes and joined in. In the laughter that ensued, the groundwork for healing was laid (personal communication 1994). Patch describes his individualized approach:

> When I saw a patient, I would spend hours learning about his or her parents, lovers, friendships, jobs, and hobbies: the entire person. This vastly expanded version of the traditional—and often truncated—patient history was the only way we could learn what affected a person's health and build a relationship between us. Most patients didn't want the level of intensity that I was willing to give, but any degree was better than nothing. I believe that my patients got what they came for and that their eyes were at least partially opened to the healing power of intimacy. (1993:19)

The value of such an individualized approach was strongly brought home to one of us (Davis-Floyd) during her mother's last two years of life. Her mother, Robbie Gildemeister, at the age of eighty-six suffered from osteoporosis and mild short-term memory loss. She had chosen, along with several of her friends, to live in the most expensive and luxurious nursing home in town. In spite of its luxury, its residents lived highly regimented lives. One day with her mother in the car, Davis-Floyd happened to turn on the National Public Radio just at the start of a special report on a nursing home that required no regimentation—at any hour of the day or night, residents could wander the halls and gardens, sit in the living room and play games or watch TV, or visit the kitchen, which was always staffed, and ask for a snack or a meal. Residents had complete autonomy over their time, what they wore, and what they ate. The report said that they were much happier, lived longer, did more for themselves, engaged in more activities, and were generally healthier than residents of other nursing homes comparable in price. Since staff members had no rules to enforce and less caretaking to do, their relationships with the residents were friendly instead of antagonistic. At the end of the show, Mrs. Gildemeister asked her daughter wistfully if she had heard of any such places nearby. (There were none.) She said she hated the regimentation of her luxurious facility, and the way the staff talked down to her and ordered her around. It was a painful reminder that the value of the individualized holistic approach can extend to people of all ages and all levels of capability.

The unexpected twists that can result from holism's high value on both individualization and interconnectedness are suggested in the theory of self-organizing systems (Wheatley 1992), which states that even the smallest event, if it happens in just the right place at just the right time, can dramatically alter the whole system. A butterfly can flap its wings in Alaska, and if that flap catches the air currents just right, the end result can be a hurricane off the coast of Florida. Holistic healers thus try not to make assumptions about cause and effect. They tend to expect the unexpected and to be prepared for healing to arise in strange places and mysterious ways. A chance remark made by a friendly janitor while he mops the floor at a moment when a patient's psychological defenses are suspended can enter her psyche, instantly transform her perception of her illness, and become the foundation of a cure. Holistic healers know better than to assume that they are the ones who heal the patient. They know that any one of a myriad of interactions over which they have no control can spark a healing process. Their genius lies in their ability to recognize that tiny flame when it is lit and help it to grow instead of extinguishing it. Such individualization of care is facilitated by their networking relationships with a wide range of practitioners.

(7) AUTHORITY AND RESPONSIBILITY INHERENT IN THE INDIVIDUAL

The idea that authority and responsibility inhere in the individual is a real sticking point in the technocracy, which insists on keeping each individual dependent on the system, and reacts, often with a vengeance, when any one person or group tries to detach. The routine use of IV lines on laboring women perfectly symbolizes this phenomenon: the IV is the umbilical cord to the hospital, graphically demonstrating that the pregnant woman is dependent on the institution for her life and that of her baby (Davis-Floyd 1992). In fact, in the technocracy, we do depend on institutions for our lives. Through that dependence, we can to some extent be controlled. Society's need for some degree of control over its citizens requires a system that places responsibility for life and death in the institution and its authority figures, for along with that kind of responsibility goes a great deal of power. Taking individual responsibility for illness and health, for death and for life, then, is equivalent to religious heresy: it reclaims the power for oneself that "properly" belongs to society. Yet that is precisely what many in the holistic health movement are doing.

A basic tenet of holistic healing is that individuals must take responsibility for their own health and well-being. No one can really heal anyone else; individuals must decide for themselves if they want to be healed, and if so, they must take action to achieve that goal—give up smoking, exercise, eat right, maybe even give up a lucrative job that makes them unhappy or a relationship that is harmful to their health. Holistic M.D.'s want very much to work with people who will assume responsibility for what they eat and the kind of lives they choose to lead. Holistic practitioners in general tend to see themselves as part of a healing team, of which the patient is a full-fledged, indeed the most significant member. The other team members are there to set up the play, as it were, but only the patient can reach the goal.

Many of our interviewees repeatedly expressed their frustration with patients who refuse to take responsibility for their own health. They may greet the new client the way Jim Gordon greeted Leslie Newman, prepared to offer her empowerment, full participation in decision making, informed choices, and so on, yet the patient may want only to be handed a prescription and told how many pills to take. In this scenario, the physician is operating out of the holistic paradigm while the patient clings to the technomedical model. Trained in the technomedical model and perfectly competent to apply it, holistic physicians are generally flexible enough to respond to the patient's lead. Although some of our interviewees refuse to revert to the hierarchical mode and may refer such patients to another M.D., most accept and work with the patient's desire to place the physician in charge. Bethany Hays writes:

> As an obstetrician I am nudged by the system to take control of birth in a thousand visible and invisible ways. My personal preference is to resist and allow control to rest in the hands of the mother. Because this is not the accepted method of care, I must know that she is in touch with her body and her inner knowing in order to have the confidence I need to subordinate my authority to hers. But women in our culture are not intuitively knowledgeable in this way. We are taught not to trust our bodies, not to listen to our bodies, and often to abuse our bodies. Medicine teaches us to trust doctors and science and to place the locus of control outside of ourselves, surrendering control to technomedical authority. When my patients choose to give themselves over to me in this way, I respond and take charge. But I realize that although they will gain

> the sense of security they seek, at the same time they will lose the opportunity to generate that sense of security for themselves. (1996:294)

During her interview Bethany revealed that, although she does "respond and take charge," she also tries over the course of their care to reeducate patients to take back the authority and responsibility they have surrendered to her.

The lawsuits that proliferate in the technocracy are the direct result of the displacement of responsibility onto institutions and technomedical authority figures. It is a given in the alternative health movement that if each citizen of the technocracy would reclaim that responsibility, the system would transform. Applying the principle of "authority and responsibility as inherent in the individual" to themselves, some of the holistic physicians we interviewed refused to allow themselves to feel victimized by the inevitable lawsuits that came their way. Instead they chose to regard each one as an opportunity for healing and personal growth. Asking, "What can I learn from this experience?" they approached their day in court with openness.

For example, one of our interviewees (a holistic obstetrician) was slapped with a major and very serious lawsuit having to do with a baby who had died during labor. There was nothing anyone could have done to save the child; nevertheless, the parents blamed the obstetrician. Toward the end of the initial hearing, the obstetrician and the bereaved mother found themselves standing face-to-face in front of the judge, who asked the mother what exactly it was that she felt the obstetrician had failed to do. Sobbing, she faced the doctor and said, "You never apologized for my baby's death. You never said that you were sorry." Of course, in true technocratic fashion, he had been afraid to say he was sorry because it might be taken as an admission of guilt that could be used against him in a lawsuit. Shocked by the irony, and moved to tears himself, he responded with a heartfelt statement of his sorrow and grief over the death and of his own feelings of guilt and remorse over the nagging feeling that there must have been something else he could have done. This healing of old and very painful wounds resulted in the parents' dropping the lawsuit. The obstetrician noted that for him the lessons were powerful beyond words. To reveal instead of suppress his feelings; to admit openly to self-doubt and remorse; to stay connected with his patients in the face of tragedy rather than withdrawing to protect himself from their pain: these were the lessons he took from this experience.

To be sure, there are no guarantees that an open, loving, and connected physician will be protected from the psychological stress and financial consequences of lawsuit any more than a cold, distant, and unfriendly one will be. Yet at the least, many of our interviewees noted, maintaining such an approach did in fact help them avoid anger and bitterness. They came to clearly understand that the technomedical model, which promises more than can be delivered, gives all authority to physicians, and denies patients a sense of individual responsibility, is itself responsible in large part for the attitudes that lead to the proliferation of lawsuits. They see the solution in the changes that result when individuals, facilitated by their physicians, begin to take back their responsibility for health.

(8) SCIENCE AND TECHNOLOGY PLACED AT THE SERVICE OF THE INDIVIDUAL

If the technocratic model of medicine can be snappily characterized as "high tech, low touch," and the humanistic model as "high tech, high touch," then it would seem to follow logically that the holistic model of medicine would be "low tech, high touch." Sometimes this is true, as in the case of hands-on energy healing for which no technological artifacts are used. (Similarly, nutritional medicine, herbal therapies, classical homeopathy, Chinese medicine, Ayurvedic healing, and somatic therapies are low or no tech.) But holistic healing can and often does incorporate high technology, from biofeedback machines to diagnostic computers. Holistic practitioners may use laboratory tests to aid in diagnosis as well as to monitor progress throughout treatment. Examples of the many technological devices used exclusively within the holistic healing domain include Voll-type electronic measuring devices used to measure subtle energy flow; dark-field microscopes used to study blood particles; machines that heal with light; and radionic devices that can be attuned to a person's vibratory field through the proxy of a strand of hair or drop of blood.

In short, we find that holistic healers in general do not reject technology; rather, they place it at the service of their clients. Instead of allowing the technologies of health care to dominate, intimidate, and lay the ground rules for treatment, our interviewees do their best to employ them both artfully and unobtrusively, in ways that empower, rather than control. Usually these technologies are not invasive, nor do they produce the toxic effects of many of the technologies of conventional medicine.

And what of science? Technocratic physicians claim to have science on their side. Certainly their journals are filled with one scientific study after another covering countless aspects of medical practice and health care. Yet, as many have noted, in medicine there is an extraordinarily large gap between practice and scientific research. Physicians are reluctant to change many commonly used procedures learned in medical school, even when evidence reveals them to be inappropriate. As we saw in chapter 2, they often become physically and emotionally accustomed to certain types of care which they use in a ritualistic sense to give themselves feelings of stability, order, and control. Are physicians who turn to holistic healing less interested in science than their technocratic counterparts? They do seem to be uninterested in using science to determine how care should be standardized; at the same time, many of them since childhood have been actively engaged with science as the most direct route to the apprehension of the astonishing beauty and intricacy of the natural world. As Alan Gaby (1994) put it in a song he called "The Long-Lost Train," his metaphor for medical school:

> Oh I was in love with genetic material, so beautiful.
> I wanted to philosophize on it.
> But my instructions were written very plain:
> "Just blacken in the spaces on the windows of the train."

Although most of our interviewees, like Gaby, found their medical school experience painful and often distasteful, this distaste did not extend to science. The 1995 Harvard manual on *Alternative Medicine: Implications for Clinical Practice* notes that "Most practitioners of alternative medicine see the label 'scientific' as an important part of their self-definition, integrity, and professional identity" (Eisenberg 1995:np). Certainly we found this to be true of our interviewees. Rather than rejecting science, they tended to find it endlessly fascinating. Many of them spent time during their academic careers doing pure or applied scientific research and/or teaching. Deborah Malka taught college chemistry for ten years before becoming a physician; Chris Northrup wanted to be a biology teacher; Scott Anderson carried out a master's program in genetics; Len Saputo was fascinated by radiology and pathology; and Olga Luchakova chose research in biochemistry and immunology over a clinical internship. Her laboratory experience started her on a path that, true to the fluidity and the metaphysical underpinnings of the holistic philosophy, eventually led her to meditation and yoga instruction. She said, "I had the strange feeling that the result of research in a laboratory depends to a degree on how the experimenter *feels*.[4] There will always be statistics to prove that these data are valid, but, within the body of scientific knowledge, the question is conceived first. You understand it first, and then you prove it, but the insight comes first. So what are the origins of scientific knowledge?"

Luchakova's experience is shared by many other holistic healers, who find that the results of scientific research often lead them right back to the principles of holistic medicine. Hundreds of studies have already been completed, within the parameters of the technomedical model, that prove the significance of many of the techniques used in holism.[5] Concerned that technomedical practitioners often scoff at and dismiss this evidence, Larry Dossey responds:

> I'd like [medicine] to walk its walk and do good science. I would like it to play science the way it says it plays science, which is to honor all data without preconceived ideas about how the world ought to work—stop skimming off the top of the data which happens to appeal to one's biases and preferences. Let the chips fall scientifically where they may. For example, if it's true that Dean Ornish has come up with a cure for heart disease . . . through diet, stress, management, and meditation, and this is infinitely cheaper than a bypass operation, let's honor it. That's good science. But do not belittle this because he happens to use meditation and group therapy and this is noninvasive and nonsurgical. If it's good science, it's good science. Quit playing favorites. Increase the dialogue, look at the data; don't filter, don't sanitize, but honor whatever pops up. I think we need to follow science wherever it leads.

French physician Michel Odent, a world leader in holistic childbirth, is fond of saying that "science will save us." He is referring to the emerging trend in Western obstetrics toward evidence-based care. Most standard obstetrical procedures, such as electronic fetal monitoring and episiotomy, are not evidence-based (Enkin, Kierse, and Chalmers 1989; Davis-Floyd 1992); in fact, plenty of scientific evidence shows that they do more harm than good. If obstetrical care in most hospitals were to become truly evidence-based, then most standard interventions, including IVs, routine use of pitocin, and the lithotomy (flat-on-the-back) position would have to be eliminated and women would give birth in upright sitting or squatting positions (Goer 1995; Rooks 1997). Here obstetrics serves as a metaphor for the wider domain of technomedicine; a 1978 study carried out by the Office of Technology Assessment of the U.S. Congress reported that "only ten to twenty percent of all procedures currently used in medical practice have been shown to be efficacious in controlled trials"; in the 1990s, it is still true that over half of the techniques physicians routinely employ have not been proven in rigorous testing.

Yet, in childbirth as in many other domains of holistic healing, a focus on scientific evidence can be a double-edged sword. Little or no scientific evidence substantiates the claims or the techniques of many alternative therapies used by holistic practitioners. Explanations for this lack include the historical unwillingness of the orthodox establishment to put money into research on alternative therapies and the fact that many of these therapies work synergistically, in ways that do not lend themselves to evaluation by the gold standard of scientific research, the randomized controlled trial. In "The Tomato Effect: Rejection of Highly Efficacious Therapies" (1984), physicians James and Jean Goodwin have dubbed the tomato effect in medicine one that "occurs when an efficacious treatment for a certain disease is ignored or rejected because it does not 'make sense' in the light of accepted theories of disease mechanisms and drug actions. [For many years] the tomato was largely ignored because it was clearly poisonous; it would have been foolish to eat one. In analogous fashion, there have been many therapies in the history of medicine that, while later proved highly efficacious, were at one time rejected because they did not make sense."

As the Goodwins point out, large-scale randomized controlled trials (RCTs) can and often do demonstrate the efficacy of the holistic approach. Yet the applicability of the RCT to holistic healing has limits. The most significant limit is technomedicine's insistence on the similarity of individuals and cases, in contrast to holism's appreciation for their differences. As an illustration, we present the following comparison of approaches to treating the common childhood ear infection.

Standard and Alternative Approaches to Children's Ear Infections: A Comparative Case Study. David Eisenberg, of Harvard and Beth Israel Hospital in Boston, is in the process of designing and carrying out RCTs on various alternative therapies that have not been rigorously and conclusively tested, including the use of homeopathic remedies for ear infections as compared to the use of antibiotics (Eisenberg 1996:24).[6] Childhood ear infections are one of the leading conditions for which antibiotics are prescribed. But there are many problems with their use. Chief among these is that children with chronic ear infections are often put on repeated rounds of antibiotics, which over time lose their effectiveness as the bacteria mutate. Because of this increasing danger, in September 1996 the FDA asked pediatricians and family practitioners to severely limit their use of antibiotics for this condition. If antibiotics fail, the next allopathic step is to insert drainage tubes in the child's ears; these tubes, in true One-Two Punch form, carry their own set of problems, including complicating the child's ability to swim and increasing the possibility of introducing worse pathogens deeper into the ear through the open tube. Thus it would be most useful to parents and their sick children if alternatives that have no side effects and do not cause bacteria to mutate could be demonstrated in RCTs to cure ear infections as effectively as antibiotics.

Within the holistic paradigm, this sort of comparison, standard in Western science, presents multiple problems. For example, a classical homeopath would be unlikely to focus on an isolated symptom and prescribe a remedy for something as vague as "an ear infection." Her approach would most likely confound any scientific investigator. She would focus on the nature of the pain—such as whether cold air or motion made it better. She would be very interested in which ear was painful and whether the child was whiny or quiet, or asked for things and then rejected them. Other clues might come from the presence of any discharge, its color, odor, and viscosity. Finally, the right remedy might be found through a casual comment made by the mother, such as "He just craves bread and butter." For this practitioner, the side of the body involved, the food craving, the aversion to cold air, and the yellow mucus are all "symptoms," one no less important than the other. A child with identical objective symptoms who craved milk might require a different remedy altogether. Similarly, in the approach of Chinese medicine, the feel of the pulse and the condition of the tongue along with other observations would lead the practitioner to the correct and unique acupuncture and herbal treatment.

A holistic nutritionist, by way of comparison, would first take a detailed profile of the child's diet, habits, and psychological and environmental circumstances. He would most likely eliminate milk products from the child's diet, as these tend to produce mucus. and many children cannot successfully digest milk; holistic healers find a strong connection between ear infections and milk allergies. He would ask the parents to eliminate the child's exposure to cigarette smoke, as it has been scientifically shown to increase the incidence of ear infections. He would address the child's relationship with his parents and other siblings, their relationship with each other, and many other factors which he would see as interrelated. An overall therapy might include changes in diet and lifestyle, counseling, exercise, a change of schools, and homeopathic remedies. Such a synergistic approach differs drastically from the separatist, isolating approach researchers must take when performing a randomized controlled trial.

Given the difficulty of scientifically assessing the efficacy of the thousands of herbs, homeopathics, vitamins, and other alternatives on the shelves of every health food store, how is an individual to decide what to use? In *Manifesto for a New Medicine*, interviewee Jim Gordon chronicles his years of experimentation on himself. In his willingness to pursue science at its most basic level, the level of individual experience, Gordon aligns himself with the ideas expressed by Willis Harman in his 1994 address to the Institute for the Study of Consciousness, during which he noted that the transformation of the scientist is one of the keys to the transformation of Western science. Harmon predicted that the new epistemology of science will be experience-based. If we would counter that subjectivity admits error, Harmon asks us to ponder whether science has ever really been objective, particularly in light of the conditioning of scientists. He also predicts that "impartial subjectivity" will come into prominence as intuition takes its place as a legitimate way of knowing (see Davis-Floyd and Arvidson 1997). Larry Dossey suggests including "areas for which there is a strong scientific basis but which we haven't acknowledged, such as the data behind consciousness-oriented approaches in health care: imagery, visualization, distant viewing, transpersonal imagery, prayer studies."

It is this partial, imperfect, emergent, experience-based science that holistic physicians embrace more than the standardized science of the large-scale randomized controlled trial, which can never account for all the subjective variables that affect human interactions and health.

(9) A LONG-TERM FOCUS ON CREATING AND MAINTAINING HEALTH AND WELL-BEING

It is easy to see why the practitioners of technomedicine are so resistant to the holistic approach: it is simpler to prescribe a tranquilizer or set a bone than to pay attention to the interconnections of the patient's emotional, mental, and spiritual states, the possibility of dysfunctions in her family life, her socioeconomic condition, the toxins in her environment. The holistic focus on creating health and well-being means that holistic practitioners must do all they can to help with all these conditions—one reason that many holistic pracititioners are also environmental activists and advocates for the poor and underprivileged. While no one person can do it all, a truly holistic approach to health care does not ignore a host of other problems in favor of focusing on a small range of symptoms that can be treated with drugs and techniques.

Technocratic physicians often express extreme frustration over what they term "patient noncompliance"—the patient's failure to take the full course of medication, to follow doctor's orders. In contrast, holistic physicians most frequently voice frustration over patients who make no long-term commitment to improving their health but want the doctor to provide them with a quick fix and let them get on with their lives as before. Knowing that a "fix" that masks or eliminates symptoms, or cures them temporarily, is a poor substitute for long-term lifestyle changes that can maintain good health, the holistic physician does not feel that meeting patients' impatient demands is practicing "good medicine."

A great deal of patience may be required to support individuals through major changes. As Carolyn Myss indicated, many patients have an unconscious fear about regaining their health. When one of us (St. John) worked as patient counselor at an alternative health clinic, she learned first-hand how unresourceful and incapable of change many patients were on their own. She helped them transform their defeatist attitude by limiting the treatment regimen of the first week to daily relaxation sessions and the taking of flower essences to achieve emotional balance. The practitioners often commented that their patients became much more capable of undertaking more complex lifestyle changes after practicing these two simple but effective techniques as preparation.

Jim Gordon's (1996b) experience with Leslie Newman is another case in point. When she first arrived in his office, she expected him to "treat her with acupuncture and prescribe some herbs." She grew furious when he started asking probing questions about her life. She insisted that her only problem was MS, which she expected him to cure. The calming and unifying effects of the breathing exercise Gordon suggested enabled her to hear his explanation that MS, like all chronic illnesses, is not unrelated to the rest of one's life but instead is a manifestation of the whole. His gentle approach resulted in her initial willingness to let go of her desire for a quick fix. He asked her to eat only raw foods for a while—a radical shift in her lifestyle right at the outset of treatment. After she had gone through withdrawal from sugar and caffeine, she herself was able to observe how addicted to them she had been and how much better she felt after she had cleansed her system. Her morning dancing helped her release years of pent-up emotions; her subsequent quiet meditations allowed her to observe the effects of her high-pressure job and her perfectionist tendencies on her body and her relationship with her lover. Little by little, over time, she made the lifestyle changes that ultimately helped her achieve both health and happiness. Through her own agency, and with Gordon's guidance, she healed the whole of her self and her life for the long term.

(10) DEATH AS A STEP IN A PROCESS

Beyond the humanist's honoring of patients' refusal of heroic treatment in a living will, beyond allowing patients to die in the place of their own choosing with the attendants they desire, beyond the humanistic view of death as "the final stage of growth" lies the holistic paradigm's redefinition of death not as any kind of final end but as an essential step in the process of living. This view stems from holists' definition of the body as an energy field, and from their deep-seated understanding of the transmutable nature of energy.

Because of their integrated views on the essential oneness of body, mind, and spirit, it is only at the moment of death that holists grant these a conceptual separation, as holistic physician and author Chris Northrup tried to explain in her interview: "We are not our bodies—I think the body is a vehicle that we have for this time around. And at the same time we *are* our bodies. . . . It's a very paradoxical thing. I believe that our biochemistry, our hormones, the chemicals in our body, our blood counts and all of that are to some degree an expression of our spirit and its connection with the body. You know, we don't *have* bodies, we *are* bodies. And we are something else at the same time. We know that from near-death experiences. So it is a paradox."

At death, in this view, the energy of the body decays and returns to earth, while the energy of the spirit or the individual consciousness continues on. Most holists seem to accept some version of Eastern philosophies of reincarnation, a processual view that allows the interpretation of death as an opportunity for continued growth into a new kind of life in spirit and then again in flesh. An informal survey that Davis-Floyd once conducted of women with a holistic philosophy who choose to abort unwanted pregnancies revealed their strong belief that they were not killing the baby, but simply sending its spirit back through the gateway for another go-round. While this positive view of death does not lead holists to rush to embrace death, it does tend to give them a strong sense of trust in the essential safety of the universe and in the wisdom and worth of its ways.

In medical practice, such trust can translate into open and empathic care of the dying, even a sense that the practitioner or the family can, if they remain open to the experience, gently usher the soul to the other side:

> Wisdom could come, for example, as a flash of light that overtakes me in the nurses' station just as old Russian Anastasia is dying in her bed down the hall. I have nursed the comatose woman for weeks, speaking low into her ear before I bathe or turn her. I treat her as if she is here, and I find myself cringing and apologizing silently to her when others talk in her presence as if she is not. The flash of light brings me into sudden communication with Anastasia, though my body remains sitting quietly in the nurses' station. I am again speaking into her ear, and helping her across a kind of gulf. To my surprise, the words that come slowly out of my mouth are instructions for the dying from the Tibetan Book of the Dead: "Oh, nobly born, do not be afraid. The time has come to set your face toward the Clear Light of Realization. . . . Go toward the light, Anastasia. Don't be afraid of it." In a few moments, the light and the words dim, and I return to the lesser fluorescence of the nurses' station—reverent, shaken, humbled, grateful—just as the orderly who has been making rounds comes to announce that Anastasia has died in her sleep minutes ago. (Roncalli 1997:181)

(11) HEALING AS THE FOCUS

To say that the holistic model focuses on healing instead of on profit is not to dismiss the role of money and the practitioner's need to make a livelihood within the system. Holistic physicians have strong views about money—both for themselves and as part of their professional identity. While they are conscious of the need to earn a living, it *follows* their personal commitment to work rather than driving it. Few of the physicians we identified as holistic practice within the framework of managed care, for example, where medicine and money are strongly affiliated. Only a few are on staffs of hospitals, where major health expenses are incurred, and virtually none are members of organized medicine (as exemplified by the American Medical Association and its regional counterparts).

Recognizing that healing occurs not in response to their actions but in the support and stimulation of the vital force, in the exchange of energy between individuals, or in the long slow progress toward health that often rewards serious lifestyle changes, holistic doctors are keenly aware of their partnership with patients. They exchange their authority for the privilege of traveling alongside a client on the journey to wellness and self-discovery. This journey is quite different from the "doing to" mechanism of the technomedical paradigm. Money is part of this exchange. Holistic doctors offer their skills, attention, and support in exchange for the commitment of their patients. Together they recognize themselves as part of the larger community, in which the healing of one is the healing of all. Unlike doctors who practice technomedicine and are, as we have described, apt to live stressful and harried lives wherein they are unable to care for themselves adequately, holistic doctors are apt to find that their own healing often accompanies that of their patients, as it is practically impossible to espouse a holistic philosophy without applying it to oneself.

Within this larger understanding, the patient—and the physician—may experience healing whether or not a cure results. Even in the absence of curing, physicians can be satisfied with their role as healers and patients can be satisfied with the outcome. When economics do not form the basis of the relationship, the subject is apt to be much less charged and the patient less likely to punish the doctor economically by withholding payment or suing. In the context of this understanding, a doctor can minimize expenses in collection and insurance coverage and pass the savings on to the patient. In the mutual appreciation that often arises between holistic doctor and patient, a deep experience of *value* replaces the focus on money.

(12) EMBRACE OF MULTIPLE HEALING MODALITIES

As we have seen, the holistic paradigm's definition of the body as an energy field in constant interaction with other energy fields makes possible its embrace of multiple modalities that remain unacceptable to proponents of the technomedical paradigm. The ultimate holistic vision entails a profound revolution in health care. Were this paradigm to gain cultural ascendance, the dominance of the technomedical model would be replaced with the cultural valuation of a multiplicity of approaches. Homeopathy, naturopathy, acupuncture, Chinese medicine, energy medicine et al. would take their places as respected and culturally legitimate disciplines. Practitioners of each modality would know enough about the others for appropriate referrral. Medical students would have opportunities to learn and become certified in these various modalities and in the specialty of holistic medicine (see chapter 8). Above all, the public would be educated in the techniques of self-care, healthy lifestyle, and the appropriate use of a variety of approaches to healing.

Holistic medicine's embrace of multiple healing modalities is gaining increasing public attention and acceptance. The clearest evidence for this statement comes from the 1993 study conducted by physician David Eisenberg and published in the *New England Journal of Medicine* (Eisenberg et al.; see chapter 1), which determined that one-third of Americans sought the services of a non-M.D. practitioner in a one-year time period—and paid out-of-pocket for three-quarters of the cost of these services. Another finding of this survey was that 72 percent of the maverick patients did not tell their doctors about their use of alternative medicine. Perhaps the center stage given to this study reflects the financial impact on medicine it uncovers, as well as the finding that the users of unconventional therapies were well-educated, middle-income whites from twenty-five to forty-nine years of age—one of the very best markets for orthodox medicine.

To the increasing public acceptance of alternative therapies, the technomedical system has responded with an increase in FDA-type policing, attacking the sale of vitamins and nutritional supplements through proposed legislation and raids on the offices of alternative practitioners. For example, George Guess, M.D., was accused of unprofessional conduct by the North Carolina Medical Board because he practiced homeopathy. After fighting for five years to no avail, Dr. Guess moved and established a practice in the more hospitable state of Virginia. However, the furious public response made it clear that this behavior from government authorities was intolerable (Janiger and Goldberg 1993:47). A similar but more drawn-out legal battle ensued after Jonathan Wright, a nationally known holistic physician and expert on nutrition, ran into trouble for dispensing the amino acid tryptophan in his office in Seattle. Some months before his arrest, a contaminated sample of tryptophan shipped from Japan had resulted in several deaths around the country, resulting in a national FDA ban on dispensing it. Wright, who relied on the substance in his practice as a holistic alternative to Prozac, found a source of uncontaminated tryptophan, had it certified as uncontaminated by the Mayo Clinic, and continued to dispense it in spite of the ban. When the FDA confiscated his tryptophan supply, he filed suit with the Justice Department against the FDA for its return. Wright's associate Alan Gaby continues the story:

> What he subsequently learned is, you don't sue the FDA! Because, shortly after that, they began making trips at night to his dumpster, trying to find something that he was throwing away that they could bust him on. They have a listing of every day they fished in his dumpster and what they found

> every day. And they found some stuff they called misbranded drugs—for example, there was an empty Vitamin B–complex box from Germany labeled "Vitamin B–Komplex" with a "K." That according to the FDA is a misbranded drug because the packaging is not readily understandable. The FDA also found in the dumpster some other materials apparently manufactured by Meridian Valley Clinical Laboratory, which is in the same building and for which Wright is a consultant. This product had mold in it, and the FDA concluded that Wright was manufacturing drugs in an unsafe manner. Yes, mold gets in things sometimes and that is why they throw it away. Then they got a search warrant and told the local police [that] they were going in on a drug bust. So they got 'em all pumped up, they got them in flak jackets—they kicked the front door down, drawn guns and all, and said "Freeze" . . . into this medical clinic! The local King County police were reported later on as saying, "We got total egg on our face; we're totally embarrassed. The FDA told us we were going in on a drug bust, but they didn't tell us the drugs were for little old ladies who had allergies."

The police raid on Wright's clinic dominated Seattle news for several days and was picked up by the national news media. A dedicated fax line to the White House set up as a result of the ensuing public outcry for a time received more than seven thousand faxes a day protesting the actions of the police and the FDA. Wright was invited to be on *Larry King Live* and other national television shows. The police had confiscated four computers and additional equipment from Wright's clinic, refusing to return them because they constituted what the police saw as evidence in a criminal case invoving the illegal manufacture of drugs. Wright was actually manufacturing trace minerals (magnesium, manganese, etc.), which was not illegal. After three and a half years, the FDA finally dropped the case against Wright and destroyed all the evidence, including his diagnostic computers (which cost more than $10,000 apiece). Yet Wright maintained a sense of humor, which impressed Gaby:

> It was amazing the way he took it. When the press interviewed him and said, "So why do you think they kicked your door down and took the vitamins out of your office?" he said, "Well, vitamin deficiency makes you very irrational." They asked, " Why do you think they had to come in with drawn guns?" and he answered, "Maybe they thought I was going to attack them with a syringe full of Vitamin B12!"

The stated motive for such attacks on holistic practitioners is the protection of the public. In reality, they represent concerted attempts to defend the hegemony of technomedicine against its many challengers. Unfortunately, the defenders of technomedicine often fail to recognize the healing benefits to the public that can accrue from these very challenges, and from holism's embrace of the multiple modalities they represent.

The Three Paradigms

With this chapter we conclude our descriptions of the three primary paradigms of medical care we have identified in the United States at present.[7] The humanistic model can be viewed as occupying a broad middle range along a wide philosophical spectrum that ranges from the orthodox technocratic approach at one end to the heretical holistic approach at the other. For the reader's convenience, we juxtapose these three paradigms in table 4.1.

We cannot stress strongly enough that these three paradigms of health care constitute ever-shifting focal points along a fluid continuum (see figure 4.1); *the boundaries between them are extremely blurry.* Many technocratic practitioners are incorporating elements of humanism. With this shift they expand their options, even that of beginning to incorporate elements of holistic thought and practice. And holistic medicine certainly encompasses many dimensions of both technocratic and humanistic practice. It is often impossible to characterize the practice of a given physician as purely technocratic, purely humanistic, or purely holistic.

As focal points for thought and action, however, we continue to find these paradigms to be useful models of and templates for the extreme variations in contemporary medical practice. Physicians themselves also seem to find them useful, in three particular ways: (1) conventional technomedical physicians with whom we have spoken seem to appreciate the opportunity afforded by our presentation of this spectrum to assess their own standards in relation to those of their colleagues; (2) our holistic interviewees have expressed gratitude for our explication of the humanistic model, as it clarifies for them the differences they perceive between themselves and other physicians who cannot be characterized as purely conventional but who do not make the same cognitive shift that holistic physicians do; and (3) humanistic physicians appreciate a way of pinpointing their beliefs that is neither as impersonal as the technocratic model nor as fluid as the holistic model. In the section that follows we will discuss the profound differences among the types of thinking that underlie these three paradigms of care.

The Four Stages of Cognition

As we saw in chapter 1, the kind of compartmentalized thinking that led to the development of the technomedical model in its present form has been classified as Stage One—either/or, black-and-white thinking that interprets the world in a univariate way, and regards itself as the sole authority (Schroder, Driver, and Steufert 1967). Stage-One systems, which include all fundamentalist religions, are generally tautological and self-

Technocratic Model >>>><<<< Humanistic Model >>>><<<< Holistic Model

Figure 4.1. The Medical Spectrum

referential—that is to say, they are closed systems. They tell a story about reality, and for confirmation of that story they refer only to the story. Thus they are constantly engaged in efforts to make reality conform to their version of it.

Any system becomes closed when its adherents cease to adapt to new information that does not fit the existing paradigm. For example, when confronted with patients once diagnosed as incurable who heal through alternative therapies, conventional physicians are apt to dismiss their cases as flukes or anomalies. When the response of one medical modality to the successes of another is to dismiss and ignore them, such dismissal indicates that its proponents have lost touch with the real world and are operating out of a closed conceptual system, one that insists on its own version of reality no matter what the facts.

While it is theoretically possible for *any* conceptual system to become closed, including all three paradigms of healing discussed in this book, the technomedical model particularly lends itself to becoming a closed system because of its general rigidity of approach and belief. It suffers at the outset from a fundamental flaw: its first two tenets, that mind and body are separate and the body is a machine, are demonstrably false; they do not match the reality of the human condition. Thus proponents of the technomedical paradigm are constrained to make them *appear to be* true, to make it seem as if reality matches their model of it. They try to do so using the same kind of separated, segmented logic that produced these ideas in the first place; the technomedical system relies on this type of purely left-brained, unimodal, Stage-One thought (see figure 4.2).[8]

The circles in figure 4.2 represent paradigms or worldviews. The four stages are steps on a continuum from very rigid, closed thinking to very fluid, open thinking. As we have seen, Stage-One thinkers are fundamentalists: they interpret the world through the filter of one narrow worldview, which functions as a closed system. In contrast, Stage-Two thinkers acknowledge the existence of other systems that cannot be explained in terms of their own. While still convinced of the superiority of their own system, Stage-Two thinkers are willing to grant some slight validity to a few of these other systems. Stage-Three thinkers, while still identifying themselves with one primary paradigm, acknowledge the value and validity of many different ways of thinking and being and occasionally modify their own belief system in response to what they learn from other systems.

The humanistic model arises from a bimodal, relational type of thinking

TABLE 4.1 THE TECHNOCRATIC, HUMANISTIC, AND HOLISTIC MODELS OF MEDICINE

The Technocratic Model of Medicine	*The Humanistic (Biopsychosocial) Model of Medicine*	*The Holistic Model of Medicine*
1. Mind/body separation	1. Mind-body connection	1. Oneness of body-mind-spirit
2. The body as machine	2. The body as an organism	2. The body as an energy system interlinked with other energy systems
3. The patient as object	3. The patient as relational subject	3. Healing the whole person in whole-life context
4. Alienation of practitioner from patient	4. Connection and caring between practitioner and patient	4. Essential unity of practitioner and client
5. Diagnosis and treatment from the outside in (curing disease, repairing dysfunction)	5. Diagnosis and healing from the outside in *and* from the inside out	5. Diagnosis and healing from the inside out
6. Hierarchical organization and standardization of care	6. Balance between the needs of the institution and the individual	6. Networking organizational structure that facilitates individualization of care
7. Authority and responsibility inherent in practitioner, not patient	7. Information, decision making, and responsibility shared between patient and practitioner	7. Authority and responsibility inherent in each individual

8. Supervaluation of science and technology	8. Science and technology counterbalanced with humanism	8. Science and technology placed at the service of the individual
9. Aggressive intervention with emphasis on short-term results	9. Focus on disease prevention	9. A long-term focus on creating and maintaining health and well-being
10. Death as defeat	10. Death as an acceptable outcome	10. Death as a step in a process
11. A profit-driven system	11. Compassion-driven care	11. Healing as the focus
12. Intolerance of other modalities	12. Open-mindedness toward other modalities	12. Embrace of multiple healing modalities
Basic underlying principle: separation	*Basic underlying principles: balance and connection*	*Basic underlying principles: connection and integration*
Type of thinking: unimodal, left-brained, linear	*Type of thinking: bimodal*	*Type of thinking: fluid, multimodal, right-brained*

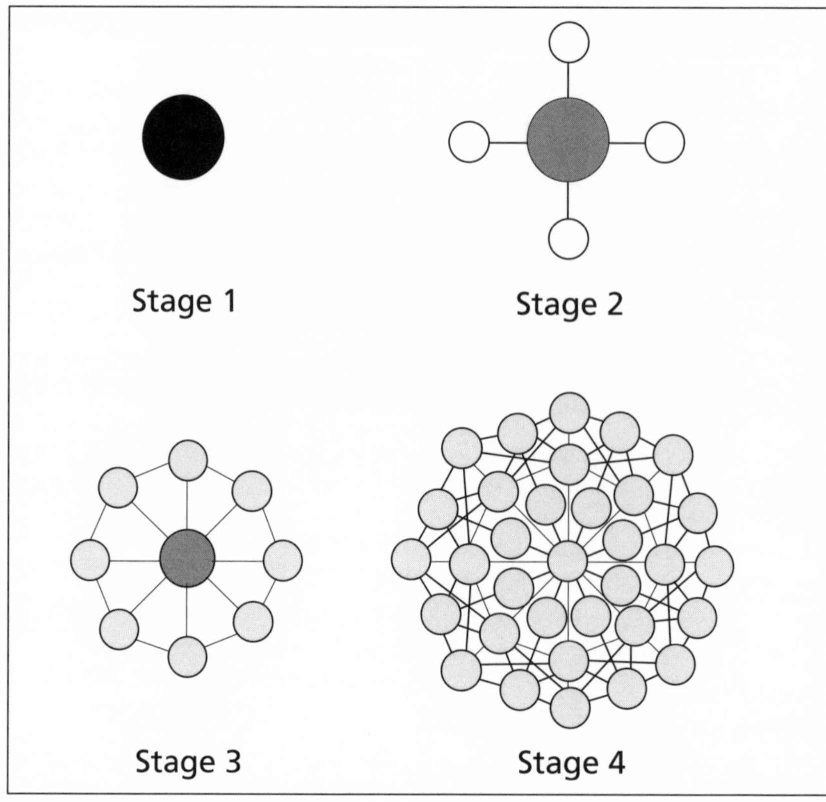

Figure 4.2. The Four Stages of Cognition. This diagram is adapted from McManus 1979b; see also Schroder, Driver, and Steufert 1967.

that is at once less rigid than the technomedical model and less fluid than the holistic model. Returning to figure 4.2, we might place humanism as ranging between Stage Two and Stage Three. Stage Two might represent those at the more conservative end of the humanistic part of the spectrum, while Stage Three might represent humanists who are moving closer to holism.

The gestalt type of thinking that characterizes the holistic model can be classified as Stage Four—fluid, multimodal thinking that fully recognizes that no one system has a lock on reality, that instead, many paradigms tell many stories, each encompassing a part of the overarching, ineffable whole. Stage-Four thinkers embrace differences and encompass their competing claims; they seek out the common threads that run between the Stage-One systems of the world, large-scale and small (e.g., Wilber 1996). They develop cognitive models that they constantly modify in response to new information, making sure that these models constitute an open system. They tend to align with the new-physics view that, at the most fundamental level of existence, we are all fluid combinations of particles and waves swimming as one in the "quantum soup" or the "energy sea" (Puthoff 1990a, b)—a place where matter, energy, consciousness, and spirit indistinguishably merge.

Without assuming its univariate truth, fluid thinkers often plunge into one paradigm or another for a time, incorporating its wisdom into their worldview. Thus physicians who spend years learning pharmacology and surgery may also study homeopathy or Chinese medicine. They may learn just enough about the new system to know when to refer their patients to another practitioner, or they may study the new system diligently, becoming an accomplished herbalist or acupuncturist or Ayurvedic practitioner. Our interviewees found these "alternative" modalities to be as challenging and complex as their medical training; many acknowledged that they had to open not only to new information, but to a whole new way of learning and of being in order to master another modality, as Jim Gordon describes:

> Years ago, when Dr. Singha suggested that the lung is the "mother" of the kidney and that somehow the kidney is connected to the back, I was incredulous. But today words and concepts like these have become as much a part of my vocabulary as the stages of embryonic and fetal growth or the physiology of the fight or flight response. I look at the coating of the tongue—if the illness is hot and acute, it is likely to be yellow; if cold and chronic, then white—and check for the tight lumpiness of qi and blood stagnation in my patient's belly as attentively as I might listen for a murmur in her heart or feel for enlargement of her liver. I ask questions that arise in both the Western and Eastern halves of my mind. I see and hear with Chinese as well as American eyes and ears, and I record what I have learned in such a way that, most often, each set of information enriches and enlarges the other. (1996:195)

In general humans have the potential to think both rigidly and fluidly, although fluid thinking usually takes more energy. (An exception to this rule may be the "aha!" experience—the quick flash of intuitive insight that generates instead of consuming energy.) Information is most easily processed in the human brain along established neuronal pathways. In order to process new information that does not match these established pathways, new pathways—along with millions of new synaptic connections—must be created. We are all capable of this but it consumes a great deal of energy. (Readers who have lived in another country and struggled to learn its language will recognize the exhaustion this effort can generate.) Even the most fluid of thinkers will lose their mental elasticity when they become tired or overstressed.

Since medical school and residency keep students tired and chronically overstressed, it is little wonder that they tend to internalize a fairly rigid version of the technocratic model, at least until the stress lets up and they are free to live as they please. Most chronically overworked technocratic physicians themselves have insufficient energy to take in the complex information offered by alternative healing systems. They are already busy trying to keep up with the stack of medical journals chronicling new developments in their specialties. At least this sort of information can be easily assimilated, since it tends to match their existing neuronal structures and so requires little energy to process.

Thus it is all the more remarkable that any physicians at all are willing to take on the challenge of learning about holistic healing, with its multiple modalities, its wide-angle focus on multiple aspects of a patient's life, its disrespect for boundaries and divisions, its touchy-feely-mushy components, and its general integrative fuzziness.[9] A walk on the wild side of holism can feel like descent from solid ground into a bog, where things mix and merge and you never know what's under your feet or above your head, and you can't see where you're going—or like a free fall down a slippery slope, with the ground nowhere in sight. Were it not for the significant limitations of both the technomedical and humanistic approaches, no doubt few would even stick out a foot! In the following chapters we analyze the motivations and chronicle the adventures of some of those who have been willing to take one tentative step, and then another, and then one more—out onto that slippery slope.

PART III

The Paradigm Shift

5 *Catalysts for Transformation*

> I was dying because I needed to make a shift and I didn't know that. I had carried the technological, the curing part as far as I could carry it, and it needed to evolve into something more spiritual. When you think of what you're going to do in life—I'm going to become a doctor, I'm going to get married, I'm going to have children, I'm going to have a big house and a nice car, and I'm going to have all of this material wealth—that will be the sign that I'm successful, that people think I'm a good doctor—that's it! And I did all of that. By the time I was forty, I had all of that. And I looked around and said, "Something's wrong. This isn't it."
> —BETHANY HAYS, M.D.

The shift from technocratic to holistic philosophy and practice involves a complete values overhaul with readily observable effects. It is fairly easy to see that holistic doctors employ techniques and subscribe to beliefs that diverge markedly from those taught in their technomedical training. Less evident to the public eye is their willingness to accept a relatively modest income, endure the stress of differentiating themselves from their peers, and risk the financial, legal, and social implications of changing their mode of practice. The most potent transformation is less visible still. It is in their worldview. The simplest way of characterizing it is to say that the doctors whose stories we will tell have shifted from a closed to an open stance toward life itself. In the course of their journeys they have adopted a far more complex worldview that provides few answers and many questions, requires flexibility and acceptance, embraces uncertainty, and completely redefines success and failure. For example, one physician commented that the greatest hurdle was to "unlearn" the patterns of belief and behavior that he had learned in medical school in order to clear some cognitive space for new information and methods. His comment bears witness to the profound nature of this paradigm shift. Participating in holism involves far more than learning terms and acquiring techniques. It is a leap from a world informed by separation to one infused with unity.

We wanted to know what prompted these individuals to change the way they practice medicine; indeed, this constituted the major focus of our research. The first few physicians we interviewed told dramatic stories of major life crises that impelled them to make radical changes in their lives. Thus we initially thought we would find such dramatic shifts in the experiences of all our interviewees. But we were surprised to learn that many of them simply knew, all the way through their medical training, that some day they would "do it differently," although they often had no idea what that meant at the time. These individuals, who did not buy into the ideology behind their technomedical training, found that this inner certainty kept them going during the long years of their training process and gave them a transcendent goal to reach for at its end. For them, as we shall see, the move away from technomedicine resembled an exciting adventure they had long anticipated more than a dramatic change in values and beliefs. In contrast, those who did buy into the technocratic model during their training often made the kind of sudden and radical paradigm shift we were expecting to find; many reported that psychological trauma and suffering often accompanied this change.

A variety of stimuli promoted such paradigm shifts. They included life crises such as personal illness, the illness of a loved one, a dissolving marriage, a profound spiritual opening. Some of the physicians in our study "hit the wall" in their practices, realizing that they were not helping their patients as much as they wished to—that the causes as well as the cures for their patients' problems lay beyond their technomedical training and skills. This paradigm shift takes different forms for those who move into humanism without fully embracing the fundamental principles of holism.[1] The humanists begin to focus on their relationship to their patients, working to make every encounter a healing encounter through the strength of that relationship—as does the nascent holist, who, in addition, begins to study and often to incorporate entirely new modalities and approaches. Both humanists and holists operate from a worldview substantially different from that modeled in their training, although many began their career with the same expectations and experiences as their colleagues.

In this and the following chapter, we will attempt to describe the transformation of the traditionally trained doctor to a holistic physician—the shift from doctor to healer. How is such a change initiated and what are the experiences of the individual in process? And how do those who have undergone this shift experience themselves and their professional lives?

What Sparks a Paradigm Shift? A Catalogue of Catalysts

Holistic obstetrician Bethany Hays insists that "if you address the belief system of the sick person and find the cure that fits, the person will heal herself." What brings a traditionally trained doctor like Hays, who has mastered biochemistry, anatomy, physiology, pharmacology, and a myriad of technological procedures, to the point of being able to say, "Anything can heal"? Terry Tyler's answer is that "the movement from physician to healer requires a personal transformation, a total or nearly total redefinition of the doctor's personhood, causing something to die in order that something may be born."

There is really no single impetus to change: each situation is unique. It is, however, possible to detect overarching themes in the transformative process of physicians seeking to expand the boundaries of their training, their practice, and their personhood. We have identified five of these themes: (1) The first encompasses the experience of doctors who invested years of service within the paradigm of their training, ultimately to abandon it when they reached a peak of frustration with its limitations vis-à-vis their efforts to heal their patients. (2) The second describes the process by which patients become the catalysts for the physician's transformation. (3) A third and particularly salient theme is that of personal injury or illness—physical, mental, or emotional. Some of our interviewees, when faced with their own personal healing crisis, had to confront viscerally the limits of Western medicine and discover the effectiveness of other traditions. (4) The fourth theme incorporates both social and spiritual awakening, from the consciousness-raising that accompanies overseas travel or an awakened feminist awareness to profound spiritual experiences that leave the individual forever changed. (5) Some of these catalysts can and do come into play during medical training; likewise, they can have major impact before the physician-to-be even enters medical school. We name this phenomenon "starting out on the other side," and include it here in our discussion of catalysts so that its complexities can be addressed.

Each of these types of experience has the power to raise fundamental questions about identity, purpose, and capability. Each can take one to the liminal space where roles must be dropped and the essential nature encountered. Of course, such existential crises also occur in the lives of individuals who are not physicians. However, for doctors, the personal and professional are intricately bound as a result of the initiatory nature of their training and the life/death intensity of their work. Major challenges to their belief systems threaten not just their personality, but their vocation, their sense of destiny, and their livelihood. They have invested heavily both personally and financially in their training; a crisis which threatens their belief system erodes not only the security of their future but their whole identity. If they are no longer the Medical Doctors they were trained to be, who are they, and who might they become?

CONFRONTING THE LIMITS OF TECHNOMEDICINE

What drives the bone-weary resident and the emergency room or primary care doctor is the belief that they are doing something worthwhile. Indeed, pulling a febrile child back from death or jump-starting a lifeless heart seem to be intrinsically valuable pursuits. The technomedical model of medicine is so thoroughly ingrained during training that physicians often must experience severe frustration with its limitations before they acknowledge that they are not satisfied with results. Years of witnessing the ineffectiveness or ill effects of the medications one prescribes, or a patient's deterioration from an unhealthy lifestyle, take their toll. An M.D. may then have a moment of epiphany like the one David Edelberg described when he suddenly realized that of the ten patients he was attending on his rounds, seven were there for diseases of lifestyle and three because of complications of treatment, and asked himself, "What's wrong with this picture?" He saw that "the man who has the epigastric burning now, in ten years will have a coronary and be in the intensive care unit. . . . If I could help him change his lifestyle and see where the problem is, I might be doing something for someone."

Doctors are understandably bereft when technology fails to deliver. Len Saputo complained, "I couldn't do a lot for a lot of my patients and a lot of what I would do would be very expensive. I was pretty disappointed at how things were going—too much morbidity, not enough successful outcomes." David Dowling said, "I started out like everybody else—wanting to be the best internist, the best cardiologist, the best general surgeon. And then I began realizing that *none of this was doing anything*. There's no medication that cures; there's no surgery that cures the patient; and I became very disenchanted with medicine as a whole."

While some physicians accept their limitations with a certain resignation, perhaps seeking more satisfaction in other areas of life, a number of those in our study used their frustration as a launching pad. Karin Montero, a plastic surgeon, became highly disillusioned by one of technology's failures: "I started practicing about a year and half before the breast implant issue hit the fan. About that time I had already decided, from observing patients with implants, that there was a problem in at least half the patients. They had to undergo very painful procedures to have the scar broken down. That led me to take a different attitude than the plastic surgeons' party line. I don't put the implants in; and I'm one of the few in this city women can come to have them taken out."

Montero's disillusionment led her to begin to think of herself as a holistic physician. She said, "I'm in the process of learning that there is a lot more I can do toward understanding prevention and how it affects body image, eating disorders, obesity. Also I'm looking at nutrition, vitamins, herbs, and things I can do for an improved postoperative result."

Several doctors told us that many of their colleagues share their frustration with the limits of technomedicine. Bethany Hays said, "There are a few that I think are doing well in conventional medicine—what I notice about them now is that they have very strong religious beliefs or they have a kind of a limited worldview, an ability to be satisfied in what seem like very limited circumstances. What I mostly see among my colleagues is that they're sort of thrashing around to try to find a way to make it more exiting or more challenging or new or—you know, it's not right for them either." David Gershan noted that his colleagues "have a soul need. They are sick, in agony because of the limitations of what they do. To do it day after day, and on top of that to be rushed—it becomes even more insulting." But instead of allowing that frustration to lead them to new learning, these colleagues often choose to suppress their frustration and pain, and to ridicule and belittle those who stray outside of conventional boundaries. Gene Ross found himself unhappy working in an emergency room: "I started feeling more and more depleted. . . . In the last several months it seemed I couldn't bounce back at all. I began to hate the patients, wishing they'd all go away. I was convinced I wasn't doing anything useful—patching up people who were alcoholics or addicts or who ate too much cholesterol seemed a monumental waste of resources. I looked around at the other doctors and they seemed fine. Later I learned that they didn't like it much better than I did, but were putting on fronts for each other."

Gershan, Montero, and the others mentioned in this section did not content themselves with putting on fronts, but instead chose to deal with their increasing frustration with the limits of technomedicine by expanding beyond its parameters into holistic care.

PATIENTS AS TEACHERS

Patients themselves often play a significant role in starting their physicians along the path to holistic practice. Although David Eisenberg's (1993) study in the *New England Journal of Medicine* showed that seven out of ten people who use alternative methods do not tell their doctors, evidently three out of ten brave souls do choose to share this information with their physicians, often with dramatic results for the physician. David Edelberg traces the beginnings of his shift to just such experiences: "After I had been practicing for quite some time, my patients began telling me about other healing methods that worked for them. They would say, 'I visited a homeopath who tied it all together. My back pain is gone and my anxiety is gone too.' *I'm* supposed to be the expert, but this other person made my patient well. My patients had found something that worked, and I knew that what I was doing was not working very well. This brought a shift in perspective."

In "Physician in Transition" (1989), Bob Anderson describes learning a cosmic lesson from a single patient:

> About five years into practice, a patient whom I treated for a duodenal ulcer became my teacher. About a year after he was "cured," he reappeared with similar symptoms. Apropros of my training, I ordered repeat X-rays,

confirming a recurrent ulcer. I instituted the same treatment as before, experiencing a slight annoyance that he wasn't well. Never once did I stop to ask the question, "Why does this man have an ulcer?" After he returned six months later with his third ulcer (second recurrence), I again repeated the treatment procedure, and he again recovered. I was ready to pop out of the interventionist model, and I began to talk with this patient, who taught me so much. I learned that he smoked, and that this predisposed him to a twofold risk of recurrence. I found that his marriage was in disarray and that he was under excessive stress. I listened, learning the lesson of the healing listener. I scheduled him for further visits, getting to know this young man, discussing options and alternatives. He did not return with an ulcer. This was perhaps my cosmic lesson in the primordial beginnings of holistic alternatives and complementary approaches.

SUFFERING PERSONAL ILLNESS

To the question "What does it take to be a healer?" Bernie Siegel (1986) answers, "The willingness to deal with your own wounds."

Aesculapius was the son of Coronis and Apollo. Unfortunately, the pregnant Coronis had been unfaithful to Apollo and was sentenced to die by fire. At the last moment, Apollo plucked the child, Aesculapius, from her womb. As he was yanked from the pyre, Aesculapius suffered burns which resulted in his being disfigured and lame for life. Apollo sent his son to be reared by Chiron, from whom he learned all that was known in the realm regarding healing. Aesculapius never knew his mother or his father. He was raised with a sense of purpose and focus which amounted to an initiatory process. His wounds as well as his great compassion bound him to a life of service. There was a monastic quality to this life. *Because of his wounds* he became a great healer whose skill was superb and whose compassion was great; he exemplifies the archetype of the wounded healer.

Across cultures and throughout human history, severe illness or injury has been the catalyst for transforming many thousands of men and women into healers. This wounded healer archetype is very much at play in the transformational journeys of holistic physicians. Physicians who have personally confronted the limitations of Western medicine through their own illnesses or the illness of a loved one, who have experienced the paralyzing fear of death or disability, and who have healed through alternative methods, are powerfully motivated to change their way of practicing. Each of the physicians who speaks in this section was healed outside the paradigm of Western medicine. This experience forever changed how they look at life and how they relate to their profession.

For example, even before attending medical school, Debra Malka experienced seemingly incurable illness. Multiple specialists failed to help. It was through body work that her condition finally began to improve.

She says, "Illness is a catalyst. Before my illness, I had never intended to become a holistic physician." Suffering from both colon cancer and an addiction to prescription drugs, David Fillmore "gambled away six months on alternative methods, trying to heal my colon cancer. I knew I couldn't mess around too long. It was like throwing dice. I had a whole lot of experiences in six months. When I came back and had another biopsy, it was normal. At that time I was very, very high, in touch with my spiritual nature. I had been to India, and was really soaking it up. The highest moment of my life was when I discovered I did not have cancer, that this stuff seemed to work" (*MetaPhysicians' Tales*). Also healed simultaneously and effortlessly was the addiction to prescription drugs that had plagued him for many years. Amazed that "there was no struggle," he began to wonder, "How is it possible that by struggling I could get nowhere, but when I didn't struggle I got somewhere by not doing anything?" With these words he expresses a strong theme that runs throughout the stories of the transformative journeys of holistic physicians—they learn, in myriad ways, about the enormous value of surrender and trust.

Like Malka and Fillmore, Walt Stoll found that his intractable physical complaints were messengers, sending signals too powerful to ignore about the need to make a change. Stoll writes:

> I was in charge of patient education at the first Health Maintenance Organization in Kentucky, and later was put in charge of curriculum development for a new primary care physician assistant program at the University of Kentucky School of Allied Health. I also taught conventional medicine in the Department of Family Practice [but] I had not applied any health information to my own life. As a consequence, I had hypertension (160/110), and high cholesterol (over 300); weighed 242 pounds; wore a brace for ruptured discs in my back; and suffered from chronic gastritis, chronic constipation, severe hemorrhoids, arthritis of both knees and my left hip, stuffy nose (for ten years), and chronic depression. In addition, the toenail of my fifth toe on each foot had disappeared.
>
> In 1977 I was exposed to applied kinesiology [a technique of testing muscle weakness or strength to identify physical conditions such as food allergies] by a dentist in Lexington. He told me that sugar and caffeine were killing me. I changed my diet mainly to prove him wrong. Immediately, my health dramatically improved. . . . Encouraged, I learned to practice skilled relaxation. Within six months, the combination of relaxation, a whole-foods diet, and aerobics totally eliminated all my chronic conditions. Now, ten years later, there has been no recurrence. An added bonus has been complete freedom from colds and influenza during all that time!
>
> The changes in my health were so obvious that patients began to ask me what I was doing for myself, and I began to share my experiences with them. Soon I was going to postgraduate holistic medical courses to find out what I was doing. And soon I began to see my patients achieving the same results. ("Physician in Transition" 1989)

Although back pain forced Peter Nunn to leave his medical practice for a time, he saw the pain as both metaphor and catalyst for change: "I went through a fairly major crisis myself. . . . I found that what I was doing for my patients wasn't even working for me. I had reached a point with my back firmly against the wall and my face in the mud. I developed such pain that I couldn't move."

The pain in Jim Gordon's back was equally effective at getting his attention. In a hurry both to learn yoga and to become the national director of a program for runaways, he threw out his back performing a challenging yoga posture. Numerous traditional orthopedists examined him and his X-rays, but had nothing to offer beyond muscle relaxants that made him drowsy and tests that led straight to back surgery, which he didn't want. Miserable and desperate, he went for the first time to an osteopath, who adjusted his back with a resounding crunch. After multiple visits he was still in despair, as the relief provided by the adjustment never lasted more than an hour or two. In a last-ditch effort to avoid surgery, he called an Indian acupuncturist named Shyam Singha in London who had been recommended to him by a friend. Over the phone, Dr. Singha prescribed hot baths with Epsom salts followed by cold showers, and a diet consisting solely of three pineapples per day. Singha explained that pineapple contains malic acid, which stimulates the lung and the colon, which in Chinese medicine are the mother of the kidney and the bladder, which are connected to the back.

None of this made sense to Gordon, but he was at the end of his rope. He followed Dr. Singha's recommendations to the letter. Three days later, he was burning with fever and the pain in his back and leg was worse than ever. Dr. Singha called this a "healing crisis," explaining that sometimes the illness must become much more acute in order to be healed. This explanation *did* make sense to Gordon. As a psychiatrist, he perfectly understood that the way to cure most mental illness is to face it and go through it. The resulting emotional crisis releases years of pent-up, repressed rage and despair, paving the way to healing. That physical healing might work the same way as mental healing was an illumination. After seven days on Singha's regimen, Gordon found his back to be "80 percent better" and himself twelve pounds lighter and "far clearer" in his mind. Singha then sent him back to the osteopath, and this time, the adjustment held. Gordon writes, "Neither my back, nor my medical practice, nor indeed my view of the world, has been the same since" (1996b:43).

Likewise, Larry Dossey's journey toward holism was sparked during his residency by the intractable pain of the migraine headaches that had plagued him since the sixth grade. These were

> very severe, classical migraines with profound nausea, vomiting, blindness, and incapacitation for twenty-four hours. I thought I would have to drop

> out of medical school at one point. I had gone through all the tests for abnormal brain function and tried all the medications that are supposed to work, but which did not, and I had a tremendous problem. In the early seventies I found that biofeedback had been successful in treating this problem. This sounds commonplace today, but in the seventies it was unthinkable that you could hook up to a gadget and learn to change your body and something as severe as a migraine would get better. [Through biofeedback] the headaches went away, not totally, but it was like a miracle. I was so convinced of the efficacy of this approach that I became certified as a biofeedback instructor, and used it in my internal medicine practice for many years. So . . . God bless our illnesses. I was a classic example of the wounded healer. Your wound is your gift in understanding illness.

Given the consensus among our interviewees that, as Dossey said, "Your wound is your gift in understanding illness," we found it fascinating that two physicians suggested that illness or other forms of dysfunction were apt to *result from* suppressing the impulse to change. Jack Travis believes "it is crucial for physicians to take this journey. The rest will sort itself out. . . . If they don't take the personal journey, they will likely seek escape in drugs, alcohol, consumerism, or the 'medications' our culture uses to hide its pain." Christiane Northrup issued a similar warning:

> Once you say you're interested in this, that you believe in it, you'd better do something about it in your life or you'll get sick. The gods will visit you in an uncomfortable form until you put your money where your mouth is. So don't read about it or get interested unless you intend to follow up. I don't know if the universe is going to give you ten years to put this together anymore. What you say you believe and how you live your life must line up. Once you start believing this, your higher power doesn't give you as much slack as when you were unconscious.

SOCIAL AND SPIRITUAL AWAKENING

Both the dawning of social consciousness and the deeply personal awakening of a sleeping spirit can set a physician on the path to holism. All growth and change is spiritual in nature in that the removal of any blocks to wholeness, whether through physical healing or emotional release, allows more of one's spiritual essence to become the operative force in one's life. Spiritual awakenings can be minor, occurring on a daily or hourly basis as we recommit to the unity which is our true self. Or they may be major, when one *satori* (in Zen teachings, an immediate, unexpected experience of enlightenment) jolts us from what passed as ordinary reality to an experience of a different dimension.

Social awakenings may involve transformed perceptions of one's relationships to one's friends, family, community, or the entire world. They may reflect, simultaneously or separately, a new ecological awareness, a shift in political perspective, the influence of living in other cultures, or the rise of feminist consciousness. Social and spiritual awakenings are so interlinked that they are difficult to distinguish from each other; thus we address them both in this section without trying to delineate arbitrary boundaries between them.

In *Spiritual Awakenings* (1995:3–15), Barbara Harris Whitfield identifies many "doorways to the soul"—transformative events that can trigger an opening to a new dimension. These include near-death experiences, childbirth, meditation, intense prayer, the death of a loved one, withdrawal from chemical dependence, overwhelming loss, encounters with angels or other guiding beings, transcendent sexual experience, spontaneous feelings of union with nature, exposure to spiritual thought, an important dream whose effects last a lifetime, *kundalini* awakening, and breath and body work. One further stimulus Whitfield describes as a series of "synchronous events" that lead one by the hand, so to speak, to various events and individuals who serve to awaken the spiritual impulse to such a degree that transformation occurs, albeit more gently and slowly. Regardless of the stimulus, the outcome is the same: "We are removed from our limited existence and come face to face with the Universe" (1995:165).

Our interviewees' "doorways to the soul" included encounters with guidance, reading an influential book or meeting an influential individual, such as a spiritual teacher, using hallucinogenic drugs, and Whitfield's "series of synchronous events." Some of these passages were primarily spiritual, some primarily social; most contain elements of each. For a "doorway to the soul" that leads an individual into a deeper relationship with oneself may at the same time lead to a deeper relationship with others; thus the doorway to the soul also becomes the "doorway to the social." In short, this section specifically deals with relationships—spiritual, social, and ecological—as the catalysts for the transformative journey.

Encounters with Guidance. The three physicians who speak next tell of singular experiences that completely changed their personal and professional perspective. Michael Greenberg, a dermatologist, experienced contact with inner guidance, after which he went on to become a radical voice in the literature describing how doctors arrive at and maintain their dominance, with his publication of *Off the Pedestal* (1990). Ultimately he withdrew from the public arena and now maintains a very satisfying medical practice, which, although it appears to be conventional, is based on a completely revamped set of values.

> I was sitting in my office, ready to quit medicine. Everybody was gone for the day. I was sitting there alone because I thought I was having a psychotic break with reality. I was looking in the Yellow Pages for a practice

broker to sell my practice when I heard a voice say, "Close the book; you're not leaving." These voice things are not literally translatable, but the message was, "Of course you hate what you're doing. You've become more of a businessman than a doctor. Not just you, not just the profession, the whole consciousness. You can stay here and listen . . . (I knew I had a choice) or choose to run away." . . . The voice said, "If you do this, you're never going to be rich or famous, but you'll always have enough." My life kind of turned on a dime then.

Julia Hall tells of a classic *kundalini* awakening which left her with psychic powers and vision not easily acknowledged within traditional medical settings.

The day before I was to interview for an OB/GYN residency, I was in such doubt and so confused that I decided to go for a reading and a healing. This encounter finished the opening process which had been going on for several years. Within three weeks I was flooded with dream material and dreaming fifteen hours a day. It was a total shift in my energy. Throughout the process I was confident that this was a spiritual healing and that something that was beyond me but was basically benevolent was in charge. But it was very, very disruptive. I developed what they now call "the *kundalini* syndrome." I didn't have flashing lights, but I did have a lot of uninvited visions. I could see energy between people and energies between *chakras*. I knew what people were going to say a second before they said it. This went on for two or three days. My spiritual eye was totally open. Along with it was a lot of pain in my heart. That period stays with me now and gives me confidence and conviction about this field of energy that most people don't see or validate. I'm hoping at some point to work in a context where people have full knowledge of my being an allopathically trained physician, but also someone who can provide a whole other dimension of care. (*MetaPhysicians' Tales*)

Anesthesiologist Walter Mueller had for many years been intensely skeptical of anyone who talked about "energy flowing." Suffering from hypertension and a heart condition, he was persuaded by a friend to attend a healing group that was just getting started.

I walked in, and that was the beginning of it all. . . . We sat around and held hands. Richard did something called resonating. I began to buzz, vibrating as if I held a buzz saw in my hand—very hard to describe. [When it was my turn to receive a healing, I lay down on the table.] They told me to close my eyes. It was a strange kind of feeling . . . like I was in a microwave oven. All around, every part of my body had electrons vibrating. It went on, the music was playing, and I had tears pouring out of my eyes.

I used to yell at my oldest daughter when she used to talk to me about "energy flowing." I would say, "Talk to me in language that I can

> understand. I don't want to hear this bullshit. What does it mean, energy flowing?!" I'd get real angry. But during that experience I could feel what they were talking about. I could feel this stuff surging into me. It was absolutely incredible. [After it was over] I walked out and went to Tilden Park and sat there for hours. It was like I was in another world. It was something I never believed could happen. All I knew was that when I came home I was terribly tired, but I was going to go on with this. (*Metaphysician's Tales*)

The exhaustion Mueller describes is typical of what anyone actively engaged in rapid and radical new learning will experience, most likely from the energy required to open up the multiple new synaptic connections needed to process new information. That, effectively, is what Mueller was doing while he was sitting in the park—allowing time for new synaptic connections to be made, new neural networks to be established. Those who do not make the cognitive effort to assimilate such experiences will end up dismissing, ignoring, or compartmentalizing them, and no real cognitive transformation will result. Medical school forced this sort of assimilation on most initiates through the rigid structuring of the ritual process. In this much more diffuse and unstructured passage to holism, the decision whether to try to integrate this new information, or to compartmentalize it, is a matter of individual choice.

Influential Book, Individual, or Group. Physicians do not seem to spend much time in leisure reading. Many lament this fact and attribute it to the pressures of practice and the need to keep up with professional developments. Nevertheless, many of the doctors we interviewed were deeply and permanently moved by reading a single book at a critical juncture in their development, most often one that took as its subject philosophy, psychology, meditation, the new physics, or chaos and systems theory. Authors whose names turned up more than once were Fritjof Capra, Bernie Siegel, Dan Millman, Larry Dossey, Hans Selye, Andrew Weil, Brugh Joy, Norm Shealy, and Carolyn Myss.

In "Physician in Transition" (1993), Jordan Goetz writes that what started him on an "alternative" healing path was a book he picked up during his medical school interview, Andrew Stanway's *Alternative Medicine*. He says, "I was intrigued by the content; I knew on an instinctual level that *of course* this works." Ed Neal, an internist who worked in an emergency room while studying other methods of healing, always felt that he had a destiny to practice medicine, rather than a particular desire to do so. He never understood why he was following this destiny until he picked up a book by Carl Jung and "felt a deep connection to what he was saying. He was talking about the soul and that was refreshing after being in medical school. And he was also talking about the self-healing function of the mind, and for me that really clicked. . . . I sensed that a lot of what was going on related to what he was talking about—about the deeper unconscious. And I had a sense that I had been compelled into medicine for reasons that related to this deeper level. I read more and then sort of had a vision that the two would go together very well."

Peter Nunn notes that reading Arthur Janov's *Primal Scream* led him to take a year off to deal with his deep-seated "fund of anger" and to study energy medicine. Larry Dossey, whose name has become synonymous with the spiritual aspects of healing, found that what took him far beyond biofeedback into unimagined realms was "a book by Lawrence LeShan, *The Medium, the Mystic, and the Physicist.* It introduced me to the modern quantum mechanical worldview. It is not an exaggeration to say that this flipped me into an experiential crisis. It became clear to me in an instant that my working assumptions about how the world works were incomplete, if not downright wrong, and that everything medicine stood for—that I had been trained to honor—was based on an outmoded view."

Sometimes the transformation sparked by a book can be fulfilled through pursuing contact with its author. Surgeon Jack Mansberger found his catalyst in Dan Millman, author of *The Way of the Peaceful Warrior*, during two intensive retreats that Millman led. Jim Gordon also found that the personal influence of a teacher who arrives at the right time can completely alter one's outlook. After his recovery from the acute back pain we described above, his experiences with Dr. Singha continued to enrich and inform his transformational journey. In the *MetaPhysicians' Tales*, family practitioner Marilyn Levinson reports the important effect of a few words spoken at a propitious time: "I was sick continuously for about two years with pneumonia and bronchitis. I couldn't stand it because I couldn't sing. The voice teacher with whom I studied was a very powerful spiritual man who participated in rituals with Native Americans. One day when I was frustrated because I wanted to be active, to do everything all the time, he told me I *did* have 'all the time.' It doesn't have to happen right now. Somehow that made an enormous impression on me. It stretched my whole vision of time, of capabilities, possibilities."

When the student is ready, the teacher appears. Sometimes, as with Jim Gordon and Marilyn Levinson, the teacher is from an entirely different cultural system. And some, like Leonard Jones, find their mentors among the pioneers of holistic medicine who have gone before:

> My actual transition began at a "Physician of the Future" conference in June 1975 in San Diego. I was inspired by a talk given by Evarts Loomis, M.D., who many consider to be the founder and original practitioner of holistic medicine in this country. Interestingly, he often refers to earlier pioneers in other countries, especially the renowned missionary physician

> Albert Schweitzer, whom he visited in Africa. Dr. Loomis had just published his book, *Healing for Everyone—Medicine of the Whole Person*. I was also tremendously impressed by Norman Shealy, M.D., Ph.D., who abandoned his neurosurgical knife and faculty position to pursue holism, broader dimensions, and better ways to control pain. ("Physician in Transition" 1991)

The individual who set psychiatrist Karl Humiston on the path to holism was family therapist Virginia Satir; he watched her "like a great flash of light" ("Physician in Transition" 1990). But individuals who profoundly influence the paradigm shifts of holistic physicians do not have to be spiritual teachers, famous physicists, or holistic pioneers. It was Humiston's mother, a psychiatric social worker, who persuaded him to take two days off to attend Satir's workshop. Other interviewees found their catalysts in a spouse, a relative, an associate, or a friend. For example, obstetrician Peter Vargas told us that a nurse he employs was extremely influential in his decision to explore the holistic approach. An internist explained that his wife "partly invited me, and partly insisted" that he attend a self-esteem workshop in 1968, which helped to start him on his journey. During her first year of medical school, Amy Saltzmann's sister handed her a copy of *Holistic Medicine*, the AHMA journal, which led her to attend her first AHMA meeting and so begin her transition to holistic medicine.

The American Holistic Medical Association (AHMA).[2] Attendance at their first AHMA meeting in fact became the primary catalyst for the paradigm shift for some of our interviewees—their doorway both to the soul and to the social. Kathy Frye "found the AHMA by reading Bernie Siegel's book *Love, Medicine, and Miracles*. On the back cover it listed him as co-president of the AHMA, and I wanted to know what that was, so I called his office and they gave me the number. I called them up and said, 'When's your meeting?' and I went and I've been coming ever since. I just love it. It's like coming home."

Founded in 1978 by Norman Shealy, Gladys McGarey, and others, the AHMA has provided a forum for interested physicians to learn about or share their experiences with holistic healing. Members come together at the annual conference, held in a different city every year, which features speakers from the famous to the unknown lecturing on a wide range of topics relevant to the theory and practice of holistic medicine. The exhibit hall is filled with vendors offering nutritional supplements, healing technologies, New Age arts and crafts, dozens of books on various aspects of alternative medicine, and authors holding book signings and chatting informally with all interested comers. The conference programs are peppered with entertainment, both scheduled and spontaneous, which can best be described as hilarious. Most noteworthy at the conferences attended by Davis-Floyd were the operatic duet sung by a female physician and a male nurse about how much they needed each other; the karma clippers (for cutting off chunks of karma that one does not want to carry around) and Buddha beeper (designed to call one's higher self from the far reaches of the galaxy) offered at discount rates by Guru Haagen-Daz (aka singer Michael Stillwater) who also—and for free—answered all the meaningful questions of life; and the clown with the big red nose (Bowen White, M.D.) who, in the midst of cracking some very funny jokes, managed to toss in a useful lesson about stool diagnosis: you know you've been eating plenty of fiber if it floats.

For many doctors, attending the AHMA meeting offers both the chance to have a lot of fun and a safe way (because no one back home need know) to meet colleagues who are a few steps further down the path and have lived to tell about it. Bill Manahan found his first meeting a catalyst for change: "My wife and I went to the first or second American Holistic Medical Association meeting. The exercise and nutrition stuff made sense to me, so I accepted the psychics and others who I would no more have listened to than jump out a window before. I thought, 'My God, these people are physicians and they're talking about this really fascinating stuff!' That's how I did it [made the shift], through this organization."

Bethany Hays, now in the AHMA leadership, describes how threatening it was for her to join:

> Here I am a conventional OB/GYN doctor in Houston and I'm going to join this organization for crackpots and weirdos that are doing Chinese herbal medicine and acupuncture and run around in costumes and do weird stuff—and they're kind of way out in left field. Then you come to the first meeting and you sit in the café to have breakfast. And the first things you notice are: (a) nobody has coffee; (b) everybody is eating mostly vegetables, no eggs or bacon, and (c) everybody pulls out a little baggie with twenty vitamins in it. It was just a scream! And now, what's entertaining to me is that there are advertisements for antioxidant vitamins everywhere. Now, if I recommend that people take four different vitamins, they go right ahead and do it; it's no big deal. What I thought, five years ago, was pretty strange behavior, is now mainstream.

Through this vignette Hays points to the rapid permeation into mainstream culture of many of the principles and techniques of holistic healing. Her experience typifies that of many holistic physicians who leave their first AHMA meeting feeling a strong sense of culture shock, only to find when they get home that more people than they realized are doing the same things in their own communities.

Amy Saltzmann's first AHMA conference during her second year of medical school catalyzed a profound shift in her values. There she learned not only about the existence of a community of like-minded practitioners, but also about the full spectrum of possibility they represented:

> It was like coming home, or waking up! . . . I don't think I had ever articulated how I wanted to practice medicine and here were these people who were articulating what I didn't even know yet. But as soon as they said it, I just went, "Yes! That makes sense and that's what I want to do."
>
> And one of the best things that happened was that I went to a preconference workshop. And there was a woman there named Deborah Glasser who until recently ran a very conventional allopathic practice with a very holistic philosophy. And then there was Patch Adams, who runs a commune health center, and he's in the process of building it and he envisions it as a place where people come to be healed and contribute whatever they can to the community. If they're healthy enough to work on a building, they do that. If they can wash dishes, they do that. And he doesn't really—I don't think—practice anything resembling the medicine I've been taught to date. And so I had these people, you know, who were just defining the spectrum. And I realized that I can fit anywhere on that spectrum that I want to be. Patch is way farther out on thin ice than I'm ever going to go. And it's kind of nice, because I know that the ice is still holding him up, and it's OK. And Deborah, at least until recently, is probably more conventional than I'm willing to be. And I saw that I can fit anywhere in here that I feel comfortable. And that just reallly gave me some freedom, and some perspective, about what's possible.
>
> And then, there's a lot of love at these meetings. These people are actively loving and learning and to the best of my knowledge that's what we all came here to do. And to be in a group that's doing it in an active, conscious way is a real pleasure, because so many people in the medical profession walk around kind of shut down. You almost get the sense that they are automatons. They went through this training process and they lost their capacity to love and feel. But here at these meetings you find people who went through the same training, but are healing themselves and learning to help other people heal.

Although the growth of interest in holistic medicine means that at least one holistic physician can be found in almost any community of reasonable size, often there is only that one. Those physicians in our study who made the paradigm shift on their own, before contact with any professional group like the AHMA, frequently experienced a sense of extreme isolation. Learning about alternatives from books, introducing new therapies to their patients with no one to talk to who could help them assess relative value and efficacy, such physicians longed for social support from their professional colleagues. Already embarked on their transformative journey and prepared to "go it alone," as one of them put it, they experienced their first contact with organizations like the AHMA or the Institute for Noetic Sciences not as a catalyst for change but as an unexpected and welcome validation of their work. Such organizations enable them, for a period of time each year, to let go of their professional isolation and enjoy the rich rewards of a community of like-minded folks. Some we interviewed were favorably disposed to the AHMA but not actively involved; a few felt that they had moved beyond it or that it was not useful to them for a variety of reasons; and some found that it became central to their quest. Jim Gordon, for example, found kindred spirits: "It introduced me to some other people who felt and believed the way I do. I had an opportunity to meet with them and learn from them and have a sense that there are people who are on similar wavelengths. I find that reassuring and helpful." Paulanne Balch discovered a strong women's presence: "I felt at home although I had just come out of corporate America. I remember there was a gender panel. I realized it was new for this organization to have strong women who had a voice in it. Women were standing up and speaking for themselves and it's a trend that hasn't reversed."

The AHMA's holistic philosophy is inclusive, as it must by definition be, and there are many in the organization who would like to include in its voting membership any licensed holistic practitioners—naturopaths, chiropractors, homeopaths, and so on—who want to join. In 1994 the AHMA board came close to voting to open up the membership, in an effort to live up to their own philosophy, to more fully "walk their talk." In the end they decided to wait. Most of the physicians who come to AHMA find that it is the *only* place where they can talk with other physicians of like mind and spirit. So deep is their need for this kind of support that they are for the time being unwilling to give it up. They decided for the present to maintain their organization as an instrument of support and education for physicians; they also decided to revisit the issue some years hence. By that time, they hope, there will be so many holistic physicians across the country that they will be able to find the support and community they need in the places where they live, and the AHMA will be free to take its next evolutionary step.

Direct Exposure to Other Ways of Healing. Like attendance at the AHMA, simple exposure to other ways of practicing medicine, in the United States and elsewhere, can provide the impetus to change. For example, several of the obstetricians in our study were strongly influenced to move toward holistic approaches to pregnancy and childbirth by exposure to midwives, both nurse-midwives in the hospital and direct-entry midwives who attend women at home. Said one, "Watching a midwife catch a baby was an entirely different experience than what I was used to. Accustomed to intervene, to do *something*, instead I had to sit on my hands and watch in amazement while the midwife nurtured the mother and empowered *her* to push her baby out. That experience made me realize how often I took control away from the mother, and it changed my life." (The power of such exposure is evidenced by a Georgia obstetrician who refuses to even watch a video of midwife-attended home birth because, as he puts it, "I am afraid it will make me want to change the way I practice.")

Doctors who are unlikely to expose themselves to other forms of healing in the United States may be more willing to risk such exposure when they are out of their native environment, as did William Goldwag: "After seventeen years of highly orthodox family practice, serving on the hospital medical board, and acquiring a modest house, a wife, four children, two cars, a cat and a dog, a canoe, a motor boat, and espousing the AMA code of thinking, my brother asked me to look into some strange medical practices performed in Europe . . . and that started the chain of transition. I visited European centers, spoke to various doctors and found there was a whole different world out there" ("Physician in Transition" 1991).

Often strange and exotic places can facilitate openness to new learning. Richard Ivker made five trips to Fiji, where he encountered "the most spiritual, loving, and balanced people I had ever met. They seemed to have a personal relationship with God." On Fiji, supported by a populace who believed that the healer is a channel for God's energy, he practiced the power of healing touch, with remarkable results that sped him on his path. David Filmore, Barry Sultanoff, and others traveled to India, seeking both healing and the enrichment of their spiritual lives.

Maureen Longworth traveled to a rural health collective in the Philippines. Sitting on a rock with a group of women while one of the woman sang, she "went into a consciousness of the most wonderful, peaceful unity with the earth and all of life. I had never experienced anything so incredible before. As she continued to sing for everyone, I was literally in tears because I was so overcome with happiness." Longworth was trained in the Philippines to do hands-on healing, with good results. But her experiences there threw her into an existential crisis when she returned to residency; at the time when she told her story to the MetaPhysicians, she was still in residency and was just beginning to explore other options. This crisis had not been resolved, but it had started her out on the journey.

The Dawning of Social or Feminist Consciousness opened the doorway to the soul for some holistic physicians. For example, an obstetrician in Texas practiced traditionally until the army put him to work in a veteran's hospital during the Vietnam War. During months of patching up senselessly mutilated bodies, he came to question not only America's engagement in that war but also the entire sociopolitical system that led to that engagement. The cognitive distance he developed from his own culture soon led him to question its medical system as well. He stopped taking conventional treatments for granted, and embarked on a long journey of learning and discovery that eventually led him to open a birthing center staffed with midwives, and to offer the women of his city true alternatives in childbirth (Davis-Floyd 1987).

Likewise, Bill Manahan found a stint in the Peace Corps, which exposed him to other cultures, other value systems, and other ways of life to be instrumental in his opening process:

> I changed significantly after three years in the Peace Corps. I dropped out of the Catholic Church. I started to protest Vietnam. I started questioning all the values I grew up with of believing in authority. . . . Suddenly we're in a different culture and we're seeing good people who just do things differently, and so I had to question my own beliefs. [For example], the Catholic Church was saying you can't do birth control and I was over in these other countries where population was such a problem and the solution was so simple . . . and I can remember saying, "This is crazy. The Church is wrong." Then I started to realize, if the Church is wrong on that, then it must be wrong on other things. And I started questioning other things. . . . And then during residency I started to always question, and you know, that caused problems for our director because I started asking "Why?" and not always in the gentlest manner.

The dawning of feminist consciousness was a powerful catalyst for some of our interviewees, including Bethany Hays and Christiane Northrup. Women who at first buy into the Western medical system, and later learn about feminism, experience a massive values shift of their own the first time they are able to perceive and identify the patriarchal values and beliefs that permeate their training. Shocked by the overt sexism in her medical school, Maureen Longworth produced a humorous film on that topic in an attempt to help herself deal with "how badly women are treated in the whole entire health care system." From there she followed her intuition to study healing in Mexico and the Philippines in order, as one of her teachers predicted, to be able to have an impact on a system that "lacks femininity" and "was designed by men without the healing qualities women bring."

Hallucinogenic Drugs. One of our interviewees and several of the MetaPhysicians acknowledged hallucinogenic drugs as a catalytic factor in their transformation. Particularly during the late 1960s and early 1970s, when many now middle-aged doctors were in medical school, drugs were part of the larger culture and were acceptable in research circles. Many physicians who were drafted were exposed to recreational drugs in Vietnam. As Terry Tyler notes, there is debate as to whether drugs offer a valuable opportunity to explore the spiritual dimension and whether, once the dimension is entered through this doorway, it can become integrated into the rest of their lives:

> The difference between psychoactive substances being healing or harmful has much to do with the intent. The attitude that seems most useful spiritually is to see the drug as a teacher showing a possibility. Once you have seen this possibility, the hard work begins: to integrate what you have seen into your everyday life, and to find nondrug pathways to this consciousness. This may take about twelve to eighteen months. If the drug becomes the only way to access these states of consciousness, you are in danger. There are no easy ways to enlightenment. When a drug has taught you what it has to teach you, it's time to quit. As Alan Watts said, "When you get the message, hang up the phone." (*Metaphysician's Tales*)

As Tyler indicates, holistic physicians are often open to new experiences and new types of learning; they temper this openness with a strong awareness of the dangers of addiction. Tyler, a psychiatrist by training, describes how a controversial drug brought him to the experience of a state of unity and, through that, back from the cliff of despair.

> I had lost my practice, my marriage, and my kids in the divorce, and was living on a small island in British Columbia. I asked a friend of mine to do some healing work with me, and he guided me in a session with MDMA [a hallucinogen]. Three days after the session, I was processing what happened when I felt my body dissolve. It was as if I had been living with an insulation layer around me several inches thick. On this day it was as if the insulation shrank to the thickness of the finest gossamer silk. There was virtually nothing at all between me and the rest of the universe. I experienced my body as light, vibration, and energy. I went out to the farthest stretches of the universe. I was joy. I knew that that is what people meant when they talked about the spiritual experiences of death and rebirth. I thought, "If this is what death is about, what a way to go!" I suddenly understood what the words "God is Love" meant. They are simply two words for the same experience, the experience of Oneness, of Self as pure energy. (*Metaphysician's Tales*)

Another specialist, pathologist Arnold Rosenberg, joined his students in a single drug experience and found a dimension of living that required a reorientation of his whole life.

> [After a single LSD experience] into my consciousness came something like neon signs flashing words that up to that point had only been abstractions. Things like "love" (which I knew didn't exist), and "happiness" (no such thing), and "truth" and "God." In that instant I realized they were all different words for the same thing. I knew that there was God and truth

> and love and happiness and freedom—beyond a shadow of a doubt. I didn't have to defend or justify it. I knew those things existed and I knew that I knew. When I went back to the laboratory, I knew it wouldn't work. Everything in my life up to that point had been a bad trip. What I was doing in the laboratory wasn't in accord with the truth. The white coat I was wearing wasn't part of the truth; it was a lie. Everything in my life had been built on a lie, and now I knew that. (*MetaPhysicians' Tales*)

Synchronous Events. Bernie Siegel calls synchronous events, our final category of doorways to the soul, "God's way of being anonymous." A divine hand does often seem to guide physicians who declare themselves open to new experiences. Often the personal and professional merge to produce exposure on so many levels—through individuals, training events, chance meetings, hirings, and firings—that it seems as though the individual is no longer in control. In "Physician in Transition," Peter Albright (1989) describes the synchronous events that led him to holism as "a string of beads." He describes events as apparently unrelated as developing a duodenal ulcer and attending meetings of the dowsing society, where he

> learned things about people and energy that hadn't even been hinted at in all my medical training. Then the beads began to jump on my necklace even faster. I read many articles and began to attend conferences where I met all sorts of people who helped me make connections in the realm of unseen phenomena. I began to appreciate the energy of thought, emotion, and interpersonal dynamics, the energy of physiologic processes, the energy of spirit. The clinical ramifications clicked together: biofeedback, acupuncture and oriental medicine, meditation, nutrition, body therapies, yoga, spiritual attunement, the environment, and on and on.

All the physicians in our study group who embarked on this transformative journey found many elements, many clues, many helpers along the way. The traveler must be open and aware enough to notice the clues, and to receive the help from those who offer it. Understanding and acceptance of synchronicity are often the key to the passageway; those who expect pathways clearly marked with signs, or wait to be handed a road map, will be disappointed. As physician Carlos Warter points out in *The Recovery of the Sacred*, "When these events occur, we embark in search of our individual truth. Therefore, a spiritual adventure . . . does not have formal guidelines. It is the undercurrent of the mystery of life that guides us and gives us the correct timing for our actions. Thus we need to learn patience, an important element in the larger context or 'big story' of our existence" (1994:xviii).

STARTING OUT ON THE OTHER SIDE

In chapter 2, we described several physicians who entered medical school with a mindset different from their classmates. Barry Elson, for example, found that the worldview he internalized through yoga and vegetarianism before he started medical school worked to ensure that he did not buy into its values and underlying philosophy. Like Elson, Charles LeBaron also entered medical school already "on the other side." Twelve years of social work had left him scarred with memories of the abuse and neglect many of his patients had suffered at the hands of an underfunded and indifferent public hospital system. Many were the times he had run after busy physicians, trying to focus their attention on his clients' needs, only to be told, "Got to run—I'm late for grand rounds." Three months into his first year at Harvard, suffused with the pain of these memories, and aware that he had not had time to so much as leave the confines of the Harvard Medical School campus, he stared longingly at the huge Citgo sign some miles away, and asked himself,

> "For the past three months, have I been anything other than late for grand rounds?" Quick, snappy, one-phrase answers were the best I could provide to anyone. Give me two years of endless short-answer tests, then put me on round-the-clock shifts, and how many [real human needs will I ignore]? I stood up, scattering pulmonary function equations and dog lab notes and leucine degradations to the floor. My cheeks were wet with tears. "You motherfuckers!" I said . . . "I'm making it to the Citgo sign." I kicked aside the book I'd thrown at the door, slammed noisily out of the dorm room, and banged down the stairs out into the deepening November twilight. Off I went, without a coat, running past Star Market, dark warehouses, billboards, cars, garbage, a MacDonald's. I got lost in some jumbled streets, but kept pushing forward, ever forward, across an immense, roaring expressway, down a short hill—and I was there! . . . My blood was boiling with delirious joy. I dashed across the square and put my hands against the cold stone of the building that supported the Citgo sign. . . . "I made it, assholes. Find yourself another personality to reconstruct with your dog labs and nice psychiatrists and carnitine acyl transferase. Maybe you won't notice it . . . but you got one victim less."

Even though LeBaron had started out on the other side, he nevertheless found himself in imminent danger of internalizing the values, beliefs, and patterns of behavior behind his technocratic training. Through the defining moment in which he made it all the way to the Citgo sign (its physical distance from the Harvard campus symbolized the cognitive distance he was seeking to regain) as well as through the more lengthy process of writing his book, LeBaron enabled himself to resist his technomedical socialization and hold onto his own set of values and beliefs.

Confronted with the same dangers, interviewee Peter Grote found himself watching his colleagues and noticing that those with the best attitudes and greater wealth of knowledge had achieved broad life experience before beginning medical training. Fearful that his "focus was getting too narrow," Grote took the radical and effective step of leaving medical school for a year and going to Africa to expose himself to other cultures and the benefits of the public health approach before he completed his medical training.

Amy Saltzmann took a different approach to maintaining conceptual distance. After attending her first AHMA meeting during medical school, she began applying holistic principles to herself on a daily basis. She got up an hour earlier than her classmates every day to run, managed to eat a reasonably healthy diet, and started a daily meditation group in which others, including her mentors and teachers, eventually began to participate. This twenty-minute meditation practice not only helped her to stay centered and maintain her holistic values, but also ensured her better treatment by those above her in the medical hierarchy who meditated with her and thus found it difficult to speak to her curtly on the hospital floor. And in these ways, she became a catalyst for their transformation.

The level of self-awareness exhibited by Elson, LeBaron, Grote, and Saltzmann during medical school—all four of whom, in a sense, "started out on the other side"—is atypical of most physicians, who simply identify with and internalize the technomedical model until one of the catalysts we have described above begins to work its distancing magic.

In the following chapter, we will share with our readers the deep intimacy of the interview process by allowing some of our interviewees to tell in their own words the full story of their transformative journeys. For the sake of analytical clarity, we have described the catalysts that sparked their journeys as separate and distinct. But that is not how they are experienced in the flux and flow of daily life. All of them may play a role, simultaneously or at different moments, in order or out, in the transformational journey from doctor to healer. As Peter Albright put it:

> It's hard to say when "it" started to happen—the transition, I mean. It's not like one day I woke up and suddenly something was happening. But certain experiences that I had come to my mind. At the time they happened, they didn't seem like steps in a process, but rather like meanderings in the desert, stumblings in the dark, or even steps backwards. They seemed like anything but great flashes of inspiration, or thunderbolts of revelation, which was what I often hoped would be given to me! But as I look back, I can pick out a few events and situations and string them together like a necklace. They have a natural relation to each other and make up a kind of whole. ("Physician in Transition" 1989)

As we mentioned above, some, but certainly not all, of the physicians we interviewed suffered during this occasionally synchronous and often confusing and bewildering process of change, which as we have seen in many cases was motivated by a major life crisis. Terry Tyler notes that "Crisis has the power to push a person through a developmental stage, allowing them to emerge in a more integrated state." One aspect of crisis is "disintegration," in which major belief systems are challenged and ultimately fall away. As in many rites of passage, you must die to your former self in order to be born. As Larry Dossey put it, "This is agony—to really put your worldview on the line and say to yourself, 'I've been to one of the best medical schools in the world . . . and in spite of that, there is something deeply flawed about my education.'"

Terry Tyler explains one source of this agony: "In the resulting void, there is chaos, uncertainty about what is real or true, or even one's own identity. In the void your thoughts may be different than usual, as if you are measuring things by a new standard. It is as if you are shining a powerful light on your life and seeing things in a new way . . . deciding what to keep and what to let go of." The void and its accompanying disorientation are reminiscent of the liminality of the medical school rite of passage. Although both technomedical training and this transformative journey toward holism can be classified as rites of passage, there are important differences between these processes. Unlike medical training, the process we are describing here is not defined by any sort of externally imposed structure; it unfolds free-form, in highly personal and individualized ways. In contrast to medical training, which often shuts down self-awareness, this transitional process is experienced with a high degree of reflexivity, a growing awareness both of self and of the experience of change. "There comes a time when the vision of where you want to be requires you to let go of something. . . .The void teaches you about your attachments. It is a time of examining your relationships, feelings, attitudes, and values, replacing those that no longer serve you with those that do" (Roman 1989:130). Michael Greenwood and Peter Nunn name this emptiness "the point of phase transition"; to reach it, "we must be willing to let go of our concept of reality and wait without particular expectations for a new and different experience. We must trust that this new awareness will emerge, because we will never be able to glimpse a new perspective without first letting go of the old one. Phase transition, then, is a place of seeming nothingness, and, paradoxically, the place of new possibilities" (1992:41).

When the crisis resolves, there is a new and more highly developed way of understanding which is greater than, and yet may include, the old. This new consciousness accounts for the high level of satisfaction among physicians who have made the shift and explains why turning back is out of the question. The new stage has more options and possibilities. Physicians who successfully pass through such a transformational crisis expand their range of responses in order to nurture the nascent impulse to heal. Let us listen now to their stories.

6 *The Transformative Journey*

> I was in my late thirties, I had reached all my lifetime goals, and yet I found to my dismay that I was dissatisfied. "Is this all there is?" I began asking myself. The answers came from many directions. I found myself thinking more about Hippocrates' words, "Physician, heal thyself." The words "heal," "health," and "holy" all mean "to make whole." I knew that if awareness of God were essential to health, then I had a long way to go toward experiencing that sense of wholeness.
>
> —ROBERT IVKER, D.O.

Near the end of his medical training, in 1940, Evarts Loomis found himself serving in an "itty bitty hospital on the northern coast of Newfoundland," and interspersing that service with two-thousand-mile trips inland by dog sled to bring health care to isolated Canadians. During that time, "the words kept bombarding my mind: 'Treat the whole person. Treat the whole person.' So I began to visualize with each patient I saw the physical, mental, emotional, and spritual person that they were." Loomis came to this inspiration through the combined influences of the spiritual studies of both Eastern and Western traditions that he had shared with his mother, a Quaker mystic who was his teacher in college, through the poetry of Walt Whitman, and a pamphlet by Albert Schweitzer he chanced to read one day. Finding no one in the United States to talk with about his ideas, in the late 1950s he and his wife undertook a journey around the world in search of teachers who could show him the way. In Switzerland, Germany, Jordan, Israel, and Tibet, he found and talked with innovative physicians, scholars, and healers of like mind. He went on to open the first holistic healing center in the United States, Meadowlark, in California, which he directed for thirty-two years, and to become one of the holistic medicine's great pioneers.

In this transformative journey from doctor to healer, each physician traverses a landscape that is unique, yet shares qualities and feeling tones with other landscapes crossed by other travelers. In the five representative stories that follow, the frustrations with conventional medicine, the experience of learning from patients, the books, the attendance at AHMA meetings, the appearance of a teacher—all the themes and catalysts uncovered in our interviews and research—appear in the interwoven form they take in real life. As the first story, David Dowling's, indicates, these catalysts work seamlessly and synergistically to speed the nascent holistic physician on his way.

Journeys of Transformation: Five Stories

TRANSCENDING THE LIMITATIONS OF TECHNOMEDICINE: DAVID DOWLING

I started out in medical school [at Harvard] like everybody else, wanting to be the best internist, the best cardiologist, the best general surgeon. And then I started to realize that none of this was doing anything. There's no medication that cures, there's no surgery that cures the patient. I became very disenchanted with medicine as a whole. And then I delivered my first baby, and I realized that this was a way that I could effect change. And at the time I thought it was a cure, you know—delivering a baby was a "cure" for a "condition." In going on from there, I realized that it wasn't a cure for a condition, but it *was* a way for me to effect positive change in a relationship, in a couple, in a person. I can help them achieve a healthy and successful pregnancy. And for me this was the most important time in a family's life—it was a privilege to be a part of that. . . .

Once I got into practice, I became confronted with a lot of women who were having problems with PMS. . . . They had gone from doctor to doctor and were being told it's all in their minds, that they were crazy, there's nothing wrong with them. And they had various kinds of symptoms related to what we now call PMS. I had done some reading and I was looking at ways for self-growth for myself. And so I started manipulating diet and manipulating vitamins and I became known as the vitamin pusher. From there I kind of on my own did some reading, looked at different journals, listened to different people, and I started using more nutritional and vitamin therapy.

And then through my own self-growth, you know—getting involved in meditation and exercise and just other ways of dealing with my own emotional difficulties, I started helping patients—I saw a mirror of myself in them. I figured it could help me, could be something that fostered my own growth, maybe I can tell the patient and help them grow on their own.

So from there I just started incorporating all the things I was using in my own life—meditation, visualization, imagery. I became acquainted with Carl Simonton and his visualization experiments in cancer, and with some of the work with preanesthetic suggestion that they were doing in California—giving patients preanesthetic suggestions to decrease blood flow as they come out of surgery. I started to tell patients to visualize certain things so the surgery would go better—to visualize golden light, turn off blood vessels. The residents and the nurses would be snickering behind me. I didn't care—I was getting good results.

And I just became more spiritually involved with my patients. The more I was giving of myself and getting back from them and getting into the spiritual realm, the more I loved what I was doing.

Q: Why did you start making these changes?

A: Because I came from a very dysfunctional family, to use the current term. I was very depressed and unhappy through most of my adolescent and early adult years. . . . And I was going through a very difficult time. My relationship with my wife was not working and I was very unhappy. And I knew people who were having harder times than me and who managed to be happy—even some bums in Manhattan have a contentment about them. And I saw people who were much more materialistically successful who were profoundly *un*happy. And I decided that I have the innate capability to be happy and content with my life, despite all the things that were going on around me. And I decided that I was going to get on that path, that I wasn't going to sit in the morass of my life but was going to create happiness around me. I knew that I had the power to do that.

Q: And you decided that on your own? Or did you read something?

A: I read a lot and I'm still reading. Carl Simonton's book was probably one of the first that intimated to me that I had the power, that people had the power. And I read [Barry N.] Kaufman's book on happiness and choice, and John Kabat-Zinn's book *Mindfulness Meditation*. These are books that I give out to my patients. And I eventually learned to meditate on my own. . . . I started out just staring at nothing and letting my mind go blank. But it was John Kabat-Zinn's book that really projected me into the structured meditation technique that I'm still doing on my own. I know that it has helped because I can release stress and negative energy very much easier than I had ever been able to in the past.

Q: So how did that spill over into your practice?

A: I just started using all the techniques that I was using for myself in my practice. Meditation techniques, nutritional techniques—I would just see which patients seemed to fit into those categories and start using them. . . .

You asked how I got into the AHMA—it was an interesting sequence of events. A patient was referred to me by the chief of pediatrics at my hospital. I was amazed because I really didn't think I was that visible. We developed a great rapport, and she introduced me to an internist who now only does acupuncture. She just felt the two of us would click immediately, and we did. And this internist was a member of the AHMA. He said, "You know, you've got to join this organization," and I said, "Fine." I was a loner. I was totally alone until then. I was doing this stuff all by myself, without any encouragement from anybody. And I joined, and from the moment I got the first bit of information—I think he even gave me one of the journals he had—after the point of even just opening the journal, I was more confirmed on my path. I suddenly felt like I was connected to something. I went to my first conference last year, and it was mind-expanding for me. . . . I really feel at home here.

Q: What was so mind-expanding about that first conference?

A: That there were so many people who felt similarly to me. It was easy for them to express it. It was just *easy* to express love, and spirituality, and connectedness, and people didn't look at you like you had six heads when you said those words. . . . And I could take things away from there and help people to help themselves. Since the convention last year, I've just mushroomed. I was going on a slow upward incline in terms of what I was doing in my practice, but since last year, it's been a mushroom, a flower opening. I'm going to blossom even more when I get home after this conference, and I can't wait till next year!

Q: Can you describe the mushrooming? What specific things did you do differently after that first conference?

A: Well, I started doing a lot more nutritional and metabolic things, like Alan Gaby does. The metabolic aspects, treating people for hypothyroidism and becoming more aware and more involved nutritionally, in terms of vitamins. It also legitimated, validated what I was already doing. Because up until then I was reading it in a book, or just trying things. But here at AHMA, there were other people I respected who were doing it and getting good results. I was able to go back and be much more comfortable in what I was doing. The patients even got a better feel for it and maybe got better results. But the other thing was my ability to relate to people. . . . I had always been shy and withdrawn and had difficulty talking with people. After spending a week at AHMA relating and connecting, it was easier to open up, to hug, to listen. . . . Techniques—no, not techniques, but just ways I hadn't thought of that enabled me to deal in a more spiritual way with my patients, with people that I'd come into contact with. I don't even like calling them patients. Because I'm a patient too. I feel that in relationship with these people, I'm a patient. Most of the time, unless I'm really tired or tensed out, stressed out, to me it's a mutual relationship.

And that was the major thing I came away from my first AHMA conference in Virginia with—the ability to much more spiritually interact with the people I was dealing with—people who came to see me professionally, friends, loved ones, even my children. . . . They've both started telling me that they're so lucky to have me as a father!

Q: How would you define holistic?

A: It's looking at the whole person. It's how you do what you do, not what you do. You can be a cardiac surgeon, and the last thing you might see yourself as is holistic. But if you see the person in front of you in the context of their life, in three-dimensionality, and if you practice your craft considering who they are to the best of your ability, then to me you're a holistic doc.

Q: As an internist, what do you do in your medical practice that makes it holistic?

A: I try to see who the person is in front of me—just being with them and observing them and feeling them, if you will—what emotions I receive as I'm holding a space for them, asking medical questions. So there are a lot of channels going on at one time for me. I try to both see who the person is, what their expectations are, what their medical problem is, *and*

> to do a thorough medical evaluation. And then try to combine that into a therapy that will lead the person upstream, as it were, toward a sense of a more causal relationship of where this problem is emanating from. And give them a way to address that problem in a language and a series of therapies that they can accept. And that can be using modalities that I use or refer to. I refer, because I think that the paradigm is that you want to include other people—naturopaths, body workers, acupuncturists, Rolfers, chiropractors, osteopaths, physical therapists, et cetera.
>
> Q: You don't do any of those yourself?
>
> A: No. Where I live there are so many of these people who do all of that very well, you don't need to be a one-man band. In fact, I think that you are much more effective if you have communication with people who do that kind of practice.

David Dowling's story demonstrates the synergistic interrelationships of the catalysts we described in chapter 5. Becoming "disenchanted" with conventional medicine, confronting personal illness—which in this case took the form of emotional problems—learning from his patients, reading books, discovering the AHMA: all of these are interwoven in his transition experience. Each catalyst plays its role in his transformational journey.

David's story is classic, in a sense—the structure of his experience parallels that of a number of other physicians in our study group. His story describes particularly well one of the themes involved in the transformational process—the development of emotional resonance. It is as if the person who went to sleep in order to let the somnambulant medical student survive comes to life at a later time and becomes acutely aware of his limitations, if not his pain. The dawn of relational ability, the courage to explore unified systems thinking, the ability to learn from the "bread crumbs" of synchronous events begins with an appreciation of self. The same exquisite discomfort which threatens to end the medical career ultimately becomes the pearl of compassion for the doctor who learns that surrender does not mean giving in.

Another classic feature of David's story is the fact that his first ventures into alternative practice were in the realm of nutrition. This is a quite common first step, as it presents less of a threat to the technomedical belief system than taking a sudden interest, say, in homeopathy. And it is a very compelling first step, as any significant improvements in patients' diets, such as taking them off of sugar and caffeine, often result in rapid and dramatic improvements in their health, thereby encouraging the practitioner to want to know more. David exemplifies many of the characteristics of holism, including a focus on healing the whole person in whole-life context, on spirituality, and on the mutuality of the practitioner-patient relationship; an emphasis on long-term life-style changes, an embrace of multiple modalities through a referral network, and awareness that the essence of holistic practice lies in applying of all of the above to himself and his own healing process—a theme that Jack Mansberger's story takes up.

"UNREASONABLE JOY": JACK MANSBERGER'S STORY

After completing his five-year surgical residency at the University of Georgia, Jack Mansberger taught there and at the University of Maryland. He described those years as "more of the same—you taught what you had learned."

> Q: When did it start to be different?
>
> A: Three or four years after I entered private practice, I stopped and looked at myself, and what I saw was this tremendous box around my emotions. And I realized that I wasn't feeling anything anymore. I couldn't even enjoy my wife and children, much less anything else. And that's when I said, "I'm not going to do this. I want to enjoy my life. I want to be able to feel everything. Something has got to change here." . . .
>
> It had started all the way back in residency. I was kind of saying "Stop and look." I was kind of stopping for a brief second, and taking a glance. I kept saying, "What the hell are you doing here? What the hell are you doing here? What the hell are you doing here?" But you're so busy doing it, you don't stop. And I was trying to stop myself, trying to stop myself, trying to stop myself, and it wasn't working. You know, "You better stop now. You better stop now. You better stop now!" Until four years ago, I'd been doing that for six or seven years. Until finally you reach a point where one day you listen and you say, "Yeah. You'd better stop."
>
> Q: What happened?
>
> A: Well actually I had read some books that touched me. The first was a book by Dan Millman, *Way of the Peaceful Warrior*. And then a series of books of his, the third one called *The Sacred Journey of the Peaceful Warrior*, which has to do with finding your own heart. And basically that's what I wanted—to find my heart. And one day it dawned on me, sitting in my office, that what I needed to do was to go out and see him. I had read his first book five years before. So I had spent five years telling myself that I needed to do that, and never doing it. So finally I said, "Well, I'm gonna do it." And so I did it. And I went out and spent time with him, and things changed and were a whole lot better. And—
>
> Q: Wait a minute. You went out and spent time with him. What does that mean?
>
> A: I spent four days with him. It was a martial arts retreat in California. I had no experience with martial arts. He gives a martial arts course, a four-day intensive, in which he teaches the art of knife fighting. Nothing's quite as scary as the idea of getting slashed with a knife, so the whole experience carries an intense emotion. . . . You know, people talk about "the

zone," kind of like a Zen experience or something like that. His whole purpose is that the only way you can pass that course is if you go into that zone, 'cause there's no way you could learn to protect yourself from three people attacking you with knives in a four-day course. You work on it from seven in the morning to eleven at night, so it's real intensive. And you'll fail, because unless you go into that zone, and allow your body and heart to take over—anyway, that was the start of it. He also teaches an advanced five- or six-day course which he calls "The Great Leap to Your Heart." I did that one shortly after I did the first one.

Q: What did that have to do with the box you had been carrying around?

A: The whole purpose was to destroy the box.

Q: Did it work?

A: It worked like a charm. And it was gone!

Q: Tell me more about what you did in that course that helped you destroy the box.

A: Well . . . for example, one night he decided it would be a great idea for all of us just to face everybody's death one time, so let's all go jump out of an airplane tomorrow morning. No instructions. Let's just go jump. So everybody went. Parachutes at 12,000 feet. Something is going on every minute of the day. He has a way of killing your ego. I mean, he starts off killing your ego, right from day one. And he has a way of allowing you to kill the box. You know, break down the box.

Q: So what did that mean for you, to destroy the box?

A: Well, for the first time I was able to go back and to be with my family. To enjoy every moment of my life. To take the small things. To really love my children. My wife said it was a damn miracle. That I was a completely different person. I mean a totally different person. For the first time in her life, she was able to truly feel my love. My children went from never asking "When is Dad gonna be home?" to saying, "We're not a family until you're here." That kind of stuff. And you can see how that would change my medical practice.

Q: How?

A: I went from "professional" to someone who could sit down and hold somebody's hand, to hug somebody, to not have the fear. There's no fear if you knock the wall down and go to that extreme—you lose the fear. You can hug somebody. You can shed a tear with a patient. I mean, you can really go an extra step with the patient as another human being without fear that somebody's going to do you in, or think bad of you. Because the last book Millman wrote is called *No Ordinary Moments*. And it dawned on me on the plane coming here [to AHMA] how lucky I was in the past couple of years to be able to have so much joy—"unreasonable joy" is what he calls it—to have unreasonable joy. Because no matter what's going on in your life, you can have unreasonable joy. To have that with my family, to have found that after so many years of destruction, of being boxed in, is just amazing. Just to find value in every moment. Truly, there are no ordinary moments.

Q: At what point did you start using the word "holistic"?

A: Well, I started with a more humanistic approach. You lose the dogma, you think there's got to be some other things here. And then I read Bernie Siegel's book *Love, Medicine, and Miracles*. And I thought, "Wow!" And then I read Deepak Chopra's first book, and I thought, "Here are some guys you can really respect who are saying something different here." I haven't really gone into alternative therapies, although I do recommend some kinds of semi-mainstream sorts of things. Which aren't very mainstream for south Georgia, where meditation and things like that in some people's minds almost lead to satanism!

Q: If a patient came to you with a problem, would you do everything you used to do, only adding maybe more touching and more communication?

A: I always do that. But I also now—it used to be that I'd think, "Well, they don't want to hear me, they don't want to see me except for surgery." Now there are people that I get a feel for. Knocking down the box opens up your intuition. And I've had people come in with some questionable test results—maybe their gallbladder is abnormal—and I really get an intuition that they have something else going on, that they really don't want any surgery. So I spend extra time talking with them. "What's going on here?" I start talking with them about emotions and stress and diet and just getting a feel, as another human being, for what the hell is going on here. And instead of saying, "We need to get that gallbladder out," I say the opposite—"Why don't you try doing these things and thinking about this stuff and come back and tell me what you think later on?" Some of them come back and say, "Please take my gallbladder out." Some of them don't. . . . People with a gallstone that big around, in pain, don't want to hear crapola. But after I get their gallbladder out, I say, "Hey, now that you're feeling better, let's talk about—"

And if I operate, I talk with them ahead of time to make sure they are calm. I play a lot of meditational kinds of music in the operating room, like Pachelbel Canon in D and things like that, where I used to play rock and roll. I talk to them when they're going to sleep and even during the surgery. I say things like, "Everything's going fine. You're doing real well. You're going to wake up feeling hungry." And of course everybody looks at me like I'm a nut.

Q: How comfortable do you feel with all of this, with being called a nut?

A: Well, like I said, this is all kind of new to me. As far as I'm concerned, I'm just at the beginning. There is a little fear, a little trepidation. Nobody has *no* fear. But I have a whole lot less. And the object is not to have no fear, but to just to have courage and warmth. I add daily to what I do. I've changed the music, I've changed the time I spend with each patient, I've changed the way I see them in the office, I've changed what I felt. You know, change is a process. It's all a journey, you know. I don't know where I'm going. Five years from now I may not even operate on people. Who the hell knows?

In this story we see a humanistic physician still in the process of transitioning toward holism. Jack Mansberger learned the hard way that healers must be wounded in order to develop the skills and the instincts necessary to heal others. But to truly be effective, they must first heal themselves. Most especially in the arena of holistic healing, it is impossible to pretend that you can prescribe for others what you are unwilling to prescribe for yourself. As one physician put it:

> When you do healing, it's a two-way street. You have to be constantly addressing your own path and your own healing and you have to share significant pieces of yourself with patients. You don't establish a communication with another human being and then expect the energy to flow one way. It flows both ways. . . . Because when you establish that link with somebody, if you haven't dealt with your own healing, the energy that goes from you to them is not good energy. It's sick. I think it's really important for healers to be addressing their own healing.

Thus, as Jack Mansberger's story powerfully illustrates, the transition to even the beginnings of holistic practice involves self-exploration and healing. Unlike the conventions of technomedicine, which treat the doctor's own habits or condition as irrelevant, or of humanism, which allows doctors to be kind to their patients without changing anything profound in their own lives, holistic doctors expect themselves and are expected by their patients to exemplify their values and beliefs in an immediate and personal way. To those who want to know how to begin, Deborah Malka recommends: "Have some complementary treatments and experience it: it's not just a philosophy! Doctors are always sick; they all work too hard. Begin to walk in the alternative world. I recommend nutritional counseling, acupuncture, or massage for a beginning, but everything works. I think to break extremely ingrained patterns, whose extent we are not conscious of, you need to have some pretty concentrated exposure and experience with alternatives. At first, you don't have to teach it or practice it, just experience it."

Bob Anderson, a past president of the AHMA, insists that "learning about alternative medicine and what it offers is a tremendous healing for the doctors themselves because they will learn that they cannot only heal themselves, but move people in the direction of authentic healing. Heal themselves first, though. That's a top priority if you're going to be healer. You got to have some if you're going to offer it. You've got to walk the talk."

Healing enough to be able to "walk the talk" must go deep, far beyond the surface personality. Doctors who open to new learning find themselves in new situations, interacting on a collegial level with individuals who are also changing. In order to succeed within these circles and be acceptable to a new type of patient, they need to become fully integrated human beings. To achieve that goal, they must first work on their "shadow" side, as osteopath Richard A. Tuscher learned: "The transition has not been all joy and happiness. To be truly present with people, including myself, I had to do 'my own work.' That included being willing to look at my own stuff—my anger, arrogance, being right. I'm aware that the work of transformation is never done; I expect I'll be doing [it] forever. Sometimes it's as pleasant as a root canal or passing a kidney stone, but it does get easier. I have met my shadow and he is I" ("Physician in Transition" 1993).

After years of imprisonment in an emotional box, Jack Mansberger fearlessly faced his shadow. With Millman's help and his own determination, he was finally able to crack open the box. This personal healing catharsis opened him not only to a new kind of connection to himself and his family, but also to new ways of practicing even so technical a form of medicine as surgery. Thus he exemplifies one of the defining characteristics of a holistic way of being—the profound and intimate connections between the personal and professional realms that result from developing a profound and intimate connection with oneself.

TAKING A YEAR OFF: BETHANY HAYS

In earlier chapters, we have heard Bethany Hays describe the rigors of her OB/GYN residency at Baylor in Houston—"It was just do it, and do it, and do it some more." Fifteen years of practice at Baylor and a specialty in perinatology left her able to "do medicine differently because I did it so well, they couldn't criticize, they couldn't question my outcomes." Asked, "What were you doing differently?" she replied, "I had developed a philosophy of childbirth that said that birth was normal and the women's bodies knew how to do that work and that technology was not key. In fact, the technology was potentially very dangerous and needed to be used only as a last resort. That women were supposed to get something more out of childbirth than a baby."

> Q: Where did you get that philosophy?
>
> A: Probably from having children myself. I think you can't have that experience without changing what you know. . . . I remember not only did I view having my children, the experience of being pregnant and giving birth, as part of my education, like I'm going to need to know this in order to help women do this, but I also knew that while I was pregnant, everything else that was coming in was being altered through my pregnant body and if it didn't make sense in my pregnant body, it just didn't get in. So I think the education that I took away from Baylor was quantitatively very different than my colleagues'.
>
> Q: Why did you leave?

A: I was dying because I needed to make a shift and I didn't know that. I had carried the technological, the curing part as far as I could carry it, and it needed to evolve into something more spiritual. I had a very limited view of what my life was about and I had sort of "gotten there." When you think of what you're going to do in life . . . I'm going to become a doctor, I'm going to get married, I'm going to have children, I'm going to have a big house and a nice car, and I'm going to have all of this material wealth, that will be the sign that I have succeeded, that I'm successful, that people think that I'm a good doctor, that I'm contributing and then I will have . . . that's it! And I did all of that—by the time I was forty I had all of that. And I looked around and said, "Something's wrong. This isn't it!"

Q: Why wasn't that it?

A: It wasn't it because it didn't address why I'm on the planet. It didn't address why I learned to do these skills. It didn't address why I had children. It didn't address why I drew to me the people I was in relationship with. It didn't address my connection with the great mystery. It didn't address anything!

When I realized that I was in trouble, that I was dying, I finally said, "I can't practice medicine and address the issues I'm coming up against. I'm going to kill somebody." When I decided to take time off, I took a year off. I walked away from it. And when I did that, what fascinated me was how many of my colleagues came to me and said, "Gosh, I wish I could do that. I *wish* I could do that." And I would say, "You can. When it becomes a high enough priority for you, you can." And I began hearing stories about colleagues who had had breakdowns and colleagues who had changed careers. . . . The other thing that fascinated me was the rumors that went around about *why* I was taking the year off. That was also very instructive because it was clear that no one could acknowledge the possibility that I could be taking the time off just for myself. That wasn't in their vocabulary.

Q: So what would they make up instead?

A: That I must have cancer, a drug or alcohol problem. To this day when I make application to a hospital or when I made application to the Board of Registration in Maine, what they really zero in on is, What did you really do in that year off? So I just say, What you want to know is was I in a drug or alcohol treatment program? And the answer is no. There was one rumor that I had become homosexual and that it had something to do with that. There was a rumor that I was getting divorced, which, of course, I did do in the year I took off, but I had no intention of that when I took the time off. What I learned is that many, if not all, of my colleagues are suffering in that way.

Q: What did you do during that year off? What was that all about?

A: I read and traveled and slept and I learned to want again. I would get up and take my kids off to school and go run in the park and then say, "Now, what would I like to do today?" I could read a book, I could go back to sleep, I could watch TV, I could call a friend and go to lunch. What would I really like to do? What do I feel like doing? I did that for about two weeks before I sort of turned around and said, "Something feels different. What's going on here?" And I realized that for years and years I hadn't had a chance to ask what I wanted to do at any given moment. It was prescheduled. I might want to go to a movie, but I had to go home and take care of my kids. I might want to rest, but I had to go to work. I might want to do something, but I was on call. . . . My time was completely scheduled, between trying to be Supermom and trying to be a good doctor.

My husband said that my career came first, my children came second, and he came somewhere way down the list. And I of course said, My children come first, my career comes second, and he came—because he was adult, I figured he could take care of himself. What I really think is, he was more right than he knew, but it wasn't my career, it was my life path—what I was here to do—that came first. My children were part of that. I always knew I was going to have children, and my children came from a very deep place in my soul. I didn't have children for frivolous reasons, but what I realize now is that I needed the experience of children to do what I'm on the planet to do. Whereas, I think my husband—what he's on the planet to do is to raise children. So in a funny way, I think he was right.

It's interesting to me how many times in the last few years I've noticed that things people said to me or about me that I absolutely resisted as totally wrong, I've had to turn around and look at again and say, "They're probably right." Not in the way that they meant it when they said it, but what they said was fundamentally true. So now I try to listen for those messages.

Q: How did you support yourself?

A: I didn't even think about how money was going to happen. I made the decision. So then I sat down with my checkbook to figure out what we were going to have to do without. My husband came up behind me and said, "What are you doing?" I said, "Well, I'm looking at my checkbook to see what we're going to have to do without if I take time off." And he said, "You don't need to do that." I thought, What does he mean, he's going to support me or what? I said, "Why not?" He said, "Well, you've got that stock that your father gave you when he died and it's still sitting in the bank vault and the stock price has gone way up. You could sell that stock and live on it for a year without any problem."

Q: So how did that year lead to the paradigm shift that you apparently made?

A: I began to read and study things other than medicine. I studied psychology, religion, feminism, New Age stuff, alternative medical practices, things that I wouldn't have had time to do if I had been working full time. One thing led to another. . . . I used to spend a lot of time in the Aquarian age bookstores looking at the books on the shelves and picking the things that looked interesting. And then a lot of those books would lead to other books. . . .

And then one day when I was really at the bottom of my despair, a friend handed me an audiotape. She said, "You might be interested in this. This tape is by a woman obstetrician from Maine, Christiane Northrup." So I took the tape and threw it in my car. It was probably months before I listened to it, and then one day I thought, "I'd better listen to this so I can give it back to my friend." So I put it in the car tape deck and all of a sudden I'm hearing somebody telling me the story of my life, and I got it! Whatever it was that was about to happen to me, this person had been through it and was on the other side of it. And I thought, I've got to find this person and find out what it is that's coming down the road. I knew something big was about to happen, but I just hadn't got a clue as to what the next step was. . . . And so I sojourned to Yarmouth, Maine, to talk to her. Because I have to talk to people directly.

Q: What happened while you were in Maine with Chris?

A: We sat out on the pier at the cannery and had lunch and talked for about two and a half hours about everything that two women doctors can talk about. We talked about white male pediatricians, our children, the practice of medicine, feminism. . . . I said, "I don't know what's happening and I don't know where I'm headed," and so she said, "What you need is a road map." I said, "That's what I need, a road map, exactly." She said, "OK, I'll give you the name of somebody." And she gave me the name of a woman who does some combination of astrology, numerology, and the kabbala. And I thought, "All right! I'm going to go to an astrologer to get this roadmap. Uh huh, you know." It was very funny. I would have done what she said if she had told me to stand on my head and spit gold nickels for five minutes each day—I'd probably have gotten right up on my head and tried. . . .

Somewhere right in there, I made a conscious decision that for me to make this transition, I was going to have to let in some information that I had discounted. And that it was time for me to simply allow the possibility that anything could be legitimate. So I went to see the astrologer, and I went with the idea of, Whatever she tells you, accept it as though it were true, and you can sort it out later. And I began to read books with the idea that this might be the truth, and the fact that you don't understand it doesn't mean it's not the truth. . . . [Chris was the] guide who kept handing me the next book. . . . Just about every time I talked with her, the conversation would be punctuated with, "Have you read this, have you read that?" and I would just scribble the names down, and go get the books.

Around this time, Bethany joined the American Holistic Medical Association. This was a "scary thing" for her to do, as she still felt herself to be a "conventional OB/GYN doctor"; dealing with the unconventionality of many AHMA members stretched her to the limit. Ultimately, Bethany's year off was thoroughly transformative. Reading, listening, learning, growing, she finally realized that what she needed as a physician was "to stop beating my head against the walls of the system" and instead to practice in a place where she and her colleagues could define reality in a different way.

After my year off, I left Houston and came up to Maine to practice with Chris at Women-to-Women. And I went to interview at the hospitals in Portland. At one of them, I talked to the chief of obstetrics and gynecology and he couldn't figure out how a perinatologist who had trained at Baylor, was board certified in OB/GYN, and had done a fellowship in maternal and fetal medicine could wind up with the granola doctors in Yarmouth! It was just too much; he couldn't find a niche to put me in. He was trying to figure out, "What am I going to do? This woman is well trained and she's highly thought of in her community and she's gonna come up here and be with the granola doctors; what am I going to do with her?" It was really funny. He was very relieved when he found out I had taught breastfeeding on the Baylor faculty, because he needed somebody to do that.

Q: Describe Women-to-Women to me.

A: Women-to-Women is a holistic women's health care clinic. We do conventional obstetrics and gynecology in unconventional ways. The organization is committed to health and growth on a personal level as well as relationship with our patients. It started as two physicians and two nurse-practitioners who work in partnership. We each have our areas of interest and expertise and our own personal philosophies of caring for patients, but we share a philosophy of helping women take responsibility for their lives and their health care and we feel that it's important for us to set an example in our own lives of continuing our personal growth and health.

Recently Bethany's partner, Chris Northrup, author of the best-selling *Women's Bodies, Women's Wisdom*, has left one-on-one practice to write and to teach. Bethany is now associated at Women-to-Women with two holistic nurse-practitioners, Marcelle Pick and Dixie Knoll, and with Dixie Mills, M.D., a surgeon with a speciality in breast health. Confronted with the medical takeover in her town by managed care, Bethany has declined to participate, trusting that her patients will be willing to pay out-of-pocket simply because they value the holistic, woman-centered care that she and her colleagues provide.

The catalysts that sent Bethany Hays on her way, from her pregnancies during residency to Chris Northrup's tape, started her on a journey of transformation that she now feels is complete. At peace with herself and her life, Bethany has integrated who she is with the way she practices. While many challenges remain, she has successfully passed through the life-crisis challenges of healing what she described as her addictive tendencies to overwork and to fight battles that don't belong to her, and of finding a path to healing that both pays the bills and nurtures her spirit.

AGONY TO ECSTASY: VERNON M. SYLVEST

Vernon M. Sylvest told his remarkable story in the "Physician in Transition" column in *Holistic Medicine* (1991), the journal of the AHMA:

As I look back upon my life, I realize that I had an intuitive feeling, even as a child, that if I knew who I was, I would be happy. Since I thought of myself as a living body, I had an avid interest in biology. At the undergraduate level, this extended into biochemistry, physiology, and embryology. After an internal tug-of-war, a career in medicine finally won out over a career in basic science research. Since I, like all other humans, experienced illnesses, I felt that understanding the disease process was part of knowing myself.

The early phases of my study of self included spiritual and philosophical considerations; however, the sources of information I had available at that time, integrated with my level of understanding, only led to contradictions and confusions. . . . Thus I gravitated to the more scientific aspects of medicine. I considered specializing in internal medicine but found, as an intern, that the specialty was laced with too much futility for my taste, and I tended to take the hopeless cases home with me. Surgery was also a consideration, because I liked the idea of being in "control" and physically doing something. In the end, pathology was my choice, for although my quest for the understanding of self in health and disease was as confused as ever, at least this specialty seemed to be closer to a direct search. Also, as a diagnostic specialty, pathology was less futile, for we could always put a name on a condition, and our job was successfully completed.

I found the study and practice of pathology interesting and intriguing. I began to lose track of my desire to understand myself and to put my focus on experiencing myself in the world, accepting the predominant cultural beliefs. I became an average, ego-oriented person, defining myself in my experiential interface with the outer world, including work, relationships, physical and material experiences, and cultural codes of worthiness. The end result of all this was more confusion. . . .

My confusion became manifest in strained and broken relationships and physical pain. In 1977, I developed a severe, crippling arthritic disease. For the next four and a half years, I was in constant pain in spite of the best rheumatology consultations available in the English-speaking world. Except for a few weeks here and there when the disease put me to bed, I continued working as a pathologist. My physical pain, however, brought my attention back from experiencing life to an attempt to understand it. . . . Still there was only confusion, which was augmented by my constant observation of the elderly, sick, and dying in the hospital. People who, I realized, had once been in their prime, as I should have been then, were shriveled in various stages of paralysis, contracture, and senility. Was this what life was all about? Nature seemed to be some sort of cruel practical joker. The living dead had more impact on me than the dead I dissected on the autopsy table.

The result of this confusion and the worsening arthritis, which began to include some visceral involvement, was severe depression and a state of desperation that led to a different, last resort in my attempt to get well. It was apparent that the only thing which would save me from this living hell was a miracle. The thin thread that held me to life was a faint hope that maybe the miracles that religions spoke of might be possible. Having reached this point of desperation, I began to pray. I asked others to pray for me. I began to attend healing services at a local church. Someone gave me a book written by Merlin Carothers, a Methodist minister, who had begun to have some unusual experiences such as hearing an inner voice that gave him guidance. He also discovered that as he laid hands on some people in prayer, they experienced what appeared to be miraculous healing. At this point in my own experience of pain, I had tossed logic out the window; when I heard that he was speaking at a convention . . . I resolved to make the trip. . . .

Reverend Carothers began his sermon by describing a pathologist performing an autopsy. The description was detailed, describing the skin incision, the dissection of the chest flap, the cutting through the rib cage and the dissection of the various organs. The description seemed to be inappropriate for the lay audience in its details. To my further amazement, he was describing the technique of dissection that I used in my own practice. . . . He had no medical background, and he did not know me, nor did he know that I was present. As he made this description, he created an analogy. As the pathologist dissects the physical body to understand the physical disturbance of disease, we must dissect our spiritual nature to understand the spiritual disturbance that produces disease.

As this was occurring, I had the feeling that I was experiencing a synchronization of the type referred to by Carl Jung. But its significance was not apparent to me at the time. I returned home still in pain. There appeared to be no miracle for me. . . . [But I continued my spiritual pursuits.] I studied nontraditional versions of Christianity such as *A Course in Miracles* and *The Aquarian Gospel of Jesus the Christ.* I extended my study into non-Christian writings and teachings. To my amazement, I found that beneath the variety of forms lay the same message. I also found myself studying quantum physics and found further agreement. The spiritual teachings describe a reality with which concepts evolving from modern physics are compatible.

As I began to accept and practice the spiritual teachings that I was learning, I began to feel less fear, less anger, less despair, and less guilt. In other words, I began to feel a sense of love and oneness with everyone including myself. My arthritis totally disappeared without any residual deformity within a year of my beginning prayer activity. My depression lifted. Broken and strained relationships healed. . . .

This transformation was obvious to the people around me. Many began to come to me for advice. Although as a pathologist, I was not seeing patients except to perform biopsies or nuclear medicine procedures, I found some patients coming to me for counsel. On several occasions, people came to me with aches and pains and would actually ask me to lay my hands on them. I did, and their pain disappeared. I then began to study therapeutic touch . . . as well as other alternative approaches to healing, now understandable to me based on my study of physics and my new understanding of the physics of consciousness and spirituality. I too began to have mystical experiences and received guidance that was quite clear. . . . One of the goals that was described was a healing center which I could organize if I so chose. I did, and the Institute of Higher Healing was founded. Although initially I planned simply to be chairman of the board of this organization and to restrict my activities in it to lectures and teachings in the evenings and on weekends, it ultimately was made clear to me that I was to leave the practice of pathology and become one of the practicing holistic physicians in the clinic.

With excitement and a sense of freedom, I changed my career in midstream. I left pathology and became a general practitioner at the Institute. The futility I once associated with clinical practice was no longer present. I began to incorporate spiritual principles and techniques into my practice. Alternative ways of working with the body's energy were introduced. I found that much of my practice fell into the realm of psychotherapy, but now without confusion. This psychotherapy is accelerated by incorporating intuitive tools. Attitudinal training and teaching perceptions that reflect truth and thus foster love rather than fear are an important part of the practice. Patients are taught the importance of prayer, meditation, vigilance over their thoughts and feelings, and the importance of being willing to love, trust, and forgive.

Guiding patients in the release of repressed emotions and negative beliefs is important not only in emotional healing but also in physical and situational healing. All healing ultimately occurs at the level of the mind, for it is in the prephysical energy of mind from which the physical is manifested and affected that disturbance occurs. The disturbance is fear produced by false perceptions—perceptions of inequality, attack, and loss. These are perceptions of separation. The truth is loving, for God is good. Thus with truth we experience love, which is the most powerful force in the universe and creates like itself. This leads to an underlying principle: there is nothing to fear.

I now have a clearer understanding of who I am. I am happy, and I have something healing to share with my patients.

In Sylvest's language, we can hear the attitude of the holistic physician who shares information instead of managing patient care, and we can celebrate with him this transformative culmination of his journey. It is revealing that when he first went to hear Reverend Carothers, what he really wanted was a sudden and miraculous healing, the spiritual equivalent of the medical quick fix. The path he ultimately took was longer but its greater rewards are evident. It is in the pain and the struggle of the journey and the profound learning that takes place en route that real transformation occurs. Sylvest's story is unusual in that he healed a chronic and debilitating disease first from the spiritual side, rather than taking the more usual route through changes in diet, exercise, and life-style. His experience clearly illustrates the holographic nature of the holistic model. Each part of it contains the whole, so that no matter which side you enter it from, you may end up encompassing it all.

STARTING OUT ON THE OTHER SIDE: ALAN GABY

Q: Why did you want to become a doctor?

A: Well, I really didn't! My father wanted me to become a doctor and he had it ingrained in me from an early age that medicine was the best profession—indeed, the only profession. He was a surgeon and he used to take me with him to the emergency room to watch him sew up cuts. And you know, I just wanted to be with my dad, so I went down there with him to watch what he did, but to me it was gross. I thought, "I don't want to do anything like that." And I also didn't like the idea of giving people drugs all the time—I did not like the idea of being a doctor that way. But I also knew that medicine was a desirable profession. People who went into it were successful and respected, and medicine would give me an opportunity to exercise my brain and my intellect. So while I didn't find anything about medicine that appealed to me, I felt it would be nice to discover something about it that I did like.

After college, I managed to get myself rejected from medical school despite having gone to an Ivy League school and despite being in the top one percentile on the Medical College Admission Test. At my interview, when they asked, "Why do you want to be a doctor?" I replied, "My father thinks it's a good profession."

Q: That's why they rejected you?

A: Right. It was obvious that I didn't really want it. Anyway, I went off and taught school for a year—taught math and coached wrestling at my old high school and sort of thought about what I wanted to do with my life. And I just happened to pick up a few books on nutrition. I read Linus Pauling's book *Vitamin C and the Common Cold*, and Carlton Frederick's book *Food, Facts and Fallacies*. And what I discovered was that there can be a nurturing way of practicing medicine where you actually give people things that are good for them and help people take care of themselves. In addition, it appeared that a great deal of the research in this area was being ignored or suppressed. So my interest was piqued. On the one hand, the nutritional approach to medicine called to the healer in me. On the other hand, it spoke to my political side (I majored in political science in college), because the controversy surrounding nutritional medicine made it, in a sense, a very political science. So I saw an opportunity to practice a type of medicine that seemed interesting, but also to be a pioneer, someone who could help change society for the better. When I read those books, something just clicked and I knew that this was my life's work. I was twenty-three. So I went back to graduate school to show them that I could do good work when I was serious about it—and got a master's degree in biochemistry with a 3.9 average and good recommendations.

Q: Where was this?

A: At Emory University. And then I went to medical school at the University of Maryland in 1975. By the time I got there I'd already read a great deal about alternative medicine and was oriented strongly in that direction. That interest created difficulties for me, though, because I was very vocal about my beliefs and many of the students and professors thought I was a weirdo. When I would raise my hand in class, the professors would sometimes make a face like "Oh, God, what's he going to ask this time about something we've never heard of?" Some of my friends called me Dr. Ascorbate—a loving but disparaging nickname. So, after a while I realized that the way to stay out of trouble was to keep my "alternative" ideas to myself and to focus on being good at the type of medicine that was being taught. Whatever else I thought was important I learned on my own time. I was sure I would be in a position to apply that information at some time in the future. Still, it was often a lonely road.

Q: Tell me about your residency.

A: I did an internship in internal medicine. Internship was physically traumatic . . . almost intolerable for me . . . because I believed that a lot of the things they were doing were dangerous, or at least that there were safer approaches that could be tried. I remember one time I had a patient with gangrene of her foot as a result of diabetes. I ordered brewer's yeast, one tablespoon per day, because published research had shown that it helps to control blood sugar. A few days later, the chief resident called me in and warned, "I just want you to know you're being watched. Because, you know, people are really concerned about the types of things you're doing here."

Q: Did the brewer's yeast help?

A: It's hard to know. I mean her foot was half rotted off from the gangrene. So brewer's yeast was not going to be enough by itself, but it was a logical thing to use to help bring her blood sugar down. The problem was that the hospital didn't have brewer's yeast. They had to go down to the health food store to get it, so they were aggravated.

And then for another diabetic patient I prescribed a high-fiber diet, which ended up being an imposition on the dietetics department. This was in 1979, before high-fiber diets were generally accepted as beneficial for diabetes. The dietitician found some peanuts—some really salty ones—to give her, and a few other foods that had a little fiber in them. But I felt like I was being resented and ridiculed for doing what I believed was perfectly appropriate.

The main reason I didn't stay for the full three-year residency was that I did not want to continue giving combinations of toxic drugs when safer, more natural alternatives were available. Also, I did not like some of the high-tech aspects of the program, like sticking wires into people's hearts. I stayed until I thought I had an adequate foundation in the basics of conventional medicine—enough experience to handle the common problems and to know when I was in over my head.

And you know, most common illnesses are just that. They're very common. Practicing good medicine requires you to be conscientious and attentive, but you don't have to be a specialist to know how to deal with most cases of, for example, high blood pressure, depression, obesity, arthritis, fatigue, and migraines. When I went into private practice, I was confident that I could diagnose and treat the common conditions. I was also willing to refer if I felt like I didn't know what was going on, or if the patient needed a complex combination of potentially toxic medications. And as it turned out, once I was in private practice, I only had to refer one or two patients per year. In many cases, the patients had actually referred themselves *from* the specialist. They had already been worked up, and they had already failed to respond to conventional treatments or had experienced intolerable side effects. So then I would try my treatments, and more often than not the patients got better.

I guess the most important thing besides being conscientious is knowing your limitations—knowing when you're in over your head. I was fully aware that my training was not adequate to deal with certain situations and that I would have to consult a specialist in those situations.

When I finished my training, I came to Seattle and went into practice with Jonathan Wright, M.D., one of the pioneers in nutritional medicine. I practiced three days a week and spent about three full days a week in the library going through medical journals. I had a strong interest in digging up all of the nutrition research I could find, both old and new. I was also interested in critically evaluating that research . . . separating the legitimate work from the hype . . . in order to make myself a better doctor and in order to become proficient in an area that I believed would shape the future of health care. I went throught the table of contents of each journal. I mean, *Journal of Urology*, Volume 1, *Journal of Urology*, Volume 2, all the way to Volume 123. I did that with each journal, and photocopied the articles that interested me. It was amazing how much important research had been completely ignored by conventional medicine.

After five years of going to the library three days a week, I began hiring medical students to continue the project. I have now entered more than twenty-five thousand citations into a computerized database and have written summaries for more than half of the articles. I have passionately studied this material for more than twenty years, because long ago I became convinced that nutritional and herbal medicine would be in the mainstream one day. I wanted to get a head start on learning about it, so that I would be ready to teach it when others were ready to learn.

Q: And that's exactly how it's working out.

A: Yes, it is. I have more requests to speak and write articles than ever before.

Like Alan Gaby, some physicians seemed to know all the way through their training that at some point in the future they would design their own approach to healing, and that it would incorporate alternative methods. This knowledge sustained them through the rigors of training and the early years of their practice. They managed to achieve balance while inhabiting two realities (or paradigms) in their thinking. Eventually, and without the suffering that characterized the other types of experiences we have described, they shifted rather easily into a new mode, as though it had been waiting for them all along. Their life path continued smoothly, more calmly than those of the doctors who experienced more definable openings. They tend to be unaffected by criticism and content with their contribution to the realm of healing, which, as in Gaby's case, is often quite significant.

After fifteen years of private practice, Gaby has stopped practicing to spend four years writing a massive book, *Nutritional Medicine*, which will contain more than fifteen thousand references and will synthesize the results of his years of research and practice. He and his colleague Johnathan Wright periodically offer seminars in nutritional medicine for physicians, who attend by the hundreds from all over the world.

On the Other Side of the Transitional Process

> I've become the kind of person I used to warn people about!
> —MERLE MOSKOWITZ, M.D.

Barbara Harris Whitfield (1995:161) describes the qualities of arriving at "the other side" of a spiritual awakening: "There is no one ideal state of being or one destination. This process varies as each individual varies. There is, however, one ideal we all share and that is unconditional love. Unconditional love is happy doing many things that ego is bored with. It is blatantly different from egotistic love, with its desires and power plays. It leads in a different direction, toward the goodness, the value, and the need of the people around us."

In "Physician in Transition" (1990) Ken Hamilton writes that a primary hallmark of a physician's successful transition from the orthodoxy of his or her training to an openness to natural healing techniques is the development of a sense of trust in and surrender to the process as it unfolds. These qualities of trust and surrender appear in the young doctor just beginning to feel the pull to other sources as well as in the reflection of the seasoned elder. They both know that trust and surrender are the right attitudes, the only ones that work and that lead to deep satisfaction. Trust and surrender allow doctors to move forward without the sense that they have to control everything; instead, they learn to be responsive to subtle messages and to opportunities that present themselves in ways they might previously have ignored or overlooked. Whether they choose to develop a clinic, return to school, or redesign their practice, their actions will be informed by the certainty that they are aligned with their true sense of purpose.

For many, as we have seen, the process includes a complete revolution of their belief systems. They no longer regard themselves as powerful interventionists in a war against disease and death. Their major identity has changed. Softer, more fluid, they now see themselves as helpers, assistants, supporters of their brothers and sisters during painful episodes, episodes they themselves have often experienced. Far from being able to rely on any standard, learned approach, many find that each patient encounter requires the utmost creativity. In fact their patients, formerly objectified, often even disliked, are now a source of learning and tremendous personal satisfaction. These physicians are committed to the human skills of communication, empathy, feeling, and emotional expression. Nothing other than an abiding sense of wholeness and satisfaction in the new paradigm could sustain an individual through such a values shift.

Once through the narrow passage of medical training, most doctors are eager to begin reaping the fruits of their long years of preparation. The average doctor can look forward to entering professional life in a pinnacle position with a well-defined career path and every expectation of success. Doctors occupy some of the most respected positions in society by virtue of their education, income, and personal power. For most new physicians, the future, though characterized by long hours and the responsibilities of patient care, will consist of steadily increasing income and the opportunity to experience the American dream to the fullest. Rather than putting income first, many of our interviewees prioritize their relationships with their patients and the ability to practice as they believe best. (In spite of the risk of losing patients, they often refuse to join HMOs, which many of them feel are ruining medicine by severely limiting what the physician can do for the patient.) They tend to value the contributions they may be able to make toward legitimizing and expanding holistic medicine over financial rewards.

Doctors who have made the transition to holism in practice become seekers in virtually all aspects of their lives. They open up to systems and experiences that they once would have avoided or scorned. They stretch their own mental and emotional boundaries through continuous learning, and their physical boundaries by incorporating into their own lives the same principles of health they recommend to their patients, as Robert Ivker explained:

> I'm learning that love in its infinite manifestations is our most powerful healer. I've changed my own dietary and exercise habits and established new dreams and goals. I now believe that anything is possible. . . . I've also begun to recognize and express my feelings, learned to better trust the feminine energy in my life both within and without, and developed a much greater sense of intimacy in my marriage. I feel much more alive and [feel] much less fear, have a far greater awareness of God, and have become a much better friend and nurturer of my playful inner child. My wife captured that essence as we left the theater after seeing *Dances With Wolves* for the second time. "You should have an Indian name too," Harriet said. "I'll call you 'Plays With Kids!'" ("Physician in Transition" 1992)

As they become more intimate with the process of their own healing, holistic physicians develop insight into the process for their patients. Robert Ivker notes that since he began his own healing journey, and began to apply the same principles to his patients, all of whom had some type of chronic ailment, "every one of them has gotten better." Chris Northrup defined this level of integration as "a way of being in the world," which she said is "a way of seeing that the whole is greater than the sum of its parts. It brings in mystery. We don't always know what's going on. The spiritual component is the most important. Edgar Cayce said, 'The spirit is the life, the mind is the builder, and the body is the result.' If I look back on all the things we've discussed—my childhood, college, residency—if I didn't have a sense of greater meaning, a sense of spiritual purpose, none of the rest would have made a whole lot of difference."

Stages of the Transformational Journey: An Overview

We describe the stages of the transformational journey to provide points of orientation on a map that may help a foundering traveler. They are not graven in stone, but like towns along a web of interconnected roads, may be passed through and returned to again and again. A given traveler may make many stops, may skip straight to the end—or indeed, as we have seen, may start out there! Structurally, the stages reveal the similarities between the transformative journey of holistic physicians and all human transitional processes everywhere, as they mirror the three stages that Arnold Van Gennep ([1908] 1966) identified for rites of passage in general: separation, transition, and integration.

SEPARATION

The beginnings of psychological detachment from the technomedical worldview mark the first essential step on the journey. Any kind of cognitive distance enables physicians to perceive the boundaries and beliefs of the paradigm in which they have been trained. If you can see the paradigm in which you are entrenched, then you are free to "think beyond" its limitations. As we have noted, this distancing move can be sparked by a myriad of catalysts, which, to recapitulate, include confronting the limitations of technomedicine, learning from patients, suffering from personal illness, and social and spiritual awakenings—sparked by encounters with guidance, by a book, individual, or group, by direct exposure to other types of practice, by hallucinogenic drugs, and/or by synchronous events. These catalysts almost never operate in isolation and are rarely perceived at the time to be the turning points they become; instead, as Peter Albright put it, they are experienced as "meanderings in the desert," "beads on a string."

And it is important to remember that many physicians have no need of such catalysts to help them achieve cognitive distance from the technomedical worldview; they start out "on the other side." These physicians often find medical training more of a struggle than do their classmates who buy into the system. Like these classmates, they have to cope with long hours and extremely hard work; unlike them, they also must cope with policies and values that they find personally offensive and often just plain wrong. Knowing that there is a better way, they have to toe the party line just to get through. People who violate their own value system on a daily basis to achieve a larger goal suffer added depression and stress. Physicians in this position often experience their entire training process as a core violation of their essential being, and it can take them years to recover their psychological equilibrium and health. But at least they have little trouble shifting into holistic practice, their goal all along; they simply move in that direction as soon as they complete their residencies. Some, like Patch Adams and Alan Gaby, choose not to complete residencies at all, preferring to go quickly into the kind of practice they wish to establish, and referring those few patients who need the technomedical care they know they are not qualified to provide.

We described how Charles LeBaron and Peter Grote kept their perspective—by taking a year off in the middle of med school in Grote's case, and by making it all the way to the Citgo sign and writing *Gentle Vengeance* in LeBaron's. We also found that some physicians who enter medical training already "on the other side" *do* eventually lose their detachment as a result of the socialization pressures they experience during training. If they do, they find medical training less stressful than it might have been. It is always easier to go through a process that you believe in than one you don't. And it is ultimately easier for such physicians to later regain the cognitive distance they lost, as the neural templates for "thinking beyond" have already been laid down in their brains, and alternative philosophies, values, and beliefs are already part of their mind-set.

TRANSITION

Cognitive distance from the technomedical model opens the nascent holist's mind to alternative ways of thinking about healing and health. If the initial catalysts are powerful enough, he may find himself leaving the practice of medicine altogether or simply taking some time off—a month, a year, or more. He now enters an entirely liminal space that contains none of the attributes of the past or coming state. Those who know where they are going when they start usually experience this time as stimulating, exciting, a phase of rapid growth. Those who do not may plunge into the depths of depression and despair. They may even have to "hit bottom" before they find within themselves something that pulls them toward a transcendent goal. Once they can see the goal, the path suddenly becomes clear, and what was all darkness and confusion is transformed into a series of steps that present themselves to be climbed.

As the preceding stories indicate, synchronicities abound. Many of our interviewees told us that during this time, it is extremely important to stay open and aware. If someone gives you a book, read it. If you walk into a bookstore and a book falls off the shelf in front of you, buy it. Listen to the tape your friend hands you one day. Go to the lecture you happen to see advertised. Synchronicity can only happen if you let it. Stay open, they say.

Whether or not our traveler chooses to take time off, her first tentative steps toward holistic practice usually involve reading books and talking with patients, friends, or alternative practitioners about holistically oriented therapies and techniques. Venturing to refer a patient or two to such practitioners, the physician is often impressed when they achieve good results where her own therapies have failed. Most of our interviewees began their shift into holistic practice with a new attention to diet, nutrition, vitamin, and exercise therapies—areas where they could feel that they were still walking on solid ground. Since most chronic ailments improve rapidly when the sufferers give up sugar and caffeine, eliminate foods to which they are allergic, and begin some type of regular exercise, the rewards of such a shift are often immediate.

And here begins what may become a long series of confrontations with what the nascent holist now perceives as the conventional—and highly limited—medical system. Encouraged and enthused by the good results he is getting, he begins to tell his colleagues, thinking that surely they will want to know. Usually he is at first laughingly tolerated, later perhaps actively rebuffed. He may be warned that he is being watched. His orders may be questioned, his cases brought up for review. He now has two options: He can confront the system head-on, writing letters to hospital administrators and demanding the right to practice as he sees fit. Or he can go underground, focusing on his own patients and letting the system do as it will. Many of our interviewees ultimately left their positions in large hospitals or universities in favor of private practices that allowed them more freedom with fewer battles to fight.

Feeling isolated and beleaguered, our traveler may decide the time has come to reach out. Attendance at conferences organized around holistic principles usually takes her journey through a quantum leap. Holistically oriented conferences such as those put on by the AHMA, Common Boundary, and the Institute of Noetic Sciences are full-body experiences, with lectures to engage the intellect; dancing, yoga, tai chi, and the like to stimulate the body; lots of hugs, intense conversations, and free-flowing love to activate the emotions; meditation to calm and center all the senses; and an open celebration of spirituality to free the soul. Few newcomers who participate in this kind of atmosphere for three or four days go away unchanged; from then on, they know where to go whenever they feel in need of a revitalizing dip in the holistic spring. And they know what books to read, what tapes to buy, and most importantly, whom to call when they need help or advice. Returning from such conferences with armloads of new information, nascent holists often find a particular modality of special interest and appeal. Through attendance at weekend workshops, they may learn enough about this modality to begin to incorporate it in their practice. They may decide to study it intensively, or simply to refer to its best practitioners in their city or town.

Somewhere along the way, the physician in transition will realize that she has passed the point of no return. The holistic paradigm does not throw out conventional medicine, but rather transcends and includes it as well as many other healing systems. As we have seen, medical holism is a Stage-Four system: one that can encompass multiple stories about reality, multiple options and alternatives. In other words, it is a cognitive system with both greater depth and greater span (Wilber 1996) than the technocratic model. To take the journey to holism is to become a fluid thinker. Once you have deepened and broadened your cognitive system to that extent, it is impossible to go back to the narrow confines of the unimodal technocratic way.

INTEGRATION

As in most rites of passage, the integrative phase in the passage from doctor to healer happens gradually, as the individual reincorporates herself into society in her new identity or role. There is of course no arbitrary point at which one can say that the transitional phase of this transformative journey has ended and the integration phase has begun. All of our interviewees agreed that growth, learning, and change are by now constants in their lives. Nevertheless there are some telling indicators in our data that can help a given individual to understand where he is on the path to holism. Two particular questions that we asked our interviewees are helpful here: "Do you experience your personal and professional lives as integrated?" and "What do you think should be done about the American medical system?" To the latter question, those who were still very much in transition tended to respond with grand schemes for health care reform. They were idealistic, optimistic, ripe with enthusiasm, full of plans to make a full-scale difference.

But those who had completed the paradigm shift had a very different response. In general, they did not think about the American health care system as a social or political phenomenon against which they had to battle. They recognized that it would evolve, and that they might be somehow limited or even attacked in the course of this evolution. Yet this was not their focus. They had learned that systemwide reform is up to the handful of people who play at the national level.[1] Rather than beating their heads against unyielding walls in the old addictive way, they had recouped and regrouped. They carefully and realistically assessed the possibilities that lay within their purview, and, as we will show, were completely fulfilled in their chosen path. In "Physician in Transition," Terry Collins wrote: "Over ten years ago, I became totally frustrated with physicians who were practicing in the disease paradigm not recognizing that there was a health paradigm. Finally I concluded that the ability to change this behavior on a large scale was a monumental task to which I was not suited. It became evident that my efforts to make change would be focused on my own field."

Unlike Voltaire's Candide, who, bitter and disillusioned, chose to withdraw from the world to cultivate his garden, these physicians reached out to create and develop programs that helped dozens, hundreds, or many thousands of others in their communities—a drug rehabilitation center, a wellness center that doubled as a community meeting place, cancer support groups, physician support groups, school programs in health education, and on and on. Although no one of them will change the world, their cumulative efforts are indeed "shifting the paradigm"—one patient, one doctor, and one community at a time. As Bill Manahan, who started a wellness center in Mankato, Minnesota, expressed it:

> Life is just great. Every day is such a joy for me because there aren't many things that faze me very much. And that's happened more since 1992, coming back from Africa; it's like it's just lightened the load. I somewhat would carry the load of the earth on my back—I had to save it. In fact, I remember saying that I'm on this world to save it. It's a real messianic complex and I think a lot of physicians suffer from that. . . . And of course, it's our best characteristic, it drives us forward to do the right things, but it also weighs us down. . . . It gets exhausting. That's why I felt so energetic and vibrant and free this last year, because I know I'm not going to save the world. I'll just do my thing. I have felt much more content in Mankato because after the kids left, it's like, "Man, what are we doing in Mankato?" This little rural town, very conservative—but it doesn't matter now where I am. I can do just as much right there and probably more than I can in an inner-city ghetto or in this squatter village out in Kenya where I lived.

Answers to the question "Do you experience your personal and professional lives as integrated?" were equally telling. Those just beginning their journey often responded like obstetrician Peter Vargas, who said, "Not really. My personal life isn't really what I think it ought to be or should be. I don't have a lot of time for myself." Those who seemed, as best we could tell, to be well on the way often responded that, while their personal and professional lives were not integrated, at least they were balanced; the latter no longer subsumed the former. And those who had completed their transformative journey often did experience the personal and the professional as one.

As they do their work in the world, whatever that turns out to be, holistic physicians who have completed their journeys find community for themselves in relationship with others. Constantly tempted to return to their old workaholic ways by the rapid growth of their practices and the ever-present demands of their patients and their communities, they often succumb. But when they start to experience the symptoms of stress and overwork, they listen to their bodies and slow down. For they know that to withhold from themselves the nurturant and careful attention they give to their patients is both inconsistent and self-defeating. As they extend holistic healing to others, they find over and over that they cannot deny it to themselves. Patients cannot be well served by a physician who is sick, no matter how loving that physician may be. Forced into dealing with their past, their bodies, their emotions, and their spirits by their own holistic philosophy, over time and with much hard work and many relapses, they heal themselves and their relationships. They search for and ultimately find that healthy balance of work to leisure, patient care to self-care, professional to personal, ultimately achieving a wholeness of living that brings them the happiness for which they ceased to strive when they began to learn, at some point along with way, the extraordinary healing power of surrender and trust.

"Follow Your Heart": Advice from the Travelers to Those Thinking about Making the Trip

We asked these satisfied doctors what advice they would offer to physicians contemplating such a change. Without exception, they advised their colleagues to "go for it." Olga Luchakova, a physician-turned-spiritual-teacher, expressed her respect for physicians and pointed to their potential: "There are developmental stages in consciousness, and many doctors are highly developed people. . . .The fact that they get the education, that they are successful, grows from the level of energy they have." Most of our interviewees did not advise taking it slow, but rather suggested applying this energy in a focused way to move rapidly in a chosen direction, even if the outcome was uncertain. They emphasized the self-healing and the satisfaction inherent in following one's heart.

The advice to "follow your heart" demonstrates a radical shift in how doctors on the threshold of change behave. We recall the completely outer-directed experience of medical education, where the curriculum was often bereft of connection and meaning and the personal needs of the student for community, for balance, for sleep, for self-respect were repeatedly violated. In contrast, physicians who embark on this transformative journey go deep inside; the required wisdom is there and is available for the asking. Paulanne Balch insists: "You've got to follow your heart, because the path of allopathic medicine is not only so narrow, it's unrewarding. Reach out. Pick up something in the bookstore. Follow that instinct. Follow the inner path that's leading you. Don't just stand in the elevator and think about it!"

In addition to advising interested doctors to experience natural healing methods, several physicians urged them to open up and be ready to learn from any source—friend, colleague, or patient. The ability to do this requires a tremendous amount of trust from individuals who were taught to mistrust sources outside of orthodoxy, even to the extent of ignoring their own experience in favor of the expected response. Sandra Kamiak suggests that

> people need to follow their deepest convictions, to go to a calm place and see where their heart is leading them. Proceed, not running off in an egotistical way, but just following their heart, sharing what they are learning with patients and colleagues. Put more life energy into what you want to do. Maybe scale down in terms of rent, what you need to live on personally. Trust—some of the details tend to take care of themselves. Talk to people who have had good experiences with other systems, even patients. Then start to inquire. If you have a friend who has had a good experience with acupuncture or homeopathy, this may be more convincing than a dozen research papers.

Allowing the process to unfold in its own time is essential. Henry Hochberg compares it to natural germination: "Like all seeds, you cannot rush the germination period without getting some kind of abnormal or unnatural product, although the tendency today might be to bring in artificial light and heat and try to get the thing growing before nature intended it to grow" ("Physician in Transition" 1990).

The advice to open to many different sources of information came from a number of our interviewees. Peter Grote recommends: "Listen to your heart and go with what feels right. Talk to other people who have the sort of practice you'd like to have. Learn as much from them as well as patients as you can. That's a source that might be overlooked—the people who are asking for something other than pharmaceutical drugs." Barry Elson says, "Read. Be open-minded. Don't close your mind to things that are new just because they're new." Jim Gordon suggests that you "go within. Find out what you ought to do. Learn what interests you. Know that you can do anything you want. Don't worry about what other people have to say and, on the other hand, listen to anybody who has anything to teach you. Have a good time!" And Karin Montero encourages physicians to "go for it, absolutely. I think it's what the future medicine will be. We need to learn it so we can teach it."

You won't be alone. Bethany Hays reminds you that "there are other physicians out here—many courageous, brilliant, ethical, responsible people—making these changes. Most of the people who have made this transition are not running away, they're running toward. They are not in trouble; they're highly respected. It's not as scary as it looks." Barry Elson recommends that you "talk to people who have been doing it for a while. There are thousands of us out here doing that kind of medicine. They're generally people with integrity and intellectual honesty who care about their patients." A final word of support comes from Bill Manahan: "If you're ready, go for it! It's really fun and exciting and I will be whatever help I can."

We found many of the holistic doctors we interviewed to be both holy and whole, and we experienced awe again and again in their presence. We felt privileged to encounter examples of what human beings can become when they employ their intelligence, courage, and compassion in pursuit of a vocation of service, under the aegis of a paradigm that is both specific enough to allow for focused action and broad enough to encourage unrestricted individual creativity. The telling qualities of their successful completion of this transformational journey include their respect for all of life; their forgiveness and tolerance of their critics; their unqualified belief in the generative powers of the human spirit; the utter joy they find in their work; and their strong sense that the process is never finished. As Peter Albright put it, "There is always more learning, more growing, more evolving to come." Many expressed such ineffable pleasure in their work that heaven on earth seems to describe their daily experience. We will share some of that joy in the next chapter.

PART IV

Living Holism

7 *Practicing Holistic Medicine in a Technocratic Society*

I love my patients and have compassion for them. When I connect with them on that loving level, that's when I'm happiest. That's when I feel in the state of grace.
—KATHY FRYE, M.D.

What happens to the men and women who break ranks with the medical establishment to design their own career in healing? How do they approach the practice of medicine? What are their financial expectations? Their levels of satisfaction? These pioneers must respect the laws that govern medical practice. What are their concerns and precautions about malpractice and professional discipline? From the joy with which these physicians pursue their vocations as their destinies, we can find hope for the future of American medicine, which we will venture to predict in chapter 8. Throughout this chapter, we draw heavily on our interview material to allow the physicians who both practice and live holistically to describe the quality of their everyday lives.

What Is a Holistic Physician?

According to the "Principles of Holistic Medical Practice" adopted by the American Holistic Medical Association in 1993, "Holistic physicians embrace a variety of safe, effective options in diagnosis and treatment, including education for lifestyle changes and self-care; complementary approaches; and conventional drugs and surgery. . . . Holistic physicians encourage patients to evoke the healing power of love, hope, humor, and enthusiasm and to release the toxic consequences of hostility, shame, greed, depression and prolonged fear, anger, and grief."

When we asked our interviewees if they considered themselves to be "holistic physicians," most offered an unequivocal assent. Kathy Frye said, "I sure do. I always have." Chris Northrup affirmed, "Yes, absolutely, I am a holistic practitioner. I like the word." Scott Anderson said, "Basically I consider myself a holistic physician because I take the whole person into account. Due to my years of yoga and meditation, I feel that I have an unusual background from which to consider the whole person." Both Sandra Kamiak and Bethany Hays said, "I'm a holistic physician; I look at the totality of the person." Bill Manahan articulated the link between his practice and his life: "I consider that I am trying to be a holistic person; so if I'm a holistic person, whatever I do with respect to practice is, I hope, holistic."

Several physicians found the label problematic, among them Jim Gordon, who said, "I think the label carries with it a kind of flaky air. I don't advertise the word, but I accept it. I am a physician, and if you want to call me an alternative doctor, I'll say that's true. I work with complementary medicine; I'm a holistic physician." Ed Neal said that he "could never figure out what it means to be a holistic physician. Those I encountered at the AHMA were nicer and listened to people's problems more and used herbs, but the idea of holistic is much more fundamental, much more being able to move in and out of paradigms. I would consider myself a budding holistic practitioner—evolving."

The ambivalence expressed by Neal and Gordon about the label "holistic physician" seems to turn on whether one is talking philosophy or technique. Michael Greenberg thinks that "very few people use the term 'holistic' appropriately . . . it's a buzzword. What many people do in holistic medicine is take nonallopathic therapies and plug them into the medical model. Holism is embracing life as it is, embracing our illness." Alan Gaby makes this distinction: "Alternative medicine is technique . . . whereas holism is an attitude—an attitude that you will spend adequate time with a patient and help them with all aspects of their health—body, mind, and spirit; and that you will work with them as partner in taking responsibility for their health."

In spite of some disagreement over the label, one commonality that unites the physicians in our study is that they have deviated intentionally and significantly from the norms and values inculcated in medical school and reinforced by organized medicine. None of them, for example, held membership in the American Medical Association. Most belonged to no state, county, or local medical group; yet their lives were characterized by study, inquiry, and service. The direction of these activities was radically different than the concerns of their cohorts within orthodox medicine. Since this book is based on interviews, not on ethnographic observation of actual practices, here we can only take them at their word. It remains for future researchers to conduct on-site ethnography to determine to what extent holistic physicians do or do not live up to the philosophies of practice they articulated so clearly to us.

Definitions of Holistic Medicine

We received much richer information and a high degree of consensus when we asked our interviewees to define holistic medicine. According to Bill Manahan, "Holistic medicine is looking at the whole system—body, mind and spirit and environment. When you come to me as a patient, I have as much to learn from you as you have to learn from me. It's adult-to-adult interaction." Jim Gordon defines holistic medicine as "using those modalities which are least harmful first; it works with people in their context and creates other kinds of healing contexts. It sees each person as unique and it understands the spiritual dimension of health care as well as of each person's life unfolding." Bethany Hays sees holistic medicine as "a philosophy which considers the whole person and all of the possibilities for healing. It is inclusive rather than exclusive."

The doctors we interviewed ran the gamut from those who broadly accepted the philosophy of holism to those with a high degree of training in the practice of a particular holistic modality. Although the holistic model as articulated by the physicians in our survey varies from person to person, regardless of its form, it represents a long and courageous walk away from the orthodox model. And although for many the impetus to shift from doctor to healer was clear, dramatic, and compelling, the outcome—the eventual working-out—was a journey through uncharted territory. What began as a soul impulse for many of these physicians now requires the attention to detail and worldly matters that any other career shift entails. Len Saputo points out that "doctors need to put in a lot of study before they start doing new things. It's not simple stuff. It takes a whole different mentality to shift from left- to right-brain integration." One doctor we spoke to who is now actively employing alternative methods described a need to "unlearn what had been learned" before learning the new techniques.

In 1993 the board of the AHMA developed and adopted a list of "Principles of Holistic Medical Practice" (see table 7.1). Presently this organization is leading the way toward the definition and certification of a medical specialty known as holistic medicine, which will be further discussed in the following chapter.

One model for holistic practice was the intense study of another modality. Several physicians in our study undertook this type of study. Sandra Kamiak explained: "I wouldn't go out and do something I had no training in. So, while homeopathy is really on the edge, I went through a very good three-year training program, and have the guidance of other physicians who are practicing this way. I feel it is important to have training and experience to practice complementary methods, and not to just 'wing it.'"

Others designed courses of self-study that prepared them to add new therapies to their repertoire. Len Saputo takes them one at a time: "I respect the integrity of other traditions and try not to be a dabbler. I respect acupuncture, Chinese medicine, homeopathy, naturopathy. When the time comes to learn one or the other, I will go into it whole hog." Scott Anderson

TABLE 7.1 PRINCIPLES OF HOLISTIC MEDICAL PRACTICE ADOPTED BY THE AMERICAN HOLISTIC MEDICAL ASSOCIATION, 1993

1. Holistic physicians embrace a variety of safe, effective options in diagnosis and treatment, including education for life-style changes and self-care; complementary approaches; and conventional drugs and surgery.
2. Searching for the underlying causes of disease is preferable to treating symptoms alone.
3. Holistic physicians expend as much effort in establishing what kind of patient has a disease as they do in establishing what kind of disease a patient has.
4. It is preferable to diagnose and treat patients as unique individuals rather than as members of a disease category.
5. When possible, life-style modifications are preferable to drugs and surgery as initial therapeutic options.
6. Prevention is preferable to treatment and is usually more cost-effective. The most cost-effective approach evokes the patient's own innate healing capabilities.
7. Illness is viewed as a manifestation of a dysfunction of the whole person, not as an isolated event.
8. In most situations, encouragement of patient autonomy is preferred to decisions imposed by physicians.
9. The ideal physician-patient relationship considers the needs, desires, awareness, and insight of the patient as well as those of the physician.
10. The quality of the relationship established between physician and patient is a major determinant of healing outcomes.
11. Physicians significantly influence patients by their example.
12. Illness, pain, and the dying process can be learning opportunities for patients and physicians.
13. Holistic physicians encourage patients to evoke the healing power of love, hope, humor, and enthusiasm and to release the toxic consequences of hostility, shame, greed, depression, and prolonged fear, anger, and grief.
14. Unconditional love is life's most powerful emotion. Holistic physicians strive to adopt an attitude of unconditional love for patients, themselves, and other practitioners.
15. Optimal health is much more than the absence of sickness. It is the conscious pursuit of the highest qualities of the spiritual, mental, emotional, physical, environmental, and social aspects of the human experience.

These principles appear in the AHMA brochure.

has a similar plan: "I did not hang up a shingle saying I practice nutritional medicine until I had sufficient understanding of it to do so. In a few years, feeling really grounded in nutrition, I may take the time it requires to learn another modality."

Len Saputo described the tremendous span of the general field of holistic medicine and his struggle to deal with its vastness:

> In the physical plane, I like to look at cellular metabolism as a primary base, rather than at disease syndromes which have special names. I think the cause of disease is one thing, and that's cellular malfunction. And that's caused by only two things: too much of something—which is toxicity—or too little—which is deficiency. When you think that way, you get to a more primary biochemical level, and altering the metabolism of the cell has an outcome on how you are. On an energetic plane, however, it has nothing to do with biochemistry. It may have to do with vibrational frequencies, with thought. A variety of spiritual disciplines are on a whole different plane, and I have not made that transition as much as I'd like to. I'm focused on the cellular stuff, and that has been enough of a stretch—coming from my medical training.

As Saputo so clearly explains, the field of holistic medicine stretches from the microscopic level of the cell to the macroscopic level of spirit and energy. David Gershan extends Saputo's argument: "The materialist paradigm is only a fraction of the really real. How we think we are scientific involves such a pure, narrow corridor of data gathering. You will find in every case the necessity to use the person, the soul, as a player in scientific work." Ed Neal, who is a Jungian analyst as well as a physician, unites these micro- and macrocosmic perspectives: "Now I see things holographically. When I look at someone, instead of seeing their body, I see a pattern of distortion which is reflected in their body, and in their words, and in their thinking, and in their spirituality." Ideally, the physician in holistic practice, at first bewildered by the complexity of this emergent field, will eventually reach such an integrated view.

Healing in Practice: Diagnosis and Treatment

The underlying tenets of the paradigms we described in a somewhat abstract way come alive when we examine how medical treatment differs for a doctor in the technomedical paradigm compared to a holistic physician. To recapitulate a portion of our earlier discussion in a more integrated form, we call on the work of physician Dean Black (1993:2–5), who explains that technomedicine's underlying goal is to *substitute* for the body. It does this in three main ways. If a physiological function, such as immunity, is weak, an antibiotic may be prescribed to substitute for the immune system. A second type of substitution may entail mimicking normal chemical processes—for example, using pharmaceutically prepared insulin. "In principle, these substitutes 'cure' the body by providing mechanisms that relieve the body of portions of its normal challenges." Surgery is the third means of substitution and is used when the challenge is mechanical—for example, when the body cannot dissolve a tumor, it is surgically removed.

The holistic doctor's objective, in contrast, is to *normalize* the body and restore it to a condition of unaided health. "Proponents of natural health argue that if you create artificial environments (through drugs) for patients, you create artificial health which prevails only so long as the artificial environment persists" (Black 1993:5), and that if you treat all patients the same, you ignore differences in their situations which may provide the very key to their health. The doctor using natural means works with the vital principle and has an abiding faith in the ability of the patient, in cooperation with his or her environment, to assume or resume a state of balance. Natural doctors, knowing that each case is unique, are not so concerned with *how* the outcome is achieved, since it will never be precisely the same with another patient. They are also aware of the synergy of various therapeutics and may simultaneously prescribe multiple approaches such as nutrition, somatics, herbs, and energy work, as Jim Gordon did with his patient Leslie Newman. The vital force responds to subtle, consistent care and support. Providing this is beyond the capacity of the practitioner alone, but must be done through a change of consciousness within the patient. When a physician is working to support the vital principle, the breadth of lifestyle modifications required of the patient can be extensive.

Thus, healing in the holistic model means designing and adopting new ways of working with patients that are radically different than the actions in a conventional medical encounter. The following series of quotations describes how several holistic doctors approach what might have been called "diagnosis" in the technomedical model.

> Some of the history-taking I do looks like Western medicine, but actually I'm covering a much broader range in trying to understand the person. I see every experience as valuable for people. I start off with the sense that everything we're going through has something to teach us. . . . I have a sense that there's a process of transformation going on in both the patient and in me, and that we're engaged in a dance together—partners in a sacred dance. My role is to help the person learn the dance and, ultimately, dance on her own. (Jim Gordon)

> I think a good physician taking a medical history from a patient must allow time for all the little details to come out, to . . . form a kind of holo-

graphic picture of what's really going on—in three dimensions. You need to follow patients where they lead you, and at the same time you've got your agenda. . . . It's the most fun part of my job. A patient-oriented diagnosis really requires being able to accept ambiguity and take the patient's symptoms at face value, not just the ones that fit into your little sieve so you can filter out the rest. That's the exciting part of the history. The exciting part intellectually is solving a difficult chronic problem and uncovering the interweaving factors—metabolically, nutritionally, and environmentally—that provide the key to unlock the person's problem. (Barry Elson)

My view is really different, but if we were going to use the mechanistic model, I'd look at the car from head to tail and say, "OK, I see the carburetor has a problem, but what's *causing* the carburetor's problem?" I try to look at things causally rather than symptomatically. (Ann McCombs)

Suppose you come in for a sinus problem. And I look through your chart and I say, "Do you get sick much?" "No, it's the first time I've been sick in five years." I'll give you an antibiotic and you're out of there in five minutes. But if I glance through your chart or you say, "Yeah, I get this two or three times every year and this is my fourth time this year," I just go, whoa!! And I'm amazed, in twenty-five minutes, we literally can get right to the core. It doesn't take very long. Because everybody knows what's going on. I'll just say, "You know, you're a healthy thirty-five-year-old woman and you don't smoke and you're not living in a very polluted area. So what do you think's going on? Why would your body be doing this to you?" And she'll say, "Oh, my family has some allergies, and it's just common." And I'll say, "Did you do this when you were fifteen or eighteen?" "No." "Well, then why the last two or three years are you getting sick three times a year? It doesn't make sense to me. Your immune system's great—I can tell by looking at you." And then they'll just pour out this stuff, which they have been thinking about all along. "Well, I've been working two jobs" . . . or "My husband is this" . . . or "My thirteen-year-old is driving me crazy" . . . or "My mother-in-law died and now my father-in-law is living with us for the last six months." They get right into it. It doesn't take very long. (Bill Manahan)

What is it that determines health? That has more to do with attitudes and beliefs than with lack of access to health care resources such as hospitals and the like. . . . So I've specialized in exploring with my clients limiting beliefs that can stay in the way of thriving beliefs, such as "I don't deserve to be healthy," or "I'm supposed to be this way. I owe it to my parents . . . to follow this script.". . . Having seen and identified these beliefs, we can move past them. Whatever can be named, can be tamed! (Barry Sultanoff, "Physician in Transition" 1993).

As these examples demonstrate, diagnosis in holistic healing ranges from attention to the biochemistry of cells to a focus on the roles of emotion, attitude, belief, and spirit. These physicians express an appreciation for the emergent, ongoing nature of the holistic diagnostic process, which Jim Gordon describes as a "sacred dance" between physician and patient. They stress the importance of looking beyond symptoms to find the *cause* of the problem, of being willing to "follow the patients where they lead," and of the individual's social, environmental, emotional, mental, and spiritual context. In every case, context is critical, as Peter Grote explains: "Nobody has a medical problem or some symptom without having some emotion attached to that and some emotional response, and it's often the emotional response that creates the most disruption in their daily life. You also have to think about how the rest of the family is dealing with the person who is anxious about their headaches."

Where conventional medical education emphasizes the similarities among persons and situations and advocates diagnosing medical problems in a standardized way, holism focuses on the patient's uniqueness and differentiating qualities, and advocates a free-form, highly individualized approach.

The treatment approaches our interviewees described were as comprehensive and varied as their creative approaches to diagnosis. Bethany Hays provides an example:

> A lady came to me who was pregnant for the fifth time after losing four pregnancies. The first loss had been due to fibroids in her uterus. Before she got pregnant the fifth time, I sent her to a fertility specialist to see if the fibroids should be removed, but he said they were too small. During this fifth pregnancy, her ultrasound at six weeks showed three small fibroids. By ten weeks they had more than doubled in size. I said to her, "Because there is so much estradiol in a woman's system during pregnancy, that's a common time for fibroids to grow. The only thing I know we can do is to block the effect of estradiol on the fibroids by using phyto-estrogen. This is how that works: the weaker plant estrogen binds with the estrogen-binding site and blocks the stronger estradiol that your body is making. Soy is the richest source of plant estrogens, so I recommend that you eat soy at least three times a day."
>
> And she did! She ate soy three times a day—even carried a Baggie with soy nuts around with her. And by twelve weeks her fibroids had stopped growing. She is currently thirty weeks pregnant and the fibroids are almost completely gone. The only evidence of fibroids I can now find by ultrasound is a thickening in the front wall of her uterus.
>
> Conventional medicine knows that sometimes fibroids grow and sometimes they don't grow, but it can do nothing about stopping them from growing. A conventional doctor would say that the reason the fibroids

stopped growing is that she infarcted the fibroids [they outgrew their blood supply and died]. But that causes pain and usually bleeding, and she had none of that.

The other thing we did was give her lots of emotional support. A woman who has lost four pregnancies doubts herself and her ability to carry another pregnancy to term. Success in this case took lots of support, and giving her a therapy she could believe in. By changing her diet under her own willpower, she created *for herself* an intervention that worked. And as a result, her confidence in her ability to carry a baby expanded exponentially.

As Hays indicates, holistic doctors work very conscientiously on their relationship to the patients and to the process of healing itself; in addition, they develop the patience and skills required to explore the labyrinth of illnesses and their possible solutions both inside and outside the technomedical realm. Barry Elson proffers a comparison of technomedical and holistic approaches to the treatment of adult-onset diabetes:

The canon you're taught in medical school for adult-onset of diabetes is to tell the person to lose weight and stop right there. Of course, they're not going to at all. So you give them a week to lose weight and when they fail, you start them on hypoglycemic medication that artificially brings the blood sugar down. When that doesn't work, you just give insulin shots. And that's the beginning, the middle, and the end of treating diabetes in Western medicine. With orthomolecular medicine, we will first help them lose weight in a very carefully thought-out weight loss program with a counselor and nutritionist and plenty of emotional support. That's number one.

Number two, we work biochemically with them in a completely different way. Sure, if the patient needs insulin we'll give it, but we'll work biochemically to reduce the need for insulin or hypoglycemic medication. We'll give chromium to stabilize the blood sugar. If I give a diabetic chromium, her diabetes will improve. I know that—it's well documented in the medical literature. But how many physicians give chromium or Vitamin E or B12? The evidence for giving those three nutrients to prevent the sequellae of diabetes is overwhelming. It's all there in the medical literature, literally hundreds of articles. . . . I've read *those* articles; I don't just read the articles the drug companies offer.

Elson's incorporation of education and emotional support with careful attention to biochemistry is typical of the approaches of many holistic physicians who take the trouble to educate themselves about the intricacies of human psychology and microbiology. Like Elson, Bill Manahan keeps his focus moving between the macro and the micro levels as he works to elicit what the patient knows:

> Let's say you have headaches or fatigue. I'd say at one end it may be as simple as you need eight hours sleep instead of seven. Or it may be that you're eating too much sugar. Those are very physical things. And then in an hour and a half or two hours, we can go through way over to here, that it may be past-life stuff or it may be cosmic stuff or it may be that you're mad at your mother. I don't care at all; all I do is help you bring out the things you already know. That's why I don't see any people at my wellness center until I've talked to them on the phone. About 60 percent I don't have come in. Only about four out of ten come to see me. Because I can tell in five minutes if I'm going to enjoy it and if they're going to enjoy it. Does that make sense? I right away say, "I won't have any answers for you but I know that *you* have the answers. And the only questions are if (1) I can help you put them into some sort of sensible form, (2) if you're ready to hear them, and (3) if we can figure out if there are helpers outside of me who can help you as well. Because I'm not going to learn cranial and sacral manipulation, acupuncture . . . you know. I couldn't learn all of it. That's why I call myself a holistic triager, you see. I can triage into "What do you think might be helpful for you?" It's fun!

In his interview, Manahan used the term "third-line medicine" to describe the way that many of the doctors in our study were working. According to him, third-line medicine "helps people who are struggling with the medical system, those with chronic pain or headache or hypertension, but who don't want to take medication. . . .Third-line medicine is needed when people have been through the system and it hasn't helped them." Jim Gordon expressed a similar view: "Basically I treat people who are completely at the end of their rope with conventional medicine and who are looking for something else—some kind of treatment, some other kind of person, some other kind of experience, some kind of hope."

Manahan, Gordon, and our other interviewees feel strongly that what is now "third line"—the medicine of last resort—should replace the technocratic approach as "first-line medicine"—a medicine of first resort, of healthy living and illness prevention that, most of the time, would preclude the need for cures. Bethany Hays points to the role of the physician in helping her patients make this conceptual shift: "I can now come up with enough data to convince most people that there is a connection between the mind and the body. They develop a different attitude about the illness. Instead of being angry or frustrated, they begin to work with it, and that opens up a lot of possibilities for healing. They may still decide to have surgery, but they ask, 'How did I get into a situation where surgery is the only option? How can I avoid this in the future?'"

Financial Considerations

None of the doctors we spoke to had become physicians because of the potential to earn above-average incomes. Terry Tyler pointed out that "medicine is not the right path if one's main interest is to make a lot of money. There are faster, less painful, and more effective ways to get rich. The depersonalizing process is not worth it." Len Saputo asks, "Who should be making half a million a year? If you're really dedicated to what you do, why would you want to do that? It doesn't need to come with it. I've never made a lot of money; never made six figures."

The physicians we interviewed ranged from those who no longer practice medicine by choice (for example, Luchakova, Travis, Dossey, Gaby) to those who practice a specialty (for example, Tyler, psychiatry; Greenberg, dermatology; Montero, plastic surgery; Hays, obstetrics); to primary care physicians who incorporate several alternative modalities (for example, Saputo, Anderson, Edelberg, Haas), and those who have chosen to concentrate on one (Frye and Kamiak, homeopathy). Each situation is likely to produce a different financial reward. The physicians who slowly incorporated their new approaches into an existing practice, like Saputo, Northrup, and Hays, seemed to have maintained a fairly consistent income level.[1] Several doctors, including Malka, Neal, and Gershan, split their time between their holistic practice and another medical job in a traditional setting that provided more income. In fact, we found that a surprising number of physicians, like Alex Cadoux, whose story introduced this book, work in emergency medicine or trauma centers while developing a holistic practice on a part-time basis—presumably because emergency medicine allows doctors to use Western medicine most effectively, which reduces the values-conflict of the doctor beginning to question technomedicine. Also, emergency medicine provides a reasonable income without the burden of a patient load.

A number of the physicians we spoke with consciously and contentedly lived modest lives. It is doubtful whether alternative medicine will ever return the same type of financial rewards as conventional medicine, due to two factors: the greater amount of the physician's time it requires, and the unfortunate effects of the current insurance and reimbursement systems.

For many physicians, time is money. Yet studying a person from a whole perspective requires more time than does the standard technocratic appointment. Questions must be asked about the emotional, spiritual, and social processes and context of the patient, and time must be allowed for a meaningful dialogue to develop. In addition, since the holistic approach is predicated on the uniqueness of each person and situation, assessment and treatment cannot be standardized but must be tailored to the individual. In addition to the time required for the consultation, holistic doctors need a certain quality of attention and deliberation in order to activate their intuitive abilities. This type of attention operates both inside and outside of linear time.

The impact of this is that the time when intuition may present information is uncertain. It may precede the patient's visit or come unexpectedly days or weeks following the visit. Homeopaths routinely "study the case," which means that they will not prescribe a remedy if they feel that they need to think about the person or even await a revealing dream to direct their work. Working with intuition requires a constant receptivity to information that might bear on a problem, as Deborah Malka suggests: "My psychic and intuitive skills are highly developed and I use them all the time. If I have a choice about making a rational, logical or an intuitive decision, I always go with the intuitive. My rational part does not have access to as much information as my intuitive."

Holistic physicians who integrate their intuitive abilities with their rational mind generally allow for longer initial visits in which to apply the art of open-ended questioning as well as active listening—two techniques designed to activate intuition. They may also take additional time to reflect before arriving at a plan for the client. Taking time and appreciating the uniqueness of each situation can provide a model for patients to work toward their own healing, but can also mean less income for the physician.

The second limiting factor on holistic doctors' incomes relates to the insurance and reimbursement debacle. Holistic physicians work within a framework wholly different from the one insurance companies base their rates on. As more and more primary care is provided within managed care settings, where the ideal patient visit is completed within a few minutes, the potential for reimbursement of holistic doctors' work diminishes. The fact that the holistic approach, while time-intensive in the beginning, offers a possibility for long-term resolution of chronic problems that otherwise would be very costly to treat has thus far had little impact on the insurance companies. According to Deborah Malka, "Insurance companies do not cover the time we spend with clients. They pay a hundred dollars for a new patient, and I spend two hours with them. Sometimes they do not even cover the diagnoses. They don't believe in chronic fatigue and food allergies—they would rather spend thousands on surgery than a few hundred to prevent it by helping people identify deficiencies in their diet."

Although it has become extremely difficult to practice outside of managed care's many organizational forms, most of the physicians we interviewed were unaffiliated. Three who were part of health maintenance organizations are not holistic physicians but humanists according to our definition—Masterson, LeManne, and Singer. They did not practice alternative techniques, but respected them. Two were frustrated and one, a subspecialist, was at peace in the situation. The holistic physicians in our study who were not part of managed care had quite original observations about it. Ed Neal does not even recognize it: "I ignore it. I don't need to make a lot of money. When I see so much pain, I'm not worried about being paid or not. The managed care thing . . . it's not a real thing." Len Saputo rejects managed care because of the constraints it would place on his ability to give effective holistic care: "I don't belong to any HMOs or PPOs. Frequently I take a half-hour for a follow-up visit [for which an HMO would not pay] because the holistic approach is much more comprehensive and people don't understand it all the time—it's important that they take responsibility for themselves. I don't want to assume responsibility for making choices for people when they are capable of doing it themselves." Most, like Michael Greenberg, feel that HMOs and holistic health care are incompatible:

> You can make a decent living. The people who are getting [paid a lot] are the docs who are very financially focused to begin with, who panicked initially when all this HMO stuff became fashionable. They felt if they didn't join these groups they were going to be left out in the cold. They deserted their colleagues. They did not collaborate. They unilaterally went out and made a decision to save their own skin and now that they have managed care, they are working very hard and they are not giving their patients much in the way of quality of service. They are not doing complete health care; they couldn't possibly do comprehensive or complementary health care like we are talking about.

Ann McCombs is less interested in making holistic medicine compatible with managed care than with offering patients a choice: "I think managed care is a joke, frankly. It's like saying, 'Let's do what we do more efficiently and get paid less for doing it.' . . . The average medical visit is seven minutes long and they want to bring that down further and have it cost less. Well, it's not going to happen, not if you're doing holistic medicine. So I'm not interested in bringing the holistic paradigm into managed care. I'm interested in opening it up as an *alternative* to managed care, so people have a choice."

David Edelberg quips about the absurdity of the managed care economic system, which collects money for health care services and realizes a profit if the services are not used:

> We got good at dealing with HMO patients. There were two thousand enrolled, which caused the offices to be mobbed. My downtown office had four exam rooms, and I moved from one to the other and I said, "I'm not really treating people anymore; I'm putting out fires. Let's just get this

> symptom taken care of and get the patient out." It's insane, this strange system. It defies all economic common sense that if you walk into your office and have an empty appointment book, it's a pretty good day economically because it doesn't use up your capitation. Imagine a beautician who walks in to an empty appointment book and says "Wow, no clients today; I'm really going to make some money!"

Finally, Saputo sees in the managed care phenomenon a healing crisis for medicine: "This is a wonderful thing to have happened. We learn from our mistakes. From catastrophe is where possibility develops and now that this disaster [managed care] has happened we are going to learn from it, to grow from it. And it's not going to be within our control as much as it is the community's."

Two trends seem likely to provide holistic doctors with the opportunity to support themselves from their work. First, more and more individuals are willing to pay out-of-pocket for health care provided by a skilled and compassionate holistic doctor, especially in view of the fact that the total expended may be far less than that required as copayments and deductibles, and the potential for long-term resolution of their problems is greater. Second, some insurance plans now specialize in reimbursing the work of various types of alternative health practitioners, although it is premature to speculate on the long-term stability of such plans. Predictions about them are especially problematic since they represent a mixing of paradigms, applying the financial structure of technomedicine to the holistic world. The underlying philosophies of the two approaches are too divergent to allow a happy marriage between insurance reimbursement and holistic medicine. Insurance companies are based on the sickness model and their financial structure reflects that. Healthy individuals are unlikely to pay premiums for care that they do not want and may not need. Holistic modalities do not translate well into the standardization of insurance terminology.

Because of the high degree of satisfaction they experience, most of the holistic doctors we interviewed have come to terms with the money issue, demonstrating, at yet another level, that a paradigm shift includes inner changes that prompt and support the outer changes. In short, these physicians have redefined the meaning of success, as Michael Greenberg explains:

> For those who became doctors to make money, great. Go for it. But for the majority who want to help people, they need to keep their focus on that. Don't get seduced. We live in a world where there is a strong belief that having more money will make us more happy—that happiness comes from getting money from somebody else. These people [patients] are our brothers and sisters. I make a very good living. I think that I deserve it from

> all the energy I put into life. But I don't go after it. It's not my focus. It just shows up as I need it to pay the mortgage. I don't chase after it. It finds me from what I do. It just works. It worked for me because it *is* me. I and my practice are one.
>
> I used to believe that a successful doctor had appointments booked six weeks in advance. I really like the fact that now anyone can call my office and there is space to see them that day. I always have just enough patients. My schedule is filled sometimes just a few days in advance. . . . I run a practice where people pay what they can afford—I tell them this in a letter. My colleagues told me I would go broke in six months. But I haven't. I cut my fees down before I had to. My standard of living has not changed through managed care at all. I *am* my practice. My beliefs become my reality. And so, the office just runs. . . .The patients just show up. They are parts of me showing up in the office. It's the most fun game I've ever played.

Bill Manahan illustrates how service in a larger context complements his medical practice as a way to give back what he has received:

> My philosophy [has been that] it's a privilege to be a physician—every patient we see, it's such an honor. It's hard to not make money as a physician, so my wife and I—she's a therapist—decided long ago that whenever I got close to making $100,000, we'd do something else. Therefore, every five or six years we stop practice for six to twelve months and do volunteer work of some sort. And then your salary goes back down. . . . We were in the Peace Corps for three years after my internship and then we went to a rural Hawaii site in '78–'79 and then in '88–'89 we went into inner-city Boston on a community health staff and then a year ago we went to Africa for six months and worked in a village clinic. That's sort of a guideline for how I say, "Am I getting too entrenched in the system?" Somehow $100,000 always seemed like more than enough.

And Kathy Frye has some advice for her more conventional colleagues: "So many of my colleagues at the hospital are miserable. They're all worried about the bottom line. . . . They're saddled with material processions. They've got a huge mortgage, a boat, a cabin, a couple of kids in college, and they're trying to find rewards outside of themselves by accumulating possessions. I tell them to sell the boat and have more fun!"

The Legal Environment

As practitioners of the art of healing, the doctors in our study have to some extent removed themselves from the economic thrust of medicine. Where do they stand, however, with respect to the law? What is the responsibility and right of doctors who no longer practice the type of medicine they were taught and licensed to practice? And what are their concerns? Although many of the doctors in our study had been sued, they had been sued not for anything related to the practice of holistic medicine but rather for events within their allopathic practices.

Practicing natural medicine or using any of the alternative methods requires that doctors use techniques and approaches outside the scope of their training. This has personal, social, professional, and legal implications. How do they know, and how does the public know, that they are competent? If challenged, against what standard are they to be measured? These are a few of the legal ramifications doctors need to consider when they change the way they practice medicine. As we shall hear from our interviewees, most feel protected because of the understanding that develops between practitioner and patient. As patients assume more responsibility for themselves, they no longer expect godlike infallibility from their doctor. Doctors who practice holistically also tend to communicate more fully and to explain not only the options, risks, and benefits, but to lay the choice squarely on the shoulders of the patient.

SCOPE OF PRACTICE

When medical doctors practice medicine as they were trained to do, they are said to be practicing within the "scope of their practice." When M.D.'s practice another healing modality, such as herbology, nutrition, acupuncture, or homeopathy, they are practicing within the scope of that discipline, whether or not it has been codified or recognized. (Acupuncturists, for example, are licensed while nutritionists, at this writing, are not.) Physicians assume they are able to use various therapies because they are licensed to diagnose and treat disease. A generally unexplored area in need of systematic research is physicians' assumption that they can use various therapies because they are licensed to diagnose and treat disease. Although the substances and techniques of the so-called alternative practices are not part of physicians' training, it is generally assumed that they may be used under the medical doctor mantle.

One authority who has studied and written extensively about these questions is attorney Jerry Green (1985, 1988), who concludes that holistic doctors are best protected legally through two strategies. The first is to distinguish between "the treatment of pathology and the maintenance of health. With this clarification, the doctor can determine when s/he is operating within the scope of practice of an MD and when s/he is within the scope of practice of another type of practitioner" (1978:np). Green believes this distinction may provide a basis for defense in the event of a malpractice suit. For example, a man may sue his doctor because the herb lobelia did not relieve his asthma. A medical doctor would be expected to prescribe medications and inhalers to relieve asthma. However, for an herbalist, lobelia is an excellent choice. Expert testimony from the field of herbal healing might be more relevant in a case like this than testimony from medical doctors who know nothing about herbs. The question of culpability would turn on whether the doctor was practicing as an M.D. or as an herbalist, which would depend on how the doctor described him- or herself at the time of the consultation and recommendation, and what expectations and level of responsibility the patient had.

CONTRACTS WITH PATIENTS

Green's second strategy by which holistic doctors may legally protect themselves is to develop a contract for shared responsibility between doctor and patient—a verbal agreement between the person seeking care and the one providing it.

> It would greatly clarify the doctor-patient relationship if people had a better understanding of what they legitimately can expect from their physicians. Medicine as it is currently defined and practiced is actually a science of pathology, designed to treat illness, injury, and disease. . . . The treatment of pathology is far different from the maintenance of health. . . . We have come to believe that medicine and health are synonymous and have grown to expect health from our doctors. This assumption has remained implied [and] has led to unrealistic expectations which go unfulfilled and lead to litigation. *This misunderstanding, not medical negligence, was the common denominator in most of the malpractice cases I was exposed to.* (1978:np; italics in original)

The contract Green recommends should contain the three standard elements of contracts: first, state the purpose of the relationship; second, outline the responsibilities of each party; third, designate the term or length of time the contract is in force (1982:367–368). Green suggests that courts might look to these agreements in adjudications rather than to the "standard of care" required by medical convention.

Christiane Northrup describes her own take on the physician-patient contract:

> I have developed an intuitive feeling about which patients can own their own will. Can they make some of these decisions on their own? I used to push the envelope a great deal, give them more credit for decision making. I don't do that anymore. Am I going to set myself up as an adversary with every patient who walks in, or am I going to dare to cross the line into a healing partnership? If I feel they are not up to this, I'll say, "Look, if you and I are operating in the paradigm where I own your breasts, and you don't, then I'm going to order all the tests in the book, and we're going to rack up a big bill."

The concept of sharing responsibility with the patient, although highly unusual for medical doctors in general, had almost universal acceptance in our study group. Interviewees felt that it freed them to be creative in their approach, to generate options, and, most importantly, to develop warm and collegial relationships with their patients. Yet not everyone who consults a holistic doctor is prepared to assume responsibility, a point Deborah Malka underscores: "The number of people who come to see me, who are very sick, but who are afraid to step out of the old program for even a moment, just shocks me. There is an awful lot of fear of taking self-responsibility."

As Larry Dossey points out, the lawsuit issue itself springs from the technomedical paradigm, which encourages both doctors and patients to seek the illusion of perfection:

> I think we, as a culture, are obsessed with assigning responsibility and expecting human beings to live up to a standard that is not humanly possible. That's called perfection. But even the best-intentioned and best-trained people make terrible mistakes. As a culture we cannot have it both ways. We cannot expect physicians to be healers and come from the heart, be compassionate, use alternative methods, and demand that they be flawless. If we hold doctors to these impossible standards, what will we see? Doctors trying to practice defensive medicine. Consumers will get a boiled-down, inhumane approach to health care.

Physicians who use holistic methods seem to have confidence in the power of communication, and, although many of those interviewed had been sued, they do not, on the whole, fear suits related to the practice of holistic medicine. "I think it's related to how you treat people," Sandra Kamiak said. "People sue for really strange reasons, sometimes not even a clinical issue, when you don't have good rapport." David Edelberg concurs: "It's a different relationship with your patients. They have my home phone number; my kids answer the phone. We get to know these people; they're family. If they've got a problem with something, we say, 'Come, let's not argue about it—we want you to get well.'"

Money is not the issue anyway, according to Dawn LeManne: "I always give my best to my patient; I give them my heart. And if I'm sued, I know I gave them my best. Of course I make mistakes; everybody makes mistakes, but I can still feel in my heart that I did the best that I humanly could. If they want to sue me . . . they can have my money. It's not what I'm doing it for." And power need not be an issue either, says Peter Nunn: "The main reason people sue is they get in a power struggle when the doctor pretends he's right, when he's clearly wrong. If you can keep talking to the patient, and particularly to their families, then you don't get sued."

In addition to practicing good communication, holistic doctors refine their ability to sense which patients are and which are not good risks for atypical procedures. Bethany Hays explained, "I make sure that I offer my patients the standard of care. I say, 'Most doctors would do this. If you're interested we can talk about other things that might work.' I don't offer much that doesn't have data to support it. If you do that, you have to take responsibility for it." Chris Northrup said that she was "not willing to order a bunch of tests that I think are ridiculous. People order MRIs for a fibroid uterus. That's an $800 to $1,500 test. I'd rather rely on my hands. We have the illusion that if we order more tests, we'll be safe. I'm not going to play those games, so my laser beam, my law of attraction beam, is much clearer."

Another strategy employed to protect against litigation is the physician's willingness to acknowledge real or potential mistakes. Ann McCombs said:

> I do everything I can do to be in relationship with my patients. The person at the front desk welcomes them warmly at the first contact. I follow through on every patient complaint. I take it to the nth degree and try to resolve it, because I don't believe the court has anything to do with justice. I really take time with my clients, and it's hard to sue people you're in relationship with even if you've made a mistake. And it's possible for anyone to make a mistake. I think we've all made them one time or another, but it's a matter of what you can do to rectify it. I suppose if I lived fully from this place, I wouldn't have malpractice insurance. But I searched until I found a company to give my malpractice money to that supports holistic physicians.

Along the same lines, Barry Elson believes that "doctors who spend a lot of time with their patients, who get to know them as people not as diseases, who do not take an authoritarian approach but a collaborative approach, generally do not get sued. Malpractice arises when a doctor gets knocked off a pedestal he helped create. The patient expects the doctor to do a perfect job, and then finds out he is a human being who botched something. Then it's too late to find the middle ground—working together as a team."

Practicing within the litigious specialty of obstetrics and gynecology, Chris Northrup had to come to terms with her risks. She states, in strong terms, what many of the physicians we interviewed had also concluded about "malpractice": "The lawsuits helped me understand what the legal system is all about. In the alcoholic family that is our culture, there's got to be someone to blame. I was willing to go to court, to sit through that, to give up my medical license if I couldn't practice the way I felt was fit. . . . There are other things I can do."

PROFESSIONAL CENSURE

While the doctors we spoke with generally felt that they were in command of attitudes and practices which minimized the risk of lawsuits from patients, they viewed the threat from the government or their own profession, although much less likely, as potentially more devastating. The government has waged several well-publicized and many unpublicized campaigns, through the courts and various agencies, against holistic physicians in the past twenty-five years. Generally, but not always, the FDA acts in concert with state medical licensing boards to build a case against these doctors. The FDA accuses and has the police arrest a doctor for using a nonapproved substance or treatment, and the licensing board follows through with accusations of negligence. With negligence defined as not doing what other doctors do (meeting the standard of care), the two policing agencies work hand in glove. The substances under scrutiny may be nutritional, as was the case with Jonathan Wright in Washington, or biochemical, as with Stanislaw S. Burzynski in Texas. Regardless of the nature of the charge, the resources required to defend oneself against an accusation take a huge toll financially and emotionally.

We have explained how the tenets of the holistic model are extremely threatening to the conventional paradigm. Guns-drawn FDA raids and seizure of records, as was Jonathan Wright's experience, are dramatic enactments of how serious this threat is. Typically, as in Wright's case, the FDA agents arrive unannounced and armed and shut down the medical practice on the spot. This interrupts any consultation in progress as well as disrupting, if not terminating, the care being given to the other patients in the practice. (Imagine a corporation suspected of polluting the environment being forced to cease operations at the time it is accused, and its chief executive arrested.) Typically, in the ensuing trial, scores of patients will appear to testify that the doctor's treatment helped them, but their testimony is not considered evidence since *efficacy* is not on trial. What is the real issue?

Canadian sociologist Murray E. G. Smith (1994:3552–3563) provided a brilliant analysis of Burzynski's systematic medical isolation in both Canada and the United States based not on his research or treatment, but solely on his violation of the social ethics of organized medicine. Burzynski's long saga involved his prosecution for the development and use of a biochemical substance that has brought about cancer remission in a large number of terminally ill people. As Smith points out, during almost ten years this prosecution lasted, the doctor was never disciplined by any medical organization. Smith maintains that Burzynski's critics have no case against his medical practice, which is the presumed basis for the accusation, but have built their case based on his violation of the medical profession's need to "promulgate and defend policies and procedures which are in harmony with dominant socioeconomic interests." Patients' abilities to choose among a wide variety of alternatives will eventually undercut "the profession's ability to shape and control its own market" (1994:356).

Patients' feelings about their treatment and its outcome are of little consequence in these types of allegations. In the technomedical model, where patients have no authority and, therefore, no responsibility, they are presumed unqualified to evaluate their medical care. Chris Northrup was reported to the medical board by a colleague for recommending a macrobiotic diet for a woman who, the doctor thought, had sigmoid colon cancer. "But the woman, herself, was thrilled with the care, and never even had cancer. The long and short of it is *she* had no complaint, but *he* did." This is a perfect illustration of the closed, tautological system at work.

Karl Humiston's experience provides another example. For years Humiston explored many different techniques in an attempt to help his psychiatric patients. After stumbling upon the role of chemical sensitivities and food allergies in mental illness, he began to test his patients for these conditions, which resulted in a complaint to the state disciplinary board about unconventional practice. "At the informal hearing it was decided that there was nothing that required further action; however my colleagues [supported] my being fired" ("Physician in Transition" 1990).

In recent decades, the rights struggles of every other group—"women, children, prisoners, students, tenants, gays, Chicanos, Native Americans, and welfare clients" (Starr 1982:388)—resulted in some gains, but that of freedom to practice and receive the healing arts of choice not only failed to make any headway, it went further and further underground. However, in recent years, the Freedom of Choice legislation movement has introduced bills to allow patients to receive treatment from the practitioner and through the modality of their choice as long as there is no evidence the treatment causes harm. The bills have passed in several states, and legislation has been proposed at the national level as the Access to Medical Treatment Act, introduced in February 1997. This far-reaching legislation offers the first legal mandate for the peaceful coexistence of holistic healing modalities and conventional medicine.

As long as the technomedical model retains its hegemony, holistic doctors, by the very definition and descriptions we have provided in this book, will be jeopardizing their careers and livelihood through the choices they make every day. In the next section we will look at how they are regarded by other doctors—those practicing within the hegemonic "standard of care."

Relations with Peers

Despite the cruelty and persecution shown by medical regulatory and government agencies from time to time, individual doctors tend to regard their holistic colleagues in a rather benign way, although often from a distance. When they do interact, however, the responses of the conventional doctors seem to range from confrontation to admiration, with a smattering of curiosity. Bethany Hays says, "I don't know how they've reacted. I don't think they know what I'm doing. Most of what's changed is inside of me and between me and my patients. We do get called the 'granola doctors' up in Yarmouth, but I don't find that very threatening. I find it entertaining." Len Saputo, whose work has attracted interest, has met mostly with admiration, "I would say the bulk of my colleagues (I'm in a ten-man call group) are in awe of the stuff I know and they want to learn about it. But it's within some limits because I've provided them material to read about the things I know and I find that they don't really spend much time reading. They say, 'It's kind of complicated. I didn't really understand it.'"

"Some [conventional doctors] are definitely supportive, some are not," Sandra Kamiak says. "Some are just waiting. It's not so much approval or disapproval, but lack of knowledge." David Edelberg finds that sometimes information helps: "I've never had any problems with physicians. This work requires diplomacy, seeing where people are having mixed emotions, focusing right in on the mixed emotions and talking about then. Like a doctor might say 'I don't really like crystal therapy.' 'That's funny,' I'd say, 'only doctors think of alternative medicine as crystals; the public thinks alternative medicine is acupuncture. How do you feel about that?' 'Oh, that's fine.'"

Barry Elson and Larry Dossey made the same discovery. "Over the years, more and more doctors have referred their patients to me," Elson said. "Perhaps some respect my practice when they see what I am doing and that I am doing it in a very careful and conscious way. Often I'll send a medical article along with a letter explaining my treatment so that the doctor can understand that I'm doing the same kind of critical thinking they are, but in a different field. I'm doing it in the field of nutrition and metabolism, but there is a scientific basis for what I'm doing." Larry Dossey said, "I appeal to my colleagues basically on the basis of data. If you talk their language, and you can point to studies that conform to good science, then they listen. They don't stand up and cheer [but] they generally are respectful of the view that emphasizes consciousness. By 'respectful' I don't mean leading the parade."

Conversely, Jim Gordon finds that some conventional physicians react negatively to new information. "Some of them are very kind of affectionate and curious and open. Others are wary. . . . When I go someplace and talk, some people get very angry. [At my last talk] most of the physicians were interested, but there were a couple of older guys who were very suspicious, and kept saying, 'There's no evidence for this.' And I said, 'There is some evidence for this. Have you read the studies?' And they were offended that I was trying to present a different point of view; they were sure there was nothing to it, and had a difficult time looking at the evidence."

Perhaps the most sympathetic, according to Ann McCombs, are "the ones that are the closet holistic types; they're responsive. . . . They start by referring me a patient, saying, 'Well, maybe you should have a try at this one.' The ones who are outright negative, I don't tend to draw those types anymore. . . . I've just made up my mind in this lifetime that this is not what I want to do. I'm not a Jonathan Wright at heart. I would rather work quietly."

The lack of sympathy from local colleagues can be difficult, nevertheless. Bill Manahan said, "The physicians in our hometown—some are against it, and some are fairly good supporters, and the vast majority is in the middle. I think one of my more painful experiences happened after my book *Eat for Health* came out. It's not very radical—it talks about the dangers of the medical diseases that can happen with dairy or sugar or things. I had maybe five or six physicians come to the book signing, but I never got feedback from even one of the ninety physicians in our town . . . even though I play bridge every month with some of them."

Power

The idea of power is central to how physicians conduct themselves. The belief that there is a right way to do things and that the answer resides within the physician contributes to a tremendous amount of power for doctors. Tom Rusk, M.D. (1993) defines this type of "positional power" as "the ability to influence others in a way that is defined by their role or job." In contrast, "personal power" is a sense of authority that flows from who one is as a person.[2] Wanting to wield only personal power, Ed Neal was forced by his patients to come to terms with the positional power that accrues to his status as an M.D.:

> Right now, "power" is a bad word because so much of it has been vertical power, power over people. But power also moves horizontally. One thing that's good about being a doctor is the power with patients. When I first started practicing medicine I didn't want that—I wanted everyone to call me Ed, but people didn't want to. . . . Patients kept throwing power back at me, and it finally dawned on me that the relationship I was in was a really ancient one, and that people needed to work out their illness with

> somebody sitting there, playing that role, the role that is transpersonal. . . . Not accepting that power was being irresponsible, even though it doesn't really have much to do with me. Now when I go to work, I put on my professional clothes and let people work out their stuff. People need to put out their illness on an archetype, so that they can chew on that and activate things within themselves. That's part of holding the healing space.

In his willingness to accept his transpersonal archetypal power, Neal is revitalizing the physician's shamanic role. Likewise, Bill Manahan describes a dawning awareness of the importance of acknowledging and using his power:

> I have a lot of power, I've found out, and I struggle with that power. I have everything just laid out. I'm white and I'm male and I'm an M.D.—I have all the advantages. And I'm an athlete, I can play any game—it's like there's never been anything that's hard for me and I've always felt guilty about that. . . . In the last year, I've owned my power. It's okay to have it—it's just a matter of how I use it, and to use it in ways that are caring and loving and are not hierarchical.

Several physicians acknowledged medical training as the source that supplied not just positional but personal power. They valued the character development that came from the same rigors of training which nearly overwhelmed them. It seems that letting go of the authoritarian and hierarchical trappings allowed them to tap into the mystery of the initiation process itself. As Bethany Hays noted, her medical training gave her the technical skills to "walk between the worlds." Barry Elson stressed the power it brought: "The M.D. degree in our society is the ticket to getting in the door. It allows me to practice the way I want to. There is a certain recognition people will give you, and they'll seek your advice because you are an M.D. It allows you to reach more people with whom you can develop a healing bond." Ed Neal added:

> I'm really proud of having done the work. It was hard work. What was really of value was being in the fire. . . . Seeing really sick people and being stressed to the max. . . . The life force is a very powerful force. Five in the morning, patients screaming and throwing up, you get a very good picture of that. That was a very good experience, but not a nice one. . . . It shows you your limitations. And the other thing which is not to be disregarded is you have the "Good Housekeeping stamp of approval." I don't have to fight with people if I want to do something. I can do acupuncture, or whatever. Power comes from that.

The Bridge

The idea of building a bridge between the healing paths of technomedicine and holism came up many times in our interviews and discussions. The bridge is a potent symbol for expressing the essence of these physicians' experience of transition from one paradigm to another, and for both creating and acknowledging the links between their training and former methods of practice and the new values and modalities they are learning. Several used the bridge metaphor to express their desire to mediate between the paradigms, to link them in practice, or to explain the exciting possibilities that arise from combining them.

Sometimes they themselves may become the bridge, as Michael Greenberg was advised to do: "It's in the belief system. I believe some doctors have left standard medicine because they believe it can't work. If they just alter their beliefs they can stay there. As a matter of fact, they're probably needed there. When they leave medicine they become outsiders and people don't listen to them. Bernie Siegel said this to me: 'It's a good thing you're staying [in medical practice] because you become a bridge, a mystic in a white coat.'" Kathy Frye too takes Siegel's advice: "I really see myself as a bridge. I do both conventional and homeopathic medicine and I'm able to kind of meet my patients where they're at. Some patients' consciousness is that they want antibiotics. . . . I can also give them the opportunity to learn other things. . . . I use a lot of nutrition in my practice I am more likely to use herbs and progest cream, less likely to put people on hormones."

Those who seek to become bridges between conventional and alternative medicine are keenly aware that they must demonstrate both competence and excellence in conventional practice in order to be taken seriously, to be effective. Amy Saltzmann said, "I'm one of the bridges between conventional medicine and holistic medicine. And I think we're still at the point where to do that, you have to know your conventional medicine pretty well." Larry Dossey agrees:

> I always felt my contribution was to be the best contemporary orthodox internist I could be, and do that as beautifully as I think that can be done, but yet try to bridge both worlds. I continue to think that is a smart thing to do. One of the reasons I've been able to make a contribution is that my colleagues trust me. They honor my credentials and know I've spent easily twenty years in the trenches. I do not think I would have been as effective if I had tried to be an expert in homeopathy or Chinese medicine or something else. I honor internal medicine approaches, although they seem very, very limited to me.

This insistence on excellence in conventional practice is typical of the physicians in our study. But the ability to serve as a bridge between conventional and holistic medicine does not come easily to all. Some interviewees who made a philosophical paradigm shift to holism have been completely unable to bridge the gap between their holistic personal philosophy and the demands of their technomedical practice. David Filmore, for example, insists that there is no bridge. Although he plunged wholeheartedly into holism in his personal life, he has been unable to extend that holistic philosophy to his work as an internist. Instead, he concentrates on being as good as he can in a purely technical sense.

> I'm sitting between two worlds in my work as a doctor. I believe that there is a world of science which does a certain job, and then there is the world of spirituality which addresses other issues. There is a beauty in science, something very elegant; at the same time, there is also something very overwhelming about the spiritual, ultimate nature of the universe. But they are just not the same thing in my mind. I have to separate the two, although it has been my desire to bridge them. I am accepting the reality that there is no bridge, just no bridge. I've been trying for ten years to find the bridge, to describe it and write about it. But more and more I am impressed with the stark reality that I can't do it. . . . There is more than one world. You can't replace one thing with another. You can't say, "We're going to replace traditional medicine with alternative medicine." And likewise traditional medicine can't say, "We are the ones who save lives." It's a puzzler for me. The bottom line for me is making a living, and I make a living doing medicine. I spend more time painting and playing music than I could do in any other field, and I fairly well enjoy a dis-integrated, not an integrated life. (*MetaPhysicians' Tales*)

In contrast, some physicians practicing in intensively technocratic settings and situations find that there are magic moments in which the possibility of actualizing the bridge that eludes Filmore suddenly becomes immanent. Anesthesiologist Walter Mueller writes:

> Some of us are interested in building a bridge between the scientific practice of medicine and this other realm. Anesthesia is a very scientific specialty, and even though I can be very scientific in my practice, and accept the fact that science is wonderful, and that knowing the laws of chemistry and these gases is very important, there are moments when this totally disappears and the other is reality is there. . . . There will be a certain moment with a patient when suddenly something will come over me and tell me, "This is the moment for the other thing," and I'm suddenly moved to put my hand over this patient's head and close my eyes. (*MetaPhysicians' Tales*)

Mueller describes a startling incident in the hospital during which he manifested the bridge. He had recently joined an energy healing group when he was called in to attend an obstetrical emergency. A twenty-year-old woman who had just given birth was experiencing severe postpartum hemorrhage. By the time he arrived, she was

> as white as that lamp over there, had a pulse that was uncountable and no blood pressure. . . . She had developed a DIC [disseminated intravascular coagulation, a disorder of the clotting mechanism of the blood] and was bleeding to death. . . . I raced around and started some huge catheters and intercaths. . . . I got blood and plasma and albumin and started pouring all this fluid into her, but she was pouring it out as fast as it went in. Then a strange thing happened to me. By then there were two more anesthesiologists, one more obstetrician, and five or six nurses in the room. . . . It was like everybody suddenly disappeared. I put one hand over her belly, not touching her, and the other hand over her heart. I closed my eyes and called on all my friends in my group to come help me. I began to channel energy to heal her, or something! . . . I had a moment's worry, "Gee, what's everybody going to think?" But I did it until I felt that it was finished. Then I opened my eyes. Everybody was still standing around. I don't know how much time had elapsed. But she had stopped bleeding. So we got her down to the intensive care unit. She was still semi-comatose, with her eyes closed the whole time. . . .
>
> In the morning my first stop was to see her in intensive care. . . . Her mother said to me, "What's your name?" When I told her, her face lit up and she said "You know, last night . . . my daughter opened her eyes and looked at you. She said to me, 'I knew as long as that guy was there that I wasn't going to die.'" That puzzles me, because she never opened her eyes and she didn't know who the hell I was. But after all my doubts, this was a reaffirmation. If you're looking for a bridge, you just have to let the moment tell you when it's there. (*MetaPhysician's Tales*)

Like Walter Mueller, Jack Mansberger, who told his story in the preceding chapter, manifested the bridge by performing his surgery while staying conscious of and attentive to the spirit of the person he was operating on. Alex Cadoux, whose story opened this book, acts as a bridge between the worlds every time he brings his orthomolecular healing into the hospital. And Bethany Hays seamlessly creates the bridge through talking with her patients:

> Q: Have you been trained in other healing systems?
>
> A: I've dabbled in a lot of alternative modalities but I wouldn't consider myself trained.
>
> Q: Which ones have you dabbled in?
>
> A: Well, I've done some therapeutic touch and some hypnosis and I'm fascinated with psychoneuroimmunology and I've done a little acupressure.

> I haven't really trained in acupuncture. I've learned a little about homeopathy, and more and more about intuitive diagnosis. You know, I come to the AHMA every year with an idea that I'll just go and learn something else.
>
> Q: Are you able to integrate these with biomedical practice?
>
> A: Sure.
>
> Q: How do you do that?
>
> A: You just walk over the bridge whenever the opportunity presents itself.

David Gershan takes a metaphysical approach to express the tension he felt between allopathy and holistic healing:

> Anthroposophical medicine does not want to supplant acute care, surgery, and many treatments which have come out of the Western tradition. There are differences in viewpoints, however, and those differences will cause angst to the student of spiritual science who is a physician. You will be torn, and the deeper you go the more torn you will be until you make a bridge between them and see that they are not different, that one is the expansion of the two. You must see this bridge. Any other approach would be arrogance, and arrogance alone would kill any sincere approach. The goal is to build a bridge between the natural, scientific approach and an expanded vision of the human being.

Acknowledging his personal limitations, Ed Neal applies an expanded vision of the bridge: "I used to have a grandiose idea that I was going to be a bridge in medicine—teach residents, write books, give talks. But lately I've been feeling like I don't need to be a bridge as much as to care for patients. I do think my experiences are very valuable—they're not common—but I've lost the desire. I don't know what happened to the bridge. My other thought is that in the collective unconscious there are movements, like a wave, and right now the whole culture is bridging."

Integrated Lives

How does it feel to practice medicine after a major shift in values? One theme expressed by the physicians we spoke to who have completed their transformative journey is the unity of their personal and professional lives. "Integration" is the word that describes their experience on the far side of the void, where the physician's life is characterized by balance, trust, harmony, and, for a few individuals, profound joy. They have tapped into their personal destiny, and the sense of separation has diminished or dissolved. Personal and professional life are one; work and income are one; giving and receiving are one. Even the dark side of the self is no longer to be feared; as Bill Manahan explained, "I have come to own my own shadow and dark side. This then helps me recognize whether or not you own yours, and to accept it if you're not at a place where you quite see it yet." Holistic physicians are charting their unique course, aware of support from like-minded colleagues, but not necessarily involved with them on a regular basis. They feel distanced psychologically from the criticism their peers might offer. Having answered the call, they have found their sense of purpose.

We saw how consumed medical students are with their studies to the exclusion of the rest of life—a way of being that many physicians continue once they enter full-time practice, one that can lead to the negative effects of workaholism and long-term imbalance in their lives. Some of our interviewees, like Chris Northrup and Bethany Hays, directly addressed what they consider their work addiction through therapy and by establishing the parameters necessary to maintain a healthy balance between work and personal life.

Others heal the professional/personal split by dropping all such parameters and thoroughly integrating the two realms. David Edelberg describes how he studies, in the evening at home, the cases of the patients he may have seen during the day. In an extreme of such integration, Patch Adams for many years invited his patients home to live with him for extended periods. Ed Neal undertook Jungian studies to continue to develop himself and, therefore, his effectiveness as a healer. Some of our interviewees, whose work has made them well known at national and international levels, found over time that they could not maintain an active practice while still keeping up with the demands of increasingly busy lecture schedules. Opting to serve the many instead of the few, Larry Dossey and Christiane Northrup left one-on-one practice and continue to gain recognition as spokespersons for the frontiers of the new paradigm.

Can work be fun? It seems that post-transition doctors, whether humanistic or holistic, have found a way to enjoy any and every aspect of their work. Just as they no longer focus on money, they no longer focus on curing at all costs or engaging in an adversarial battle with disease and death. They have a markedly expanded view of their role as healers and a significantly reduced expectation of themselves as saviors. This allows for the sense of play and of great pleasure in work, an area that formerly produced frustration, stress, and hostility toward patients.

"When I get up in the morning, it's like my work makes my heart sing!" says Ann McCombs. "I'm more rejuvenated at the end of my day than I am at the beginning, and that's what soul-satisfying work is." Barry Elson is "really happy with my life at this time. I absolutely love my practice. I'm busy as can be—booked a month or more ahead. My patients are doing well and benefiting from the work we do. It's very fulfilling to me. I almost want to pinch myself and wonder if I'm going to wake up, because it's what I've always dreamed of doing." In the same euphoric boat is George Keeler: "I reorganized to one office, one place for emergency work, and one place to teach. I began rowing for exercise, learning homeopathy as a method of alternative treatment, and sharing what I've learned through patient education in my daily work and writing. Finally I have a practice where every day is a joy with patients I love and doing what works for both of us" ("Physician in Transition" 1990).

The collaborative model of care, in which doctors share responsibility with patients, eliminates the sense of separation and effort so often mentioned by pre-transition doctors. Gone, or certainly minimized, are fears about legal liability in an environment where trust and agreements rather than obedience to the standard of care govern the healing interaction. The balance that was absent during medical school has returned and become a priority, as Joel Fort's life illustrates: "I've been able to blend my personal and professional ethics through a combination of thoughtfulness about my life and freeing myself from the quest for money and security. That allowed me to control my own time, and time is life. I decided for myself the right balance among contemplation, tennis, chess playing, music playing, lecturing, teaching, clinical work, and social activism. I have freed myself to lead a consistent life—and also a much more interesting and adventurous one."

Each finds balance it his or her own individual way. Jacqueline Wilson, in great demand as a homeopathic practitioner, limits her practice to four days a week for direct patient care, and turns away new patients in order to maintain that limit. To facilitate this balance between the personal and the professional, she keeps her overhead low, which enables her to travel. She designed her office setting of "natural light, trees, flowers, and birds" to bring balance between her work and the natural world.

Larry Dossey expresses the satisfaction with life that we often heard:

> I have gotten to the point in my life where I am blessed to do on a daily basis what I am more interested in doing than anything else in the world—fiddling with ideas about how consciousness manifests in the world. I get to write books about this. People actually ask me to give talks about my work. This is apparently valued by enough people that we get to play this game and have fun with it. Sometimes in the morning I pinch myself to make sure that this is really happening. I hope the day I die that I will have the freedom to have the fun and joy that I have doing what I'm doing right now. If nothing ever changed throughout the rest of my life, I'd be happy camper.

Two of the physicians we interviewed take additional delight in the proximity of their work setting to their families, and describe an interplay, on a daily basis, between their family and professional roles and responsibilities. "It's kind of hard to say where the personal life stops and the professional life begins," David Edelberg said. "I live only five miles away, and my kids come here and I go back and forth many times. I can't imagine doing anything else. I wake up in the morning and I say, 'Ah, yes, it's a work day!'" Chris Northrup finds that:

> It's possible to have a balanced life—where you don't have a professional and a private life, you have a whole life. Raising children, being rooted in a community, being real are all very important to me. This culture feeds us a very limited view of our possibilities and it's done specifically to make us better consumers, to keep coming back to buy more because we are not fulfilled. My office is two miles from home. I can go home to pick something up. My daughter's school is on the same street as my office. I can drop something off at the dry cleaners, pick up one of my kids, stop at the office, go though my mail, go to my house, bring my kids to the office, and have a cappuccino with the staff. My husband's office is in the same town, so basically my whole life is about two square miles. I vote in my community and I know the school committee members. I like it. It's very integrated and I'm thrilled with it.

Caring for people, the heart of healing, is not the exclusive domain of the holistic doctor. However, within a paradigm where equality and parity prevail, doctors are relieved of the burden of role-bound behavior and can more freely enter into a satisfying emotional exchange. Len Saputo says, "I get a lot of return from care-giving, making people feel better. I care a lot about how they feel. I care a lot about my patients. I get a lot back that way." And David Edelberg noted,

> What I enjoy most is the day with patients, and so what sustains me most is working with patients. At the end of the day, when my wife and kids are asleep, I take out the charts of the patients I saw that day and all my shorthand observations. Then I write my chart notes, and, as I'm writing, think about each patient, about the ramification of their illness, how it affects them, how hearing about their illness has affected me, where their illness fits in the scheme of their lives and of society. That's what sustains me. (1994:32)

The gift that comes from enduring uncertainty, in some cases criticism, while moving through one's personal transition is an unflagging sense of certainty and self-confidence once the river has been crossed. These doctors have their work in perspective regardless of how much or little time it consumes or how financially rewarding it is. They are no longer dogged by fatigue. Many experience themselves as a channel for healing energy from the universal source; they are no longer the doer. This accounts for their high energy levels. For example, Bethany Hays explained that in her old way of practicing, she gave and gave to her patients and left feeling "exhausted, completely drained." She said, "I think what I'm learning now is how to conserve my own energy and yet to provide the people I care for with energy that they need. . . . What I'm learning is to take that energy from somewhere other than my own cell tissue, other than out of me, to let that energy come through me but not from me."

As we have noted previously, holistic physicans find it impossible to make this paradigm shift without applying its principles and practices to their personal lives. They care for themselves using the same alterations in attitude and lifestyle which they recommend to their patients. Balance, self-esteem, healthy living, confidence, trust, joy. Medical school is a distant nightmare.

Another characteristic of those who have completed the paradigm shift is a certainty that what they are doing is enough, and where they are is the right place to be. Each one has found his or her niche and many have named it heaven. This contrasts with, for some of them, intense periods in the past of exploration, dropping out, dissatisfaction, and major geographic upheaval. Each person's form of practice is unique. "I think if you follow this path very seriously, everybody's practice looks different because it is the expression of their core essence," observes Ed Neal.

Noticeably lacking in these statements from all the doctors we interviewed was a concern for the future. Very few were striving for something they did not have or expressed ambition for anything beyond a sort of ripening or deepening of what they were already doing. One senses that their future will entail continued learning and refinements rather than the profound suffering and values-shift that many of them underwent in order to reach this stage. Terry Tyler suggests that once through the "big stuff," future changes occur more easily and gracefully: "In the early, awakening phases of a personal journey, transformation is often dramatic and painful. Later, when one has integrated much of life's essential purpose, transformation is gentler, simply a relaxing into, a letting go, a surrender, a knowing." In the *MetaPhysicians' Tales*, Gene Ross expresses this idea dramatically: "I started talking to people who were doing alternative medicine and having quite a bit of success. I wanted that for myself. That was facing the monster, fearing it, and taking a risk. I have many more monsters to face, but I realize they are not going to kill me. Each time I face one, a sense of cleanness results: something blocking the process has been dissolved. As I continue this, I find my capacity to love increases."

Growth and learning never cease for the holistic physician. But their earlier confusion about the direction in which they should grow is replaced by a sense of clarity about the appropriateness and the rich potential of their new growth trajectory, as Ann McCombs acknowledges: "I hope I never stop learning, I never stop growing. I hope that my mind is always as open as it is right now. We have to leave a legacy. . . . It's taken a lot of time, a lot of heartache to [get to this place], and I want to expand that, and be learning until I die." As Scott Anderson looks ahead, "Five years from now I see myself continuing to grow and develop in the process of becoming a physician, a healer, a devotee. . . . In ten years I want to be involved in serving people in spiritual growth rather than just helping them get over years of bad habits. I would like to take people into the higher reaches of wellness, the higher reaches of self-actualization and contribute to this great process that humanity is all about."

Life-Stage Culmination

Several theorists of human nature have postulated that adults pass through developmental stages just as children do, and that these stages each present certain challenges, which, when met, bring feelings of satisfaction and a sense of appropriateness. Attaining each stage in sequence gives individuals a sense of completion and fulfillment regarding their life as a whole. In his seminal work *Childhood and Society*, psychoanalyst Erik Erikson identified eight stages of human development, describing each in terms of the triumph of the developmental force over the regressive force. For example, the first stage in infancy he calls "basic trust versus basic mistrust" to describe the triumph of confidence in oneself and one's environment that ideally characterizes the infancy stage. Similarly, "autonomy versus shame and doubt" describes the emergence of the successful two-year-old psyche, while "initiative versus guilt" results when the slightly older child relaxes into his identity as a capable person. "Industry versus inferiority" reveals the choice of relationship to the world, to the community and the beginning levels of vocational sense.

At the beginning of adulthood, "identity" must triumph over "role confusion" to bring lifelong satisfaction in adult endeavors. An individual on secure footing is ready to chose "intimacy" over "isolation" in relational areas. Through procreation or involvement in vocation, successful adults will have a sense of "generativity" versus "stagnation" in leaving a legacy through children or works that will outlive them.

The sweetness of this journey manifests most completely in the eighth and final stage, where the mosaic reveals its pattern and is seen for its wonderful artistry. Based on their levels of satisfaction, we can conclude that post-transition doctors have reached this eighth and final stage of development, "ego integrity versus despair," which occurs "[o]nly in him who in some way has taken care of things and people and has adapted himself to the triumphs and disappointments inherent in being . . . only in him may gradually ripen the fruit of these seven stages. It is the acceptance of one's one and only life cycle as something that had to be, and that, of necessity, permitted of no substitutions. . . .The possessor of [such] integrity is ready to defend the dignity of his own life against all physical and economic threats" (Erikson 1963:268).

Conversely, the individual who fails to achieve ego integrity would feel despair and the accompanying "feeling that the time is too short for the attempt to start another life, and try out alternate roads to integrity" (Erikson 1963:268–269).

Carl Jung's concept of individuation, a state reached when one has sufficiently differentiated oneself from the past, including family of origin, societal patterns, and even other life influences, closely approximates Erikson's eighth stage, with one major difference. According to Progoff, individuation for Jung not only means the personal integration of the individual, but also "refers to the quest for self-actualization as an archetypal psychic process, on the principle that it [the archetype] is the essential sub-structure underlying the multitude of forms by which mankind experiences its spiritual life" (1955:144).

The journey from undifferentiated to differentiated, although painful and fraught with anguish, can have a transcendent quality if one recognizes in it the archetypal pattern of the hero's journey (Campbell 1968). Physicians, according to Jung's understanding, are destined to experience difficulty in their journey toward individuation, "due to their immersion and identification with the social and cultural forces which must be cast off." The forces Jung is referring to are "the inordinate faith in science and the stress on rationality" (Progoff 1955:146) that link the physician to the core values and beliefs of Western culture. These must be cast off as excess baggage, so that, unencumbered, the hero can complete the journey.

The journey we have walked with the physicians in this book has charted their development from idealistic medical students through a stage of disillusionment, frustration, and doubt, to a social or spiritual awakening that often catapulted them into a state of chaos and confusion, as Terry Tyler recognizes: "The transformative process can be painful and disorganizing most of the time. It feels like the world has been turned upside down or that even the world or ourselves have ceased to exist. Much in the person actually dies, because on a deep level we are profoundly changed. It often feels like physical death is imminent. People do not often do this voluntarily. They do it because they are in a desperate crisis or the alternatives seem worse" (*Metaphysicians' Tales*).

Once through this painful state, the "dark night of the soul," these physicians emerged as invigorated, individuated healers who move forward gracefully against societal norms, confident that they will be given whatever resources they require to actualize themselves through their work. In this stage, where they accept their "one and only life," their past struggle becomes their source of energy and present peace. The wound of uncertainty or disillusionment opens the place where compassion, commitment, and acceptance flower.

From the joy with which these physicians pursue their vocations as their destinies, we can find hope for the future of American medicine, which we will venture to predict in the following chapter.

8 *Visions for the Future of Medicine*

> Holistic medicine recognizes all the dimensions of the person and understands that you can't have a disruption in one aspect that doesn't affect the others. It also means that we share a global responsibility for the planet and the future of the species to begin empowering people to take care of themselves, to dismantle the hierarchies within our own profession that have been serving paternalism, and to stand up for cooperation among all the healing disciplines.
> —PAULANNE BALCH, M.D.

We have spent a major portion of this book distinguishing between the technomedical, humanistic, and holistic approaches to health care. Now we face the challenge of envisioning a future in which they each play their appropriate role. The first question that must be answered is, What relationship among these three paradigms is likely to emerge from present conditions to create the future of medicine? Will these paradigms remain separate and distinguishable points along the spectrum that ranges from hegemony to heresy, or will they merge to form a synergistic whole, the shape of which we can now only speculate about?

The holistic physicians in our study used the bridge metaphor to describe their attempts to mediate between technomedicine and holistic healing. Whether they referred to a need to build the bridge, to cross the bridge, or to become the bridge, they assumed that the paradigms would remain somewhat distinct, at least for the foreseeable future. In essence this bridge metaphor references the importance of keeping what is useful from technomedicine, such as emergency life-saving techniques and drugs, while giving the relationship- and life-enhancing techniques of humanism and holism more prominence and legitimacy.

What forces in society are powerful enough to influence the course of medicine in the immediate future? Many predict that an ever more vocal and influential public will insist on the availability of natural healing techniques either as adjuncts to conventional care or as replacements for it. There is evidence that the public is ultimately offering the greatest challenge to medical hegemony. A number of states have passed a freedom of medical treatment bill within the past few years, and a National Medical Access Bill was introduced in both houses of Congress in 1995, but not acted upon. Essentially this legislation upholds the right of individuals to seek treatment from any practitioner they choose. In a country where the rights of racists, pornographers, and serial killers are protected by law, the very need for legislation protecting freedom of choice in medical treatment testifies to the monolithic nature of the medical care empire. Many feel that freedom of choice in medical care should become an amendment to the Constitution—right along with the rights to speak, worship, and bear arms.

A force as compelling as the voice of the citizenry is economics. Since the emergence of managed care, profits, which drive technomedicine and were formerly distributed to medical institutions and doctors, are now directed toward those in the business of running medicine. As an incentive to generate more profits, the practice of offering low-cost alternative therapies within the HMO system is rapidly taking hold. This practice brings up the question of the cooption of holism by the hegemonic technomedical model. As Morris Berman has pointed out in *Coming to Our Senses* (1990), hegemonies may *seem* to be giving ground to heresies when in fact they are moving to co-opt them. We will say more about the implications of this below.

On the other side of the economic argument, Western medicine is widely acknowledged as a triumph of modern science and technology, and nearly every spokesperson on the subject wishes to see technomedicine preserved and available within its legitimate role—providing life-saving and emergency care. How to prevent it from consuming a disproportionate share of medical resources, while making it universally available as a backup for conditions that fail to respond to gentler methods, is a conundrum not yet addressed. In the future, it seems possible that technomedicine may become third-line medicine—the arena of last resort, not the first place to which people turn for health care, while holistic medicine, the medicine of preventing illness through creating wellness, may become first-line medicine, the place where people start.

How far could such a fundamental shift go? Can a reasonable person anticipate the minimization or elimination of Western technology even in the face of trauma and serious illness? In the Epilogue to *Space, Time, and Medicine* (1982), Larry Dossey described a scenario in which the mastery of self, including biological processes, can substitute for conventional care. "Myocardial Infarction 2000 A.D." tracks a man who is experiencing a heart attack through its onset, intensification of symptoms, and resolution without the intervention of any medical care. The man controls his own physiological and emotional states, presumably as a result of long practice. He sustains little tissue damage. Fully healing himself from the inside out, he regulates his blood pressure, controls the pain, and reduces his fear until he settles into a long healing nap. Upon awakening he proceeds with his activities. This vision incorporates some of the elements of shamanic healing and self-healing and offers a blueprint for moving beyond technology in managing even critical conditions.

The precedent for this blueprint, of course, is the yogic tradition, which sees mind and body as yoked in a well-functioning, homeostatic unit, capable of responding to inner and outer signals for adjustment. While we may find it difficult to imagine a whole society with the discipline and motivation to adopt these techniques, more and more individuals are undertaking the task of growing in consciousness in all areas of their lives. Self-regulation, self-help, and holistic healing have become increasingly appealing to the segment of society dubbed "the cultural creatives," who, according to a recent study conducted by the Institute of Noetic Sciences (Ray 1996), constitute at least 24 percent of the population.[1]

While Dossey gives us a peek into possibility, most of the practitioners we interviewed would agree with Len Saputo's view of Western medicine: "When the horse is out of the barn, there's nothing better." Keeping the horse *in* the barn, however, is the subject which most of our interviewees felt required more attention. More than a cry for more public health programs or medical prevention, their call is for nothing less than a revolution in social thinking in which widespread popular acceptance of the concepts of self-care, social responsibility, and consensus regarding the allocation of resources will support a holistic approach to health. A theme that ran through the comments of most of the holistic physicians we interviewed was the need for what Joel Fort calls a "societal mandate" regarding prevention. This includes everything from training people to grapple with their impulses, thereby reducing accidents, addictions, and acts of violence, to the adoption of a healthy lifestyle through nutrition and exercise, to Chris Northrup's in-depth vision:

> At present, we're still giving government subsidies to tobacco farms, and the "war on drugs" does not include cigarettes and alcohol, even though those are the things that are killing everybody. We fail to recognize that doctors are just downstream pulling bodies out of the water. No one is working upstream, seeing what's shoving them in to begin with. Unless we start working upstream, this disease care crisis will just continue. We have to have a fundamental shift.
>
> That fundamental shift means each of us has to look inside, at where we hold our pain, and how we try to medicate it, and that requires feeling that pain that ends the pain, as Steven Levine says. And very few people want to do that. They want a good time, they want a good romance, but what they don't realize is that life is so much more fun if you just do that, if you just own what's going on.
>
> I would like to see a system where everyone knew that their basic needs would be taken care of . . . if they broke a bone or had a laceration or something catastrophic, it would be taken care of and they would not lose their home trying to pay for it. But in addition, we need to understand the technocracy or addictive system or whatever you want to call it, and to under-

> stand that health does not come by buying a new outfit or a new set of tools. The only way to feel healthy is to feel connection with your community and with your own spirit. Relationships open the heart. . . .
>
> I would teach everyone to have a lifetime of looking for and being nurtured about their gifts and talents. I would teach that family history is not a script. . . . Health care can be positively transformed when people realize that their body is the outward manifestation of their emotions, their dreams, their soul, and that they have the power within them to create heaven. As doctors we must move into a partnership model where the patient is taking responsibility for health and the doctor is a consultant. That will transform health care. It will never be transformed as long as we give over our bodies and souls and minds to experts.

Northrup's vision of a transformed health care system, based on partnership models of healing in combination with individual responsibility, self-exploration, and spirituality, is shared by most of our interviewees, humanists and holists alike. The power of this vision, combined with society's growing acknowledgment of the usefulness of complementary techniques within conventional medical institutions, is working to ensure that there soon will be few remaining voices raised in an effort to obliterate holism from the future of medicine. With the battle for survival in a technocratic world close to being won, the issue becomes one of politics and positioning, as the more mainstream acceptance holism achieves, the greater the danger of its possible co-option. If holism, which focuses on healing and connection, is subsumed by the biotechnical paradigm, which focuses on profit and separation, only a discordant reality can ensue.

Will Holism Be Co-opted by the Dominant Paradigm?

A trend is in process toward incorporating certain alternative therapies inside managed care. Applying the managed care principles of cost savings and efficiency means that standardization is required of any modality within that system. This means standards for referral, numbers of visits, length of visits, treatment, and fees. We described in some detail how the underlying philosophy of natural healing lies in its understanding of each individual, each disease episode as unique. The implications of attempting to mold holistic care to a standardized approach are serious, especially within a paradigm where the underlying values are divergent, perhaps even oppositional.

Once alternative techniques become widely available within orthodox medical settings, it is questionable how viable they will be in terms of their own paradigm and its underlying tenets. For example, we were recently told by a midwife that a group of physicians in her town wanted to purchase the birth center she had founded. They figured they could increase its profitability by offering epidurals as an extra feature of labor care. Recognizing this for what it was—the forced incorporation of an element from one paradigm into another, the midwife refused their offer in the best interests of her clients. She knew that the cascade effects of epidurals—increased length of labor, increased need for other interventions, increased cesarean rates—would destroy the holistic essence of the midwifery model of care she had striven to provide.

The fate of the independent family doctor, who has long represented the essence of the humanistic approach, is another case in point. It has become close to impossible for family practitioners to remain in practice independent of managed care. Employees who have insurance must see only physicians who have been approved by the insurance company for reimbursement. To see a doctor outside of this group, the patient must pay a financial penalty. (Similarly, as acupuncturists, chiropractors, and other healers are taken into the managed care fold, fewer and fewer individuals will choose practitioners outside this framework.) The remaining mavericks who opt out of managed care (including most of our interviewees) will survive mainly through the loyalty of their client network or through their reputation for unique and effective treatment, for which their clients must be willing to pay out-of-pocket.

Unfortunately the public has become accustomed to medi-business dictating which doctor they may see, how often, and for how long. Standards that at first seemed ludicrous and unacceptable have become an accepted part of care from both the doctor's and patient's standpoints. Managed care will inevitably try to reduce the practice of healing to the same time and dollar considerations it has been applying to technomedicine. Humanistic and holistic practitioners who find themselves part of this framework may have to knuckle under to these limits regardless of how inimical they seem to their philosophy of care. Eventually, the art of healing revived in the contemporary humanistic and holistic approaches may once again succumb to the business of healing—a triumph for the principle of separation that underlies the technomedical paradigm.

Once neatly packaged, it is easy to anticipate alternative medicine's partial legitimization through further certification and licensure activity within certain types of institutional settings. From there, training programs in holistic modalities will make accreditation their major goal and will concentrate on preparing their graduates to be certified more than to be healers. In this gloomiest of all futures, holistic medicine will be subsumed by biotechnical medicine—Cinderella to its powerful stepsister forever.

As Morris Berman (1990) has shown, any system that fails to grow and change with the times will crack and crumble from its own rigidity. Hegemonies need heresies so that they can co-opt them and use their energy to revitalize the hegemonic system. Heresies, eager to make inroads into the conventional system, often unwittingly participate in this kind of co-option. Concomitantly, some movements within the holistic health community are working hard to prepare for their integration into biomedicine. Herbalists constitute a case in point. Long criticized by mainstream medicine, herbal therapy is assuming a more prominent role in the treatment of many conditions. In our sanitized, pharmacologically focused culture, herbal therapy means taking pills or capsules containing herbal ingredients. In an effort to ward off FDA critics and to prepare to fit into mainstream medicine, some herbal manufacturing companies are now ensuring that their product contains standardized amounts of the herb's active ingredient within each capsule, thereby providing the same guarantee as manufacturers of synthetic drugs. Since the amount of an active ingredient does not necessarily correlate with its therapeutic effect, nor does it indicate whether pesticides and fertilizers were used to grow or to preserve it during transport, standardization of herbs is not always helpful and may sometimes be misleading.

The difference between co-option of the heresy by the hegemony and subversion of the hegemony by the heresy often exists in the mind of the beholder. Some see efforts such as those described above as worst-case examples of the technomedical model reaching outside of its paradigm to pull in material that will never fit without being stripped of its holistic value. Others are optimistic that, since organized medicine defines medical care, securing the favor and approval of its adherents will advance the cause and increase the popular acceptance of alternatives. Some degree of co-option may seem like a small price to pay for the larger gain, for the inroads the humanistic and holistic models may make into the technomedical realm can potentially make a huge difference there.

Adherents of a heretical paradigm in imminent danger of co-option have often found that the best way to preserve its purity is to carve out entirely new cultural spaces within which the new way of being can flourish. In 1996, after years of spadework, the American Holistic Medical Association created a certifying board for holistic physicians, called the American Board of Holistic Medicine, which is specifying requirements for certification and creating an application process and a written examination. This "health-focused" specialty is intended to promulgate the scientific basis of using holistic medicine to treat illness, especially chronic conditions, as well as train physicians to refer appropriately to other types of practitioners.

Impetus for creating this specialty was generated by the increasing media attention to alternative medicine, by the accumulation of scientifically credible research evidence, and by the growing cultural acceptance of holistic medicine. For evidence of this growing acceptance, McCombs and Anderson (1996:6) point to the creation of the Office of Alternative

Medicine at the National Institutes of Health, the licensing of naturopaths and other practitioners in a growing number of states, the rise in the number of multimodal wellness centers across the nation, and increasing support in state legislatures for physicians' use of alternative modalities. They speak of these events as holistic medicine's "coming of age."

In other countries, notably Scotland and Germany, medical officials and practitioners are taking a more systematic approach to integrating alternative medicine with conventional alternatives than are technocratic practitioners in the United States. In Germany, the Federal Department of Health has directed all medical training facilities to offer courses in natural healing procedures. In the future all M.D. candidates will be required to earn credits in this area and pass an examination.

Nothing of this level of rigor has been introduced within U.S. medical school curricula, but opportunities for physicians to learn alternatives under the tutelage of knowledgeable peers are springing up. M.D.'s can now learn homeopathy as well as Chinese medicine, including acupuncture, in courses specifically designed for them inside and outside of medical schools. One question this trend poses is whether complex, experience-based systems can be taught within the framework of the technomedical model.

Such a step represents the possibility of diminished distance between orthodox medicine and holistic healing. Some see this type of crossover as an attempt to push back the walls of standard medicine and change it for the better. But critics of this approach assert that homeopathy is a highly complex, intuition-based modality whose effective practice requires a study of its philosophy and history and an appreciation of its subtlety. They are concerned that it will become diluted, limited in application to what M.D.'s can or choose to learn, and, worst of all, that these parameters may impact future regulation of the field. Many nonmedical healers have strong feelings about the potential "medicalization" of their art. If M.D.'s take over holistic healing, what role will be left for other practitioners, and what will happen to the systems of healing they treasure? Will their piecemeal co-option result in their demise?

An alternative set of possibilities has arisen in the development and spread of the wellness center in many American cities. For many years, Gladys McGarey, M.D., has quietly pioneered the systematization and application of Edgar Cayce's healing recommendations through an integrated approach, using a mix of practitioners. She is well qualified to give form to this vision:

> Medicine of the future, as I envision it, will be an integrative health care system. My prayer is that the system will consider the whole being: body, mind, and spirit. Integrating the spiritual dimension, which acknowledges

> the spiritual nature of mankind, will allow true healing to happen. . . . I see patient care of the future revolving around a center where people of all races and conditions come for healing in an environment that is ecologically and environmentally safe. A setting where like-minded healers (allopathic, chiropractic, psychologists, and massage, physical, and biofeedback therapists) as well as shamans and healers of all cultures could respect each other's abilities and work together to manifest [true holism in health care]. (McGarey 1995:2)

Around the country, many holistic physicians (like Alex Cadoux, whose story began this book), in collaboration with their alternative colleagues, are running just this sort of community-oriented wellness center. Yet such centers are still very few in number compared to the overwhelming preponderance of allopathic hospitals, clinics, and home services. What would it take to realize the blend of approaches and personnel suggested by Dr. McGarey on a societywide scale?

An Integrated System

According to Senator Tom Harkin, "Mainstreaming alternative practices that work is our next step. A dialogue between the alternative and conventional medical communities is essential and long overdue. If the health care community is not working together toward a common goal—everyone's wellness—then toward what goal are they striving? What rational excuse could any practitioner proffer for withholding an effective therapy?" (1995:71).

Achieving an integrated health care system would require fundamental shifts in the institutions that constitute what is now the practice of medicine. In chapter 2 we discussed some of the changes now under way in medical education that are designed to restore a more personal approach to medical practice and to expose medical students to the concepts and techniques of various alternative therapies. Beyond this "transformation of the scientist" as Willis Harman described it, there are several other fundamental changes which must precede the evolution of a fully integrated health care system.

INTEGRATED SCIENCE

Many thinkers within the holistic model are convinced that science, the conceptual baseline of technomedicine, will paradoxically become the mechanism for its expansion into holism. Because more and more scientific research is demonstrating that dramatic results can be achieved through alternative methods, it seems possible that established medicine will honor its own criteria and embrace those holistic modalities and treatments whose efficacy has been scientifically shown. This move would require a tremendous amount of open-mindedness on the part of technomedical diehards, since it has been shown time and time again that the science accepted as fact by the adherents of a given paradigm, especially a hegemonic one, is the science that fits within the parameters of that paradigm (Kuhn 1982; Rubinstein, Laughlin, and McManus 1984).

As we saw in chapter 4, holistic physicians tend to be strong supporters of and believers in science. Their vision of appropriate science parallels their vision of appropriate medicine: it is an expanded view of science, one that respects the double-blind study *and* grants a place to centuries-old evidence as well as anecdotal and observed phenomena. They differ from their technomedical colleagues in their understanding that different systems require different approaches. To bring them together, as Senator Tom Harkin explains,

> We must find an approach where everyone can stand in agreement on the therapies that work; where the unbendable rules of randomized clinical trials and the uncertainty of anecdotal case studies are laid aside in favor of a third approach—one that will quantify the effectiveness of various therapies without breaking them down into series of chemical reactions and physiological processes. An approach that does not declare a winner and a loser between the conventional and the alternative. An integrated approach that emphasizes prevention as a component of wellness. (1995:71)

But efforts to develop this new, integrative science are still up against some very powerful oppositional forces. "Research," which often functions not as science but as a proxy for science, underpins the whole profit-driven medical establishment. Behind this filter, according to many, stand the pharmaceutical and medical technology industries.

One of the requirements for breaking out of this bondage is a revamping of the role of research, particularly the use of the prospective double-blind study to prove or disprove the worthiness of any technique. This kind of change can be difficult when economic interests drive the protocols:

> The National Cancer Institute and Merck and Company announced large-scale tests of Proscar, a drug that is said to hold promise for preventing prostate cancer. The new study would be praiseworthy were it not for the fact that the wrong drug was being tested. . . . An extract of saw palmetto berries (*Serenoa repens*; Serenoa) has the same mechanism of action as Proscar and is clearly more effective for the symptomatic relief of benign prostatic hyperplasia. Because prevention of prostate cancer is believed to occur by the same mechanism as alleviating BPH, Ser-

> enoa should be at least as effective as Proscar while costing half as much. Unlike Proscar, Serenoa does not cause impotence in one out of twenty men who take it. It's understandable that Merck would not want Serenoa to make Proscar look bad, but the NCI is supposed to be acting purely in the public interest. (Gaby 1994:74)

"Show me the study" is the retort most often offered to dispute the efficacy of a particular treatment, lifestyle intervention, or substance proffered by alternative medicine. Yet a plethora of studies showing the benefits of various alternative therapies have been successfully completed under appropriate research conditions; the results are ignored if they do not support current prejudice. Compounding the problem is the difficulty of obtaining funding for research in the areas of alternative healing which lend themselves to this type of investigation. The attitude displayed toward alternative therapy investigation in most medical circles remains less than supportive.

For example, in "Breaking into the Old-Boy Network" (1994), Alan Gaby describes being invited to serve as a panel member in a symposium on chronic fatigue and fibromyalgia sponsored by the National Institutes of Health and the Centers for Disease Control. Because he has had good results with nutritional support for patients with these conditions, he looked forward to presenting his results. "On closer examination," he states, "it became apparent that the members of the 'alternative medicine' panel were not being offered a level playing field. Each of us was allowed five or ten minutes to speak . . . much larger blocks of time were allotted for presentations that had little or nothing to do with helping patients get well. For example, there was a forty-five-minute lecture on whether chronic fatigue and fibromyalgia are overlapping or exclusive diagnoses. . . . It is a sad state if affairs when getting well is thought of as a questionable alternative to documenting a patient's suffering" (1994:939–940).

A perhaps greater problem, as we explained in chapter 4, is the fact that alternative medicine does not, in many instances, lend itself to standard research protocol—for example, lifestyle management, a mainstay of alternative healing, does not lend itself to double-blind prospective studies.[2] This results, under the current dominant paradigm, in its being forever suspect, and what is suspect is not paid for by insurance companies. In working with their patients, many alternative practitioners design a "program," meaning a combination of lifestyle modification, diet, exercise, supplements, and other forms of treatment such as homeopathy or acupuncture for their patients with chronic conditions. Individually tailored, these interventions can never be replicated because they employ multiple agents at one time and the variables are uncontrollable.

The Office of Alternative and Complementary Medicine at NIH is at present the only public funding source for investigation of alternative modalities. Their average grant in the 1996 funding cycle, $35,000, is jokingly referred to in alternative circles as a homeopathic grant. (Homeopathy uses minute doses to cure disease.) Indeed, the entire budget of the OAM is often referred to as homeopathic. It was initiated with $2 million in funding out of the $10 billion allocated to the NIH that year. Nevertheless, like a homeopathic remedy the OAM has been catalytic; Jim Gordon has noted that upon its formation, "Overnight, doing research on alternative medicine became a worthy subject of scientific scrutiny and a route to academic advancement" (1996b:31). And in a hopeful indication of the integrated science to come, the budget of the OAM was increased in fiscal year 1996 to $7.4 million, in fiscal year 1997 to $12 million, and in fiscal year 1998 to $20 million.

INTEGRATED PERSONNEL

Health care is primarily a service industry, and the education, certification, compensation, and relations among the personnel involved have a huge impact on the shape of the service. As we described earlier, the technomedical model is characterized by hierarchical organization. Holistic practitioners tend to operate in isolation from technomedical practitioners. They form their own centers; the physicians are usually not hospital-affiliated; and their referral network may or may not extend to medical specialists. A vision for the future might include a lateral web of trained specialists, from herbalists to surgeons, with each profession acknowledged for its contribution. Appropriate communication and respect would characterize this network.

Other health personnel changes in the future might include the use of high-tech personnel, including surgeons, only when other methods fail. A major contributor to the high cost of health care is the routine use of high-tech intervention as first-line care. The public has been conditioned to expect doctors to "do something" for every complaint they present. Doctors have been trained to oblige, even if the something means prescribing drugs with side effects. Because doctors are not trained in natural methods and are not sensitized to the body's self-healing capabilities, their solutions often cause more problems, thus engaging the patient in the medical One-Two Punch, a cascade of interventions that obliges them to continuously seek help for their ever-worsening problems. The public needs to be trained in self-care and self-referral. Mainstream doctors need to understand and respect this approach, indeed to require it of their patients.

The future may see certification of training programs and institutions and credentialling of personnel free from any economic or special interest influence. Two such influences have underscored the certification of health care professionals. The first is the application of standards that define only M.D.'s as qualified to perform comprehensive diagnoses and treat disease to the exclusion of other professionals, unduly limiting their abilities to treat their clients. For example, dentists are licensed to diagnose and treat only diseases of the head and neck, and to provide nutritional counseling only as it relates directly to the teeth. Yet the hundreds of holistic dentists now practicing in the United States know that the teeth are part of the whole body system; it is impossible to separate their care from overall nutritional and lifestyle health care. The narrow focus that constrains their ability to practice puts these professionals and a host of others (for example, nurses, nutritionists, homeopaths, and chiropractors) in legal jeopardy when they give advice or treat conditions outside of their medically defined "scope of practice."

A second, and reciprocal, influence on the certification of health practitioners has been the strongly held establishment belief that the public can neither make wise choices about health care nor protect itself from unscrupulous practitioners. This belief encourages medical decision makers and others to assume that medical information is privileged, belonging only to the medical profession. Patients are not allowed to see their charts, and the public is not taught the basics of medical care, as both are considered to be the exclusive purview of the medical profession. Such withholding of potentially empowering information encourages citizens to continue abrogating responsibility to physicians.

Of course health professionals need training in order to assume responsibility for treating patients. However, they do not all need to be able to diagnose and treat all types of disease. A reasonable goal for holistically oriented professionals might be to be able to recognize pathology beyond their ability to treat and make an appropriate referral. In place of the present emphasis on costly, high-tech, highly specialized medical care, the public would be well protected and better served by holistic, non-M.D. health professionals who would stress the benefits of prevention and wellness—including nutrition, exercise, and other immune system–stimulating lifestyle modifications. Such professionals would work in tandem with M.D.'s, who could serve them as backup without imposing on them the tools, techniques, or prejudices of the technomedical model. In such a system, holistic wellness care would be first-line medicine and primary care M.D.'s would be second-line, with the high-tech specialists serving as the line of last resort.

Regarding the public's ability to protect itself from unscrupulous medical practitioners, a word about licensure is in order. Used to legitimize health professionals, licensure's purpose is to protect the public. Yet it has also protected the technomedical paradigm's interests by excluding certain classes of practitioners and limiting the scope of practice of others. It has isolated the professions from one another; a massage therapist who wishes to become a chiropractor, for example, must take the whole course of chiropractic training. There are virtually no career ladders for health professionals. Some alternatives to licensure, which serve virtually the same stated purpose, are accreditation of training programs and intraprofessional certification. Both allow the profession itself to determine what constitutes adequate training and preparation for practice while releasing the profession from the undue influence of the technomedical establishment, which dominates licensure activities at the state level.

The future for health professionals might also include new categories of health consultants and healing practitioners as required in a society oriented toward prevention and self-care, a possibility that in no way obviates the need to legitimatize the professionals now virtually unrecognized. Among these are naturopathic physicians, homeopaths, nutritionists, and many others. A society in transition to holistic values will require the assistance of socially sanctioned individuals to help them make appropriate lifestyle choices, learn self-care, and choose wisely when seeking professional help. Lifestyle consultants and coaches, patient advocates, and home health companions for at-risk populations such as the elderly are examples of categories of workers who might help to fill existing needs.

INTEGRATED INSTITUTIONS

What changes might take place in the design and operation of institutions—especially hospitals? The hospital of the future has been the focus of visionary activity among a number of thinkers within alternative medical circles. Elson Haas, M.D., predicts the development of the "healing hospital" which integrates care for "acute and chronic conditions" along with health education and lifestyle modification in a resort or spa environment. He would like to see an organic garden that produces food for the hospital and provides an opportunity for people well enough to move around to get their hands in the dirt and their heads in the sunshine. Leland Kaiser (n.d.) envisions the design of an architecturally supportive environment where everything from birth to death could occur in a healing and conscious environment. He maintains that patients' experience of their hospitalization is in large part responsible for its outcome: "If you visit patient rooms in a contemporary hospital, you will find patients showing signs of boredom, regression, loss of identity, ignorance, fear, loneliness, confusion, helplessness, and pain. These behaviors characterize poor quality medical care. With better design of the social environment, patients experience stimulation, empowerment, transformation, love, nurturance, group support, learning, independence, inspiration, and euphoria. An experiential hospital designs its social environment as carefully as it designs its physical environment." Along with other thinkers, Kaiser insists that the hospitalization should be "a special opportunity for the patient to become more empowered, experience a spiritual transformation, and take charge of his life. If attention is given only to the clinical intervention, this opportunity is forfeited."

It is our strong belief that the hospital of the future should incorporate the best of technocratic, humanistic, and holistic care. It would retain the useful techniques of technomedicine but change the philosophy that underlies their practice, defining them as third-line support in a holistic program. Surgeons, for example, would assume that anesthetized patients are conscious and treat them accordingly; pre-operative visualization would set the patient up for success; and family members would be waiting in the postoperative recovery room. In other words, the underlying principle of separation would be replaced with connection and integration, principles that the behavior of the staff would reflect.

We can envision a Reiki healer on call in the emergency room to send healing energy to each patient even as the technocratic team does its interventionist work. An hour or more of daily massage would be integral to the care of every patient able to be touched, with energy healing available for those burn victims and others who cannot. Nutritional and psychological counseling would be offered each day, support groups of all kinds would meet on every floor, and the hospital food would be the greenest, freshest, most organic, and most nutritious to be had anywhere. Much of it, as Haas suggests, would be grown in the hospital's own organic gardens, where the patients could tend flowers or rows of vegetables if they so desire, or simply stroll or sit and enjoy the view. The attractive rooms would have windows opening onto the gardens and pretty courtyards where folks can gather. Music and art would be everywhere; we envision those long bare hospital walls covered with artwork done by the patients themselves in well-equipped art rooms available to all. Staff meetings on each floor would include every practitioner and therapist involved in the patient's care, from the radiologist to the nutritionist. Their combined input would result in a truly comprehensive and well-rounded approach.

Planetree Hospital (see chapter 3) has taken several steps in this direction. But the slow and limited growth of Planetree's tremendously innovative approach to hospital care is telling. Beginning with the architecture, everything about most hospitals is designed to serve the functional needs of the staff and expedite technomedical care. It is very difficult to reorient hospitals to focus on patient needs in a comprehensive, holistic way—such reorientation must rebuild not only the physical walls of the hospital building, but also the mental walls of the paradigm that generated its design. While the addition of softer, more humanistic services will surely enhance the experience of many patients, if hospitals are to become the healing centers envisioned by Elson Haas, they must take a "zero-based approach" to planning—that is, an approach free of assumptions that allows for a total revisioning of health and healing.

INTEGRATIVE FINANCING

Since the health care system of the future will be produced by a future society, we might usefully ask how a society that would support a holistically oriented health care system would look. And how would it allocate its health care resources?

On the macro level, the government would need to invest in public education. This is quite different from the current emphasis on disease prevention. "Preventive medicine is not mammograms," says Elson Haas; rather it is "individual responsibility for health." And that responsibility, he says, is difficult to assume in the present insurance systems that are "disease oriented," in which the deductible prevents entry into the system. He would advocate first-dollar coverage with the co-pay increasing with use as an incentive to take advantage of a truly prevention-oriented system. Alan Gaby agrees: "If we are going to make an attempt to provide medical services for everyone, we should at the very least re-orient our priorities. That is, we should begin allowing third party coverage for inexpensive treatments that work . . . [and] refuse to pay for expensive treatments that do not work, which include much of what is now being done by conventional doctors" (1994:1095). During our interview with him, Gaby also argued that insurance by its very nature is a problem, suggesting that its elimination or transformation would be a huge step in the right direction:

> Get rid of insurance. Have a type of nationalized catastrophic insurance. If we're going to be in the business of insurance, do it more like medical savings accounts. Either get people [government] vouchers or have them pay for their own care. That way the market will determine what is done. At present, medicine is not a market, it's an economy. We need to turn it back into a market. And the FDA needs to have its wrists slapped so it will get off the back of natural substances. Do more research on natural substances; make them more available. Tell the medical scene to get back to its roots and stay away from high-tech, high-cost toxic medicine except in situations where it is absolutely necessary.

Many suggest that economics will cease to drive health care when it becomes a reasonably priced commodity. This can be achieved by the use of natural, inexpensive healing modalities for the majority of conditions, combined with the elimination of smoking and chemicals in food and water and the reduction in accidents and violence-related episodes that would accompany a healthier population. Within such a society, fee-for-service medical care combined with support for catastrophic costs seems adequate. Private insurance companies would be eliminated or transformed, which would restore normal consumer relations between an educated, informed, and empowered public and caring and confident healers.

The Future of Medicine and the Future Society

Shifting the responsibility for health as well as for the payment of health services will require a significant emotional maturation of our society. People will need to move into greater consciousness in order to realize that they make health choices every minute. They will need education about disease prevention, environmental preservation, and self-care. Finally, and perhaps most difficult of all, they will have to forgo magical thinking about their own mortality and simultaneously face their intense fear of death. It is this last fear that prevents people from getting really involved with self-care. Ironically the less people care for themselves, the less involved with death they can be—until it faces them squarely. Working out a life within the context of death awareness and acceptance can actually lead to a much healthier lifestyle and greater responsibility. Acceptance of the inevitability of death helps an individual to engage more fully with life and more purposefully exercise choice. Denying death allows one to justify a cavalier "eat, drink, and be merry" approach to life.

With maturity regarding personal responsibility for health will come maturity regarding financial responsibility for health. The third-party payer system encourages avoidance of personal responsibility, an unwillingness to assess value, and a reluctance to understand the processes of one's own body. Health insurance is the ultimate victim statement: "Somebody else is going to pay when things go wrong with my body, and I really don't care how much it costs if it doesn't come out of my pocket." With financial responsibility will come enhanced motivation to change deleterious habits and follow through on health-enhancement programs. Medical knowledge will no longer be the exclusive purview of medical practitioners. With massive public health education programs that teach children from kindergarten on about human anatomy, physiology, nutritional and emotional needs, and so on, people will develop greater self-knowledge and will select their health services intelligently, with an eye to wellness and prevention. For the most part, they will pay out-of-pocket for these low-cost services. Insurance, if it continues to exist, will be reserved for catastrophic events.

To date, holistic health care in the United States has been largely a middle-class phenomenon. Lack of public education about the importance of diet and nutrition, in combination with the high costs of organic foods, nutritional supplements, and initial wellness care, have made them generally unavailable to the poor. This situation must change. In our future society, understanding that paying upstream for prevention is far more cost-effective than paying downstream for illness, federal and state governments, in tandem with religious and other private groups, will ensure that the poor have access to nutritious food and to the same wellness- and prevention-oriented care as the middle class. Effective public education programs will help to ensure that poverty does not correlate with poor nutritional choices—the same budget that buys low-nutrient white rice, for example, can buy nutrient-rich brown rice, and fresh vegetables still cost less than soft drinks and chips. Individual efforts to make better health choices will be aided by many holistic practitioners who will take Joel Fort up on his suggestion that they donate a percentage of their time to caring for those unable to pay. At the level of the wider society, "what we are really after," Norm Shealy insists, "is the development and growth of the spirit. When people begin to take responsibility for their health, they begin to move toward their spiritual reality, [to focus their energy on the things that they *can* change, thus arriving] at the state of the transcendent will" (Shealy and Myss 1993:261).

Philosopher and humanist Rudolf Steiner postulated that society has, innately, a threefold nature that reflects the three primary aspects of human nature. These are the sphere of "rights," which is loosely aligned with our notion of government and law; the economic sphere, which is concerned with compensation and ownership or wealth; and the spiritual/cultural sphere, encompassing the arts and every aspect of life concerned with humankind's higher functioning, including education and medicine. Viewed in terms of Steiner's three spheres, medicine in this county falls squarely in the economic realm with an interlocking grid of laws to protect the rights of the participants, as long as the rights are quantifiable in economic terms. The *spirit* of medicine is deadlocked by the overarching power of the realms of economics and law.

One cannot envision the future of health care as those aligned with the holistic paradigm would like to see it without radically altering its relationship to money and the law. With respect to economics, the entire technomedical system must realign itself with goals that have a global focus. It must: (1) accept a level of growth that is consistent with ecological concerns; (2) restore normal economic relations between buyers and sellers; (3) develop a balanced marketplace with a choice of practitioners, services, pricing, and location.

Meeting these goals requires a social and political mandate from an electorate willing to assume personal responsibility for health and illness and to forgo unrealistic fantasies of rescue from self-responsibility. As a society we must grow in awareness of the dysfunctionality of the myth of technological transcendence; we must come to understand that technology will never transcend all of nature's limitations, including old age and death. Our attachment to this cultural myth and to the technomedical model of which it forms a part has led to extensive misappropriation of resources. As a nation, we devote too much to medical and pharmacological research and product development, and too little to prevention, health education, and improvements in the nutritional value of our food and the quality of our environment.

In the minds of many people in this country and others, medical care is a right, not a privilege, and should not have to be paid for by the individual citizen. Many Americans look to Great Britain and Canada for models of nationalized health systems that the United States should adopt. But to those in the alternative health movement, including most of our interviewees, nationalized health insurance entails technomedical hegemony and would thus severely limit the availability and accessibility of alternatives and curtail individual freedom of choice. Conceiving of health care in a free-market economy, as we suggest here, departs radically from these national and global trends toward centralized medicine—a fact that reflects the power of the technomedical industry to convince the public that someone else should pay for health care. As we demonstrated earlier in this book, the medicalization of the life cycle, from conception to death, when combined with the flagrant destruction and depletion of planetary resources and the compensatory inventions of technology, has produced a mandate for an interventionist health care system. Redistributing resources to provide a healthy planet as a backdrop for a healthy life, restoring the notion of health care as a moment-to-moment series of personal choices, and eliminating deleterious and harmful medical treatments, would make it more than possible to provide free catastrophic care for those who need it. Catastrophic care would then become the "right," with all other aspects of "health" referred either to the individual or to society as a whole. Alan Gaby notes that

> According to some, we should spare no expense to provide all Americans with the medical care they need. The problem is that we are already sparing few expenses, spending nearly a trillion dollars a year on medical care. Yet, in some ways, we have one of the sickest societies on the planet. To those who say that health care is an inalienable right, I say that clean food, air, and water, basic shelter, and a decent income for all workers are inalienable rights. Since our resources are finite, we should carefully consider how best to use them in order to promote the greatest good for the greatest number of people. (1994:1085)

On the personal level, education in the home needs to focus on the consequences of lifestyle choices and to articulate values that opt out of the American dream of processed food, sedentary life, and consumerism. The concept of self-care requires a daily conscious focus on one's physical, mental, and emotional state and the ability to take corrective action whenever imbalance is sensed. When one cannot correct the imbalance or when the condition is more serious, one might consult a practitioner as a guide to understanding the situation and arraying options, rather than as a technical expert expected to "fix it." When health care becomes self-care, it can no longer be thought of as a commodity, and the grip of economics will lessen.

As long as medical care is designed and controlled by economic forces, the legal system, which translates civil inequities into economic terms, will have free reign within this sphere. However, should this paradigm shift occur societywide, the legal system would have a meaningful role to play in the health care system. For the law to assume its rightful place as the guardian of freedom in health care decision making, the prerequisites include:

- An educated public, able to exercise responsibility in making choices
- Recognition of personal responsibility and its consequences in lifestyle choices
- Freedom restored to individuals to select healing resources
- Regulation of health care practitioners free from political (economic) agendas
- Reduced societal obligation to pay for personal negligence
- Societal tolerance for ambiguity, mystery, and uncontrollable and acausal events

The underlying value required to separate healing from legal strictures is freedom. And with freedom comes its constant companion, responsibility. Our victim-oriented society produces scenarios in which smokers sue tobacco companies rather than taking responsibility for their addiction. While the legal process moves into high gear to determine guilt and innocence, tobacco companies continue to crank out millions of cigarettes, sometimes with the help of government subsidies to tobacco growers. This situation is indicative of our pervasive reluctance to engage in radical thinking about why we have the conditions we have in health care and society in general. While it is undoubtedly beneficial to limit tobacco companies' ability to sell and promote their products, laws and litigation do absolutely nothing to promote personal responsibility. Under present conditions, expanding medical treatment of smokers to include psychological services to address the roots of their addiction would be more effective.

The fact that massive amounts of money are spent in heroic efforts to stave off imminent death and develop ever more expensive new technologies, instead of on the preventive and educative care that could have prevented the catastrophic illness and obviated the need for the shiny new machine, reflects our societal narcissism. We behave as though our resources are unlimited, refusing to recognize our intergenerational responsibility to our communities and to the planet we inhabit. Redesigning health care along more holistic lines begins with the individual's self-responsibility and willingness to express and live values that are fundamentally divergent from the prevailing cultural myth. Barry Sultanoff evokes the potentially transcendent quality of this transformation:

> We must be visionaries, and help our clients entertain possibilities, especially the possibility of the best outcome for their situations. We must be guides who nurture and coax forward the inner healer in each of our clients. Why have we clung to the paradigm of doctors as ultimate authority? We have discouraged personal responsibility and self care. We have converted into medical dogma the notion that it is somehow dangerous for patients to tinker with themselves. . . . Since dream is the language of the unconscious, if we're going to affect deep change, we must . . . seed a dream or vision that's different from the prevailing fear and paranoia; a dream of cooperation, creativity, and fun; a dream of possibility rather than limitation. (1994:484)

Hegemonies and heresies, instead of being viewed as competing claims to "truth," can be seen to represent an evolutionary process. In *A Brief History of Everything* (1996), Ken Wilber insists that the essence of evolution is that each next step must both transcend and include the ones that went before. Molecules transcend and include atoms, cells transcend and include molecules, organisms transcend and include cells, sentience transcends and includes the precognitive states that preceded it. Thus, Wilber argues, a paradigm that truly represents the next evolutionary step for humanity must not eradicate, but must transcend and include, what went before. For our purposes here, Wilber's insight means that to represent real evolution in health care, the holistic paradigm of medicine must transcend and include the other two paradigms. Holism must keep what works from the technomedical and humanistic models, yet go beyond them to incorporate what their limitations would not admit.

While we cannot know exactly what form this incorporation will take, we have tried to envision and describe the qualities it must exhibit. Earlier we noted that a society's definition of the human body both shapes and reflects that society's vision of itself and the universe it inhabits. Americans have been living out the vision shaped and reflected by a definition of the body as a machine, and we know what kind of society that vision has worked to create. If the paradigm shift we have been discussing in this book were to happen on a culturewide scale, what kind of society might be shaped and reflected by a definition of the body as an energy field?

Should that definition ever become widely accepted, we see no danger of holism taking hegemonic form, as its diffuseness will make it too difficult to control. Like the Internet, holistic healing is a Stage-Four open system, fluidly and immediately responsive to new information. In place of the current medical hierarchy, with everything else "alternative" to allopathy's dominance, health care would come to constitute a networking system of interconnections. Its multiple modalities and fiercely individualistic applications will prevent the kind of exclusivity of practitioner and method that allopathy insisted upon. The fullness of the holistic vision will be manifested by healers whose compassion and commitment enable—no, *require* them to inspire the very best from a partially sedated public in order to create the necessary conditions for health and wholeness for the individual and the community. Within this larger ethos of inclusion and transcendence, seemingly opposed values will blend to create a medicine of the future—one that reflects the will of a healing rather than an ailing world.

Appendix

Interviewees and Other Data Sources

PHYSICIANS INTERVIEWED

Board certification, if any, follows the physician's name. Additional interests and expertise are listed on the line below. All names are real unless preceded by an asterisk, which indicates a pseudonym.

Scott Anderson, M.D., Internal Medicine, San Rafael and San Francisco, Calif.
Nutritional medicine
Paulanne Balch, M.D., Family Practice, Boulder, Colo.
Alex Cadoux, M.D., Emergency Medicine, Internal Medicine, Baltimore, Md., and Tucson, Ariz.
Orthomolecular medicine, integrative medicine, cardiovascular disease reversal
Larry Dossey, M.D., Internal Medicine, Santa Fe, N.M.
Lectures, writes, publishes *Alternative Medicine*
*David Dowling, M.D., Internal Medicine, Boulder, Colo.
Visualization, meditation, nutritional medicine
Anu de Monterice, M.D., Psychiatry, Cotati, Calif.
Herbal medicine
Paul Dunn, M.D., Pediatrics, Oak Park, Ill.
Eclectic; osteopathy, neurology
David Edelberg, M.D., Internal Medicine, Chicago, Ill.
Holistic medicine; director, American Whole Health
Ted Edwards, M.D., Family Practice, Austin, Tex.
Barry D. Elson, M.D., Northampton, Mass.
Allergy/environmental medicine, clinical nutrition, chronic illness
Joel Fort, M.D., Ph.D., Psychiatry, San Francisco, Calif.
Retired clinician; organizational consultant
Kathy Frye, M.D., Obstetrics and Gynecology, Tucson, Ariz.
Homeopathy
Alan Gaby, M.D., Seattle, Wash.
Nutritional medicine
David Gershan, M.D., Family Practice, San Francisco, Calif.
Public health, anthroposophical medicine
Jim Gordon, M.D., Psychiatry, Washington, D.C.
Holistic medicine, Chinese medicine, herbal therapies
Kathleen Grandison, M.D., Family Practice, Shelburn Falls, Mass.
Nutrition, homeopathy

Michael Greenberg, M.D., Dermatology, Elk Grove Village, Ill.
Eclectic

Peter Grote, M.D., Family Practice, Seattle, Wash.
Eclectic

Elson Haas, M.D., Internal Medicine, San Rafael, Calif.
Holistic medicine; director, Marin Center for Preventive Medicine

Bethany Hays, M.D., Obstetrics and Gynecology, Yarmouth, Me.
Women's health, maternal-fetal medicine, intuitive diagnosis

Sandra Kamiak, M.D., Psychiatry, Saratoga, Calif.
Classical homeopathy

Dawn LeManne, M.D., Oncology, Hayward, Calif.
Managed care setting

Evarts Loomis, M.D., Family Practice
Holistic pioneer, founder of Meadowlark

Olga Luchakova, M.D., Ph.D., Pediatrics, Lafayette, Calif.
Instructor in yoga and Christian mysticism

Ann McCombs, D.O., Family Practice, Seattle, Wash.
Holistic medicine

Deborah Malka, M.D., Ph.D., Soquel, Calif.
Holistic modalities, energy medicine

Bill Manahan, M.D., Family Practice, Mankato, Minn.
Holistic generalist and teacher

Jack Mansberger, M.D., General Surgery, Thomasville, Ga.
Humanist

*Glenn Masterson, M.D., Internal Medicine, Vallejo, Calif.
Family practice in managed care setting

Lewis Mehl-Madrona, M.D., Family Practice, Geriatrics, Psychiatry, Burlington, Vt.
Emergency medicine, midwifery, alternative cancer and AIDS treatments, Native American medicine; author and lecturer

Karin Montero, M.D., Plastic Surgery, Austin, Tex.
Nutritional counseling, preventive medicine

Ed Neal, M.D., Internal Medicine, Portland, Ore.
Jungian analyst

Christiane Northrup, M.D., Obstetrics and Gynecology, Yarmouth, Me.
Author and lecturer in women's health

Peter Nunn, M.D., General Surgery, Victoria, B.C., Canada
Eclectic; herbs, Chinese medicine, counseling

Amy P. Saltzmann, M.D., Internal Medicine, Palo Alto, Calif.
Medical acupuncture, nutritional and herbal therapies, mindfulness meditation

Len Saputo, M.D., Internal Medicine, Walnut Creek, Calif.
Complementary medicine

*Natalie Singer, M.D., Internal Medicine, Oakland, Calif.
Primary care in managed care setting

John W. (Jack) Travis, M.D., M.P.H., Afton, Va.
Preventive medicine; author and speaker on adult and infant wellness
Terry Tyler, M.D., Psychiatry, Durango, Colo.
Breath work, Reichian energy work
Peter Vargas, M.D., Obstetrics and Gynecology, Denver, Colo.
Humanist

METAPHYSICIANS FROM *METAPHYSICIANS' TALES*

The personal stories of these MetaPhysicians appear in Tyler and St. John 1989; an asterisk indicates a pseudonym.

*Jess Carpenter, M.D., Psychiatry
*Gary Cook, M.D., Psychiatry
*Ruth Childers, M.D., Family Practice
*Karen Feldman, M.D., Obstetrics and Gynecology
*David Filmore, M.D., Internal Medicine
*Julia Hall, M.D., general practitioner
*Myron Hirshberg, M.D., Family Practice
*Mike Holt, M.D., Pediatrics
*Rebecca Lawrence, M.D., Family Practice
*Marilyn Levinson, M.D., Family Practice
Maureen Longworth, M.D., Family Practice
*"Phenix," M.D., child psychiatry
*Alex Ransonhoff, M.D., Family Practice
*Arnold Rosenberg, M.D., Pathology
*Gene Ross, M.D., Emergency Medicine
Terry Tyler, M.D., Psychiatry
*Walter Mueller, M.D., Anesthesiology

Members of the MetaPhysicians who were also interviewed for this book: Larry Dossey, Sandra Kamiak, Dawn LeManne, Glenn Masterson, Jack Travis, and Terry Tyler.

PHYSICIANS FROM THE "PHYSICIAN IN TRANSITION" COLUMN

The "Physician in Transition" column appeared for several years in *Holistic Medicine,* edited by Bill Manahan and published by the American Holistic Medical Association, 6728 Old McLean Village Drive, McLean, Virginia 22101 (703–556–9245); HolistMed@aol.com (www.ahmaholistic.com). Specialties are drawn from the stories. (Full information on the issue, date, and page numbers of each story appears in the reference section.)

Peter Albright, M.D., Family Practice
Henry Edward Altenberg, M.D., Psychiatry
Bob Anderson, M.D., Family Practice

Terry Collins, M.D., Preventive Medicine
Paul J. Dunn, M.D., Pediatrics
Jordan Goetz, M.D., Internal Medicine
William J. Goldwag, M.D., Family Practice
Sol J. Grazi, M.D., holistic general practice
Ken Hamilton, M.D., General Surgery
Henry Hochberg, M.D., Surgery
Karl Humiston, M.D., Psychiatry
Robert Ivker, D.O., Family Practice
H. Leonard Jones, Jr., M.D., Internal Medicine
George Keeler, M.D., General Surgery, Psychiatry
Gurudarshan Singh Khalsa, M.D., Family Practice
Albert Kunnen, M.D., Obstetrics and Gynecology
Roy Kupsinel, M.D., Family Practice
Alice Laule, M.D., Opthamology
Cathy Lindsay, D.O.
Evarts Loomis, M.D., holistic medicine (since the 1940s)
Judith Petry, M.D., Plastic Surgery
Amy P. Saltzmann, M.D., Internal Medicine
Walt Stoll, M.D., Family Practice
Vernon M. Sylvest, M.D., Pathology
Barry Sultanoff, M.D., Psychiatry
Richard A. Tuscher, D.O., Family Practice (deceased)
Bowen White, M.D., Family Practice
Jacqueline Wilson, M.D., Family Practice

Physicians from "Physician in Transition" who were interviewed for this book: Paul Dunn, Bethany Hays, Evarts Loomis, Bill Manahan, and Amy Saltzmann.

Notes

Chapter 1. The Technocratic Model of Medicine

Portions of this chapter have been adapted from Davis-Floyd 1992.

1. We are aware of the dangers of overgeneralization about a monolithic "biomedicine" (see, e.g., Cassell 1991; Cassell and Jacobs 1987; Gaines and Hahn 1982; Hahn 1985; Hahn and Gaines 1985; Good 1990, 1994), and we agree with Mary Jo Delvecchio Good and Byron Good that overarching analyses of biomedicine and "the biomedical model" tend to produce glib characterizations, and that "little can be expected of studies of the nature of medical knowledge unless they are situated, contextualized, and ethnographically rich" (1985:83).

Face-to-face at an anthropology meeting some years ago with Byron Good, one of the most respected medical anthropologists in the field and an ardent protester against the monolithic approach to the study and criticism of biomedicine, Davis-Floyd asked him with some trepidation if he felt that in spite of its variations, biomedicine could be accurately characterized as a system that (1) mechanizes the body; (2) objectifies the patient; and (3) alienates practitioner from patient. He replied in the affirmative. This endorsement by an authoritative figure, one known for his ethographic investigations of the variations within medicine, gave Davis-Floyd the impetus to proceed with the description of technomedicine we present in chapter 1.

2. Beth and Piaget 1966; Ley 1983; Rubinstein, Laughlin, and McManus 1984:34; Sperry 1974, 1982.

3. Lynn Payer's *Medicine and Culture* (1988) offers a fascinating analysis of the cultural differences between the medical systems of four of the most industrially advanced countries—France, Germany, England, and the United States. In Europe, where the germ theory of disease was developed, homeopathy was not eradicated by allopathy but continued to exist as a respected profession.

4. See for examples Beuf 1979; Goffman 1961; Hahn 1985; Illich 1976; Konner 1987; LeBaron 1981; Mendelsohn 1979, 1981; Nolen 1979; Parsons 1951; Stein 1967; Tao-Kim-Hai 1979.

5. Specialists are physicians whose training makes them experts in a bodily system (gastroenterology, cardiology, nephrology, orthopedics, etc.) or in a specialized mode of treatment (surgery, emergency medicine, neonatology). Subspecialists further refine their area of expertise, often combining a primary focus with a specialty (pediatric nephrology); apply their specialty to one area (orthopedics for the hand); or combine two specialty areas (cardiac surgery).

6. A survey by *Medical Economics* revealed the net incomes of physicians earning a quarter of a million dollars or more, according to specialty, as follows: 3 percent psychiatrists, 5 percent family practitioners, 5 percent pediatricians, 7 percent internists, 19 percent general surgeons, 25 percent anesthesiologists, 30 percent obstetrician-gynecologists, 33 percent cardiologists, 39 percent radiologists, and 48 percent orthopedic surgeons. On average, 10 percent of all nonsurgeons and 28 percent of all surgeons earned this amount annually (*Birth* 1996).

7. For an excellent and succinct discussion of the relative merits of various scientific methods of evaluating medical care, including the RCT, see Enkin, Keirse, and Chalmers 1989:3–10.

8. At the same time, it has trapped physicians in a vicious cycle. Aware that the information on the monitor printout will constitute the official record of a birth, they find themselves working less to enhance the birth experience for the mother and more to make the monitor strip look good, lest it be used against them in court (Cartwright 1998). They rush to perform a cesarean when the strip shows slowdowns of the fetal heart (a normal occurrence in many labors), only to find, all too often, that the baby is fine and could have had a normal (and much less expensive) birth. A plethora of randomized controlled trials conducted over the past fifteen years has shown that intermittent auscultation by trained personnel produces outcomes as good as or better than the monitors, without increasing the cesarean rate or the cost of birth. (Leveno et al. 1986; Prentice and Lind 1987; Shy et al. 1990; Sandmire 1990). See Goer 1995:131–153 for summaries of thirty-nine medical studies relevant to EFM.

9. The male bias in medicine has not only resulted in an obstetrical system that treats the female body as an inherently dysfunctional machine, it has also endangered women's lives in other areas. For example, the large-scale clinical trials on the proper treatment of heart attacks were conducted on men; for many years, women treated for heart attacks received drug dosages that had been established for men, often completely inappropriate for women's smaller bodies—a dangerous corollary of the technocratic treatment of the male body as the prototype of the properly functioning body-machine.

10. The other half of research performed is basic research into life processes, which attempts to discover or unlock secrets that may lead to improved conditions. The National Institutes of Health and private foundations and medical centers spend another $15 billion on such basic research, which has no immediately apparent profitable application (Califano 1994:41). The results of these efforts, though they are primarily publicly funded, are made available to the private sector for use in applied research and development.

11. Many physicians, holistic and otherwise, have written candidly about their views of orthodox medicine. The stories of Deepak Chopra (1991), Patch Adams (1993), Bernie Siegel (1986), and W. P. Joy (1979) are a few of the better known. A number of our interviewees, including Larry Dossey (1982), Christiane Northrup (1995), Jack Travis (1981), and Peter Nunn (with Michael

Greenberg, 1992) have published accounts of their personal experiences with traditional medicine and why and how they have moved beyond the confines of their training. A bibliography of such accounts developed by St. John and Tyler in 1992 includes more than two hundred titles. Since such maverick physicians are rarely allowed to publish in peer-reviewed journals, most of their voices have not been widely heard.

Chapter 2. Medical Training as Technocratic Initiation

Portions of this chapter have been excerpted in revised form from an article by Davis-Floyd, "Obstetrical Training as a Rite of Passage," *Medical Anthropology Quarterly* 1(3) (1987):288–318, which contains interview material from an earlier study. All direct quotations from interviewees not otherwise identified are from that article.

1. In this chapter we focus on the psychological transformation of medical students, not on the process of medical training, which has been well and thoroughly described by numerous social scientists and physicians. See for excellent examples the works of Renee Fox (1957, 1980), Nancy Stoller Shaw (1974), Diana Scully (1980), Ann Oakley (1984), Howard Stein (1990), and Byron Good and Mary Jo DelVecchio Good (1993; see also Good 1995); as well as by physicians Cynthia Carver (1981) and Michelle Harrison (1982), medical anthropologist Melvin Konner (1987), and former social worker Charles LeBaron (1982), who have recorded their personal experiences of this process (see also Buchner and Stelling 1977).

2. The role of ritual in Western biomedicine has been examined in various contexts. See Beuf 1979; Davis-Floyd 1992; Fox 1957; Katz 1981; Henslin and Biggs 1971; Miner 1975; Parsons 1951.

3. Charles LeBaron was a social worker in the New York hospital system for twelve years before he entered Harvard Medical School at the age of thirty-four. His book, *Gentle Vengance* (1981), perceptively and insightfully chronicles his experiences during his first year at Harvard in 1979, before any attempt had been made to create the present "New Pathways" program. We draw on it heavily in this chapter and elsewhere, in part to call attention to this valuable and overlooked book.

4. See Davis-Floyd 1992:7–21 for a more complete description of ritual and rites of passage; see Laughlin, McManus, and d'Aquili 1990 for a discussion of the neurophysiology of ritual.

5. It has been suggested that because the corpus callosum, which plays a major role in conveying information between hemispheres, is significantly larger in women, they are less able than men to maintain emotional detachment. In other words, while men can compartmentalize, engaging in left-brained rational thinking that completely excludes the emotions, women are more likely to think and feel at the same time, making decisions and taking actions in a more integrated, whole-brained way. (However, the whole brain is involved

in all brain functions, and the corpus callosum can be deliberately developed in either sex.)

6. The other seven research centers are based at the University of California at Davis, Columbia University, Minneapolis Medical Research Center, the University of Maryland School of Medicine, the University of Texas Health Science Center, the University of Virginia School of Nursing, the Kessler Institute for Rehabilitation in New Jersey, Bastyr University in Seattle, and Beth Israel Hospital and Harvard Medical School. For information about the research being conducted in these centers, contact the Office of Alternative Medicine Clearinghouse, PO Box 8218, Silver Spring, MD 20907–8218. Phone: 888–644–6226; Fax: 301–495–4957. Website: http://altmed.od.nih.gov.

7. The *Journal of Alternative and Complementary Medicine* every year publishes a full listing of all courses in alternative medicine taught in U.S. medical schools; to order a copy, call 800–654–3237.

Chapter 3. The Humanistic Model of Medicine

1. The physicians we interviewed who represent the humanistic model are Dawn LeManne, Joel Fort, Glenn Masterson, Natalie Singer, and Peter Vargas. In earlier stages of their medical careers, Bill Manahan and Karin Montero also classified themselves as humanists.

2. In this choice Moyers was strongly supported by the Fetzer Institute, a foundation headquartered in Kalamazoo, Michigan, and dedicated to discovering the relationship of body, mind, and spirit to human health and healing (Fetzer Institute 1995:3). This funding strategy reflects a policy decision made in the early 1990s by the Fetzer board to work with the proponents of medical humanism, which it termed "relationship-centered care" (Tresolini and the Pew-Fetzer Task Force 1994), to transform the system from the inside (Janis Claflin, Fetzer board member, personal communication).

3. A technocratic physician quoted in Biesele and Davis-Floyd (1996:310) responded this way to Siegel's message: "What Siegel is saying is that whether you have a diagnosis of a cancer or not, that should not keep you from living your life. There are still things to do, and [you] may be able to tune in to the connections you do have. Relationships are still important, maybe more important. . . . [And Siegel] is emphasizing the emotional content by shaving his head to be sympathetic with those patients having chemotherapy, hugging his patients, and being in contact, sharing their feelings." There was a certain wistfulness in this physician's acknowledgment of his own very different orientation to patient treatment, as he noted, "I haven't come to that point . . . I just recommend hairpieces instead."

4. Numerous studies support the superiority of patient-centered approaches, which, as Smith (1996:7) points out: (1) produce many of the same data about symptoms ordinarily obtained in conventional interviews (Linfors and Neelan 1981); (2) produce the personal data and emotional material, normally screened out of conventional interviews, essential to developing an accurate biopsycho-

social description of the patient (Cox, Holbrook, and Rutter 1981; Cox, Rutter, and Holbrook 1981; Hopkinson, Cox, and Rutter 1981); (3) produce some information about physical symptoms not elicited in doctor-centered interviews that is often of great value in diagnosing physical disease (Cox, Rutter, and Holbrook 1981); (4) efficiently point to the most important problem the patient has at a given time (Smith and Hoppe 1991); (5) increase patients' satisfaction with their care (Roter, Hall, and Katz 1987; Hall, Roter, and Katz 1988; Roter 1989; Smith et al. 1995a), which in turn may decrease malpractice suits (Vaccarino 1977; Huycke and Huycke 1994); (6) enhance patient compliance and increase patient knowledge and recall (Lazare 1973; Hall, Roter, and Katz 1988; Roter 1989)—all of which are associated with better outcomes; and (7) improve the confidence of residents in their psychosocial skills and increase their anticipation of positive outcomes (Smith, Marshall, and Cohen-Cole 1994; Smith et al. 1995b).

Chapter 4. The Holistic Model of Medicine

1. According to interviewee Evarts Loomis, when the American Holistic Medical Association (see chapter 5) was in the planning stages, he, Norm Shealy, and Gladys McGarey engaged in a discussion of whether to spell "holism" with a "w" or with an "h." The "h" won, he says, "because 'whole' and 'holy' all go back to the Anglo-Saxon 'hal,' which gave us in English both 'hale' and 'heart.' So it was much more comprehensive, because when you're dealing with holism, you're dealing with health, you're looking at totalities, including the heart."

2. A Harvard Medical School manual, *Alternative Medicine: Implications for Clinical Practice* (Eisenberg 1995), developed under the direction of David Eisenberg, explains:

> Most alternative medicines ally themselves with the theory of "vitalism" to explain that which makes living things different from inanimate matter. In the West, vitalism is derived from the academic traditions of Paul Joseph Barthez' "principle vital" and the alternative tradition of Franz Anton Mesmer's "animal magnetism." Manipulation or enhancement of the body's vital energy is often used to explain the efficacy of alternative therapeutic interventions.
>
> Alternative medicine's vitalism emphasizes at least four areas: a) vital energy as a force analagous to electromagnetism, but so subtle that it continues to evade conventional science's detection; b) vital energy as a psychic or mental force; c) vital energy as spiritual presence(s); and d) vital energy as an organizational principle or informational network. Examples of vital energy as a physical force include homeopathy's vital spiritual force, chiropractic's innate intelligence, and Robert Hare's psychic force.

3. For a discussion of midwives' use of intuition as authoritative knowledge, see Davis-Floyd and Davis 1996 and Roncalli 1997.

4. Recent research conducted by R. Wiseman and Marilyn Schlitz (1996) indicates that the intentionality of the researcher can have a profound effect on the results of the experiment.

5. The RCTs on the efficacy of prayer reported in Larry Dossey's *Healing Words* (1993) constitute a case in point. For summaries and meta-analyses of RTCs addressing multiple aspects of nutrition, see Alan Gaby's text, *Nutritional Medicine* (forthcoming 1999).

6. In 1991, the *British Medical Journal* reported on a survey of research on homeopathic medicine between the years 1966 and 1990. Out of 107 studies, 81 indicated positive results. The survey was undertaken by physicians in the Netherlands, whose original intention was to disprove the effectiveness of homeopathy. Their guarded conclusion is that "the evidence of clinical trials is positive but not sufficient to draw definitive conclusions. . . . This indicates that there is a legitimate case for the further evaluation of homeopathy, but only by means of well-performed trials" (Kleijnen, Knipschild, and ter Riet 1991:323).

7. Many paradigms of healing are operating in the United States that we do not touch upon in this book. These include many folk, traditional, and religious models. In addition, every alternative healing modality has an underlying belief system specific and unique to it. And every medical specialty and subspecialty has a culture and a worldview specific to members of that specialty. The public health paradigm, which is tremendously influential in this country, is not specifically addressed beyond our mention of its connections to the humanistic model.

8. As previously noted, the whole brain is actually involved in all brain functions, so the distinctions that many have drawn between "left-brained" and "right-brained" thinking are themselves somewhat arbitrary and inaccurate. What we should really speak of is a predominance of left-lobe activity in certain types of thought. For example, the left hemisphere primarily mediates language production, analytic thought, and lineal and causal sequencing of events, whereas the right hemisphere primarily mediates the production of images, gestalt or holistic thought, and spatiotemporal patterning (Bryden 1982; Ley 1983; Sperry 1974, 1982). Simplifying a bit, one could say that the left lobe distinguishes parts, and the right lobe makes possible the perception of the whole. The ability to perceive the whole makes it less likely that one will become too narrowly focused on the part.

9. Of course, many of the individual modalities considered holistic are ancient, specific, and highly precise.

Chapter 5. Catalysts for Transformation

1. As noted previously, we had intended to focus our research on holistic physicians, only becoming aware of this middle ground of humanism late in the game. Thus, our data do not speak very specifically to this issue. Chapter 3 includes some examples of what sparked individual physicians to begin to

perform research and practice in the humanistic arena. It is our impression that often such a shift toward humanism is sparked by exposure to the benefits of a caring relationship, either (1) when one physician is moved by observing another, usually a mentor, interacting in a humanistic way with patients in a setting where such interactions are rare; or (2) when a physician receives tremendous positive feedback after trying to relate, as Arthur Kleinman did as a medical student trying to help the burned seven-year-old. We further speculate that the nature of such a shift may be more gentle and less dramatic than the shift to holism, as it can simply involve the incorporation of compassionate, individualized care into an otherwise conventional technocratic practice.

2. American Holistic Medical Association, 6728 Old McLean Village Drive, McLean, VA 22101 (703–556–9245). E-mail: HolistMed@aol.com. Website: www.ahmaholistic.com.

Chapter 6. The Transformative Journey

1. Several of our interviewees do function at the national level; these include Larry Dossey, who often lectures across the country and whose many books on healing (e.g., 1982, 1993) are well known and widely read; Christiane Northrup, author of *Women's Bodies, Women's Wisdom* (1994), who has become a national spokesperson for feminist approaches to healing; and Jim Gordon, author of *Manifesto for a New Medicine* (1996b), who chairs the Advisory Board of the National Institutes of Health Office of Alternative Medicine.

Chapter 7. Practicing Holistic Medicine in a Technocratic Society

1. The financial and organizational structure of holistic clinics often does not mirror the technocratic norm. We mentioned previously that Women-to-Women, the women's health care clinic in Yarmouth, Maine, where both Bethany Hays and Christiane Northrup work, is jointly owned by one of the M.D.'s and a nurse-practitioner; the other M.D. is an employee, as is the other nurse-practitioner. Both physicians commented on how frequently they run up against public expectations that the two doctors own the clinic and are in charge. They stressed that "there is no hierarchy" in their organization; the M.D.'s and the nurse-practitioners work independently, consulting with each other when appropriate.

2. An interesting aside on the subject of power is the power that holistic physicians often ascribe to particular modalities. For example, Kathy Frye, an OB/GYN and practicing homeopath, told us: "The [homeopathic] remedy . . . works on the level of energy, at the level of primary cause. If you get the right remedy, you don't need to be on a special diet, you don't need to restrict what you eat, you don't need a bunch of medical tests, and you don't need to watch

your cholesterol. Because the remedy changes the rate at which your cells vibrate." Far from expressing a mechanistic relationship to her modality (classical homeopathy), Frye is describing its potential to actually affect not only the body, but the emotions and the mind, and, therefore, the choices an individual would make with respect to diet. In other words, taking the right homeopathic remedy can strengthen the vital principle. When this occurs, a person will naturally tend to choose the right foods and a balanced lifestyle.

Chapter 8. Visions for the Future of Medicine

1. The other major cultural groups that Ray (1996) identifies are the "Heartlanders," the bearers of cultural traditionialism, who constitute 29 percent of the population, or 56 million adults, and the "Modernists," who comprise 47 percent of the population, or 88 million adults. He divides the "Cultural Creatives" (24 percent of the population, or 44 million adults) into two groups, the "Core Cultural Creatives" (10.6 percent, or 20 million), who have both person-centered and ecologically conscious values, and the "Green Cultural Creatives" (13 percent, or 24 million), who have values centered on the environment and social concerns from a secular point of view.

2. A notable exception is Dean Ornish's (1990) seminal study of cardiac patients on the effect of diet and lifestyle (exercise, relaxation, social support) on the prevention of subsequent heart attacks.

References

Abrahams, Roger D. 1973. "Ritual for Fun and Profit (or The Ends and Outs of Celebration)." Paper delivered at the Burg Wartenstein Symposium on Ritual: Reconciliation in Change. New York: Wenner-Gren Foundation for Anthropological Research.

Abrams, Frederick R. 1997. Review of *Do We Still Need Doctors,* by John D. Lantos. *Journal of the American Medical Association* 278(13):1123.

Adams, Patch. 1993. *Gesundheit!* Rochester, Vt.: Healing Arts Press.

Albright, Peter. 1989. "Physician in Transition." *Holistic Medicine*, July, 10–11.

Anderson, Bob. 1989. "Physician in Transition." *Holistic Medicine*, January–February, 6–7.

Altenberg, Henry Edward. 1989. "Physician in Transition." *Holistic Medicine*, November–December, 11.

American Holistic Medical Association Brochure. n.d. AHMA, 6728 Old McLean Village Drive, McLean, Va. 22101 (703–556–9245); HolistMed@aol.com. (www.ahmaholistic.com.).

Babcock, Barbara, ed. 1978. *The Reversible World: Symbolic Inversion in Art and Society*. Ithaca, N.Y.: Cornell University Press.

Bach, Edward. 1931. *Heal Thyself*. London: C. W. Daniel.

Barendsen, Kristen. 1996. "Why People Don't Heal: An Interview with Carolyn Myss." *Yoga Journal*, September–October, 66.

Bastick, Tony. 1982. *Intuition: How We Think and Act*. New York: Wiley.

Beckman, H. B., and R. M. Frankel. 1984. "The Effect of Physician Behavior on the Collection of Data." *Annals of Internal Medicine* 101:692–696.

Benner, P., and J. Rubel. 1989. *The Primacy of Caring: Stress and Coping in Health and Illness*. Menlo Park, Calif.: Addison-Wesley.

Benson, Herbert. 1984. *Beyond the Relaxation Response*. New York: Times Books.

———.1987. *Your Maximum Mind*. New York: Times Books.

———.1993. "The Relaxation Response." In *Mind-Body Medicine: How to Use Your Mind for Better Health.*, ed. Daniel Goleman and Joel Gurin. Yonkers, N.Y.: Consumer Reports Books.

Benson, Herbert, J. F. Beary, and M. P. Carol. 1974. "The Relaxation Response." *Psychiatry* 37:37–46.

Benson, Herbert, and Miriam Klipper. 1976. *The Relaxation Response*. New York: Avon.

Benson, Herbert, Eileen M. Stuart, and staff of the Mind/Body Medical Institute. 1992. *The Wellness Book: The Comprehensive Guide To Maintaining Health and Treating Stress-related Illness*. New York: Carol.

Berger, John. 1967. *A Fortunate Man*. New York: Pantheon Books.

Berkman, L. F., and S. L. Syme. 1979. "Social Networks, Host Resistance, and Mortality: A Nine-Year Followup Study of Residents of Alameda County." *American Journal of Epidemiology* 109:186–204.

Berman, Morris. 1988. *The Reenchantment of the World*. Ithaca, N.Y.: Cornell University Press.

———. 1990. *Coming to Our Senses: Body and Spirit in the Hidden History of the West*. New York: Bantam.

Berry, Wendell. 1996. "The Disease of Specialization." *Food and Water Journal*, spring.

Beth, Easton, and Jean Piaget. 1966. *Mathematical Epistemology and Psychology*. Dordrecht, The Netherlands: D. Reidel.

Beuf, Ann Hill. 1979. *Biting Off the Bracelet: A Study of Children in Hospitals*. Philadelphia: University of Pennsylvania Press.

Birth: Issues in Perinatal Care. 1996. 23(2):114.

Biesele, Megan, and Robbie Davis-Floyd, 1996. "Dying as Medical Performance: The Oncologist as Charon." In *The Performance of Healing*, ed. Carol Laderman and Marina Roseman. Philadelphia: University of Pennsylvania Press.

Black, Dean. 1993. "Pigs in the Dirt: How a Little Common Sense Can Resolve the Health Care Debate." *Health and Wellness Report* 3:10.

Bohm, David. 1980. *Wholeness and the Implicate Order*. London: Routledge and Kegan Paul.

Bryden, M. P. 1982. *Laterality: Functional Asymmetry in the Intact Brain*. New York: Academic.

Buchner, Rue, and Joan G. Stelling. 1977. *Becoming Professional*. Beverly Hills, Calif.: Sage.

Buckley, Thomas, and Alma Gottlieb. 1988. *Blood Magic: The Anthropology of Menstruation*. Berkeley and Los Angeles: University of California Press.

Budd, Matthew A. 1992. "New Possibilities for the Practice of Medicine." *Advances* 8(1):7–16.

Burack, R. C., and R. R. Carpenter. 1983. "The Predictive Value of the Presenting Complaint." *Journal of Family Practice* 16:749–754.

Califano, Joseph A. Jr. 1994. *Radical Surgery*. New York: Random House.

Campbell, Joseph. 1968 (1948). *The Hero with a Thousand Faces*. 2d ed. Princeton: Princeton University Press.

Capra, Fritjof. 1988. *Uncommon Wisdom*. New York: Simon and Schuster.

Cartwright, Elizabeth. 1998. "The Logic of Heartbeats: Electronic Fetal Monitoring and Biomedically Constructed Birth." In *Cyborg Babies: From Techno-Sex to Techno-Tots*, ed. Robbie E. Davis-Floyd and Joseph Dumit. New York: Routledge.

Carver, Cynthia. 1981. "The Deliverers: A Woman Doctor's Reflections on Medical Socialization." In *Childbirth: Alternatives to Medical Control*, ed. Shelly Romalis. Austin: University of Texas Press.

Cassell, Joan. 1991. *Expected Miracles: Surgeons at Work*. Philadephia: Temple University Press.

Cassell, Joan, and Sue Ellen Jacobs, eds. 1987. *Handbook of Ethical Issues in Anthropology*. Washington, D.C.: American Anthropological Association.

Chopra, Deepak. 1991. *Return of the Rishi: A Doctor's Story of Spiritual Transformation and Ayurvedic Healing*. 2d ed. Boston: Houghton-Mifflin.

Collins, Terry. 1994. "Physician in Transition." *Holistic Medicine*, Fall, 10–11.

Complementary and Alternative Medicine at the NIH. 1997. 4(2):1.

Coulehan, John L. 1995. "Emotions in Medical Practice." *Literature and Medicine* 14(2):226–235.

Coulter, Harris. 1982. *Divided Legacy*. Berkeley: North Atlantic.

———. 1995. "Coincidental Man: An Interview with Harris Coulter." By Julian Winston and Gwyneth Evans. *American Homeopath*, summer, 38–45.

Cox, A., D. Holbrook, and M. Rutter. 1981. "Psychiatric Interviewing Techniques VI. Experimental Study: Eliciting Feelings." *British Journal of Psychiatry* 139:144–152.

Cox, A., M. Rutter, and D. Holbrook. 1981. "Psychiatric Interviewing Techniques V. Experimental Study: Eliciting Factual Information." *British Journal of Psychiatry* 139:29–37.

Crocker, J. Christopher. 1985. *Vital Souls: Bororo Cosmology, Natural Symbolism, and Shamanism*. Tucson: University of Arizona Press.

Czaplicka, Marie Antoinette. 1914. *Aboriginal Siberia: A Study in Social Anthropology*. Oxford: Clarendon.

Davis-Floyd, Robbie E. 1987. "Obstetric Training as a Rite of Passage." *Medical Anthropology Quarterly* 1(3):288–318.

———. 1990. "The Role of American Obstetrics in the Resolution of Cultural Anomaly." *Social Science and Medicine* 31(2):175–189.

———. 1992. *Birth as an American Rite of Passage*. Berkeley and Los Angeles: University of California Press.

———. 1993. "The Technocratic Model of Birth." In *Feminist Theory in the Study of Folklore*, ed. Susan Tower Hollis, Linda Pershing, and M. Jane Young. Urbana: University of Illinois Press.

———. 1994. "The Technocratic Body: American Childbirth as Cultural Expression." *Social Science and Medicine* 38(8):1125–1140.

———. Forthcoming. *The Technocratic Body and the Organic Body: Hegemony and Heresy in Women's Birth Choices*. New Brunswick, N.J.: Rutgers University Press.

Davis-Floyd, Robbie, and P. Sven Arvidson. 1997. *Intuition—The Inside Story: Interdisciplinary Perspectives*. New York: Routledge.

Davis-Floyd, Robbie E., and Elizabeth Davis. 1996. "Intuition as Authoritative Knowledge." *Medical Anthropology Quarterly* 10(2):237–269.

Davis-Floyd, Robbie E., and Joseph Dumit. 1998. *Cyborg Babies: From Techno-Sex to Techno-Tots*. New York: Routledge.

DiGiacomo, Susan. 1987. "Biomedicine as a Cultural System: An Anthropologist in the Kingdom of the Sick." In *Encounters with Biomedicine: Case Studies in Medical Anthropology*, ed. Hans A. Baer. New York: Gordon and Breach.

Dossey, Larry. 1982. *Space, Time, and Medicine*. Boulder and London: Shambala.

———. 1993. *Healing Words*. San Francisco: HarperCollins.

———. 1995a. "How Should Alternative Therapies Be Evaluated?" *Alternative Therapies* 1(2):6–10.

———. 1995b. "Whatever Happened to Healers?" *Alternative Therapies*, 6–13.

Duffy, John. 1979. *The Healers: A History of Western Medicine*. Urbana: University of Illinois Press.

Duncan, David. 1993. "Is This Any Way to Train a Doctor? Medical Residencies: The Next Health Care Crisis." *Harper's* 286 (1715):61–66.

Dunn, Paul. 1993. "Physician in Transition." *Holistic Medicine*, winter, 8–10.

Edelberg, David. 1994. "Making Room for Alternatives: An Interview with David Edelberg." *Second Opinion* 20(1):20–33.

Ehrenreich, Barbara, and Deirdre English. 1973a. *Complaints and Disorders: The Sexual Politics of Sickness*. Old Westbury, N.Y.: Feminist Press.

———. 1973b. *Witches, Midwives, and Nurses: A History of Women Healers*. Old Westbury, N.Y.: Feminist Press.

Einstein, Albert. 1950. *Out of My Later Years*. New York: Philosophical Library.

Eisenberg, David. 1995. *Alternative Medicine: Implications for Clinical Practice*. Course workbook. Cambridge: Harvard Medical School Department of Continuing Education and the Department of Medicine, Beth Israel Hospital.

———. 1996. "The Invisible Mainstream." *Harvard Medical Alumni Bulletin* 70(1):20–25.

Eisenberg, David M., R. C. Kessler, C. Foster, F. E. Norlock, D. R. Calkins, and T. L. Delbanco. 1993. "Unconventional Medicine in the United States: Prevalence, Costs, and Patterns of Use." *New England Journal of Medicine* 328:246–252.

Eisler, Rianne. 1987. *The Chalice and the Blade: Our History, Our Future*. San Francisco: Harper & Row.

———.1995. *Sacred Pleasure: Sex, Myth, and the Politics of the Body*. San Francisco: HarperCollins.

Eliade, Mircea. 1975. "Modern Man's Need to Understand the Rites of Passage." In *Rites*, ed. John Cafferata. New York: McGraw-Hill.

Ellis, Peter Berresford. 1994. *The Druids*. Grand Rapids, Mich.: Eerdmans.

Engels, George L. 1977. "The Need for a New Medical Model: A Challenge for Biomedicine." *Science* 196:129–136.

———. 1980. "The Clinical Application of the Biopsychosocial Model." *American Journal of Psychiatry* 137:535–544.

———. 1988. "How Much Longer Must Medicine's Science Be Bound by a Seventeenth-Century Worldview?" In *The Task of Medicine: Dialogue at Wickenburg*, ed. K. L. White. Menlo Park, Calif.: Henry J. Kaiser Family Foundation.

———. 1995. "For Whom the Bells Toll a Second Time: John Romano, Physician and Psychiatrist (1908–1994)." *Rochester Medicine,* summer, 10–12.

Enkin, Murray, Marc Keirse, and Iain Chalmers. 1989. *A Guide to Effective Care in Pregnancy and Childbirth*. Oxford: Oxford University Press.

Erikson, Erik. 1963. *Childhood and Society*. New York: Norton.

Farrer, Ginger. 1980. "Singing for Life: The Mescalero Apache Girls' Puberty Ceremony." In *Southwestern Indian Ritual Drama*, ed. Charlotte Frisbie. Albuquerque: University of New Mexico Press.

Fetzer Institute. 1995. *The Institute Report*. Kalamazoo, Mich.: John E. Fetzer Institute.

Ferguson, Marilyn. 1980. *The Aquarian Conspiracy: Personal and Social Transformation in the 1980s*. Los Angeles: Tarcher.

Fisher, Jeffrey. 1994. *The Plague Makers*. New York: Simon and Schuster.

Flexner, A. 1910. *Medical Education in the United States and Canada: A Report to the Carnegie Foundation for the Advancement of Teaching*. New York: Carnegie Foundation.

Flint, Janna. 1996. "Residents: From Students to Physicians." Student term paper, Medical Anthropology, Dept. of Anthropology, Rice University, spring.

Fox, Renee C. 1957. "Training for Uncertainty." In *The Student Physician*, ed. R. Merton, G. Reader, and P. L. Kendall. Cambridge: Harvard University Press.

———. 1980. "The Evolution of Medical Uncertainty." *Millbank Quarterly* 58:1–49.

Friedson, Elliot. 1967. Review essay. "Health Factories: The New Industrial Sociology." *Social Problems* 14 (Spring):393–400.

———. 1970. *Profession of Medicine*. New York: Dodd, Mead.

Gaby, Alan. 1994a. "Med School Revisited." On *About Doctors and Folks*. Baltimore: Med Lion Music. Compact disc.

———. 1994b. "Breaking into the Old-Boy Network." *Townsend Letter* 133:939–940.

———. 1994c. "Medicine as a Business Distorts Values." *Townsend Letter* 128:74.

———. 1994d. "What's So Special about Medical Care?" *Townsend Letter* 135:1085.

———. 1999. *Nutritional Medicine*. Seattle: Alan Gaby, gaby@halcyon.com.

Gaines, Atwood D., and Robert A. Hahn, eds. 1982. "Physicians of Western Medicine: Five Cultural Studies." *Cultural, Medicine and Psychiatry* (special issue) 3:381–418.

Garza, Michelle. 1996. "The Medicalization of America: How the Technocrat Came to Be." Student term paper, Medical Anthropology, Dept. of Anthropology, Rice University, spring.

Gaskin, Ina May. 1977. *Spiritual Midwifery*. Summertown, Tenn.: Book.

Geertz, Clifford. 1973. *The Interpretation of Cultures*. New York: Basic Books.

Gilligan, Carol. 1993. *In a Different Voice: Psychological Theory and Women's Development*, 2d ed. Cambridge: Harvard University Press.

Goetz, Jordan. 1994. "Physician in Transition." *Holistic Medicine*, summer, 11–12.

Goodwin, J. S., W. C. Hunt, C. R. Key et al. 1987. "The Effect of Marital Status on Stage, Treatment, and Survival of Cancer Patients." *Journal of the American Medical Association* 258:3125–3130.

Goodwin, James, and Jean Goodwin. 1984. "The Tomato Effect: Rejection of Highly Efficacious Therapies." *Journal of the American Medical Association* 251:2387–2390.

Goer, Henci. 1995. *Obstetric Myths versus Research Realities*. Westport, Conn.: Bergin and Garvey.

Goffman, Erving. 1961. *Asylums: Essays on the Social Situation of Mental Patients and Other Inmates*. New York: Doubleday/Anchor.

Goldsmith, Judith. 1984. *Childbirth Wisdom from the World's Oldest Societies*. New York: Congdon and Weed.

Goldwag, William J. 1991. "Physician in Transition." *Holistic Medicine*, spring, 18–20.

Goleman, Daniel, and Joel Gurin. 1993. *Mind-Body Medicine: How to Use Your Mind for Better Health*. Yonkers, N.Y.: Consumer Reports Books.

Good, Mary-Jo Delvecchio. 1990. "The Practice of Biomedicine and the Discourse on Hope: A Preliminary Investigation into the Culture of American Oncology." In *Anthropologies of Medicine: A Colloquium on West European and North American Perspectives*, ed. Beatrix Pflederer and Gilles Bibeau. Heidelberg, Ger.: Viewig.

———. 1994. "Medicine on the Edge: Conversations with Oncologists." In *Science, Technology, and Culture*, ed. George Marcus. Chicago: University of Chicago Press.

———. 1995. *American Medicine: The Quest for Competence*. Berkeley and Los Angeles: University of California Press.

Good, Byron J., and Mary-Jo Delvecchio Good. 1993. "'Learning Medicine': The Constructing of Medical Knowledge at Harvard Medical School." In *Knowledge, Power, and Practice: The Anthropology of Medicine and Everyday Life*, ed. Shirley Lindenbaum and Margaret Lock. Berkeley and Los Angeles: University of California Press.

Gordon, Jim. 1996a. "Call for a New Medicine." *Harvard Medical Alumni Bulletin* 70(1):26–33.

———. 1996b. *Manifesto for a New Medicine: Your Guide to Healing Partnerships and the Wise Use of Alternative Therapies*. Reading, Mass.: Addison-Wesley.

Grazi, Sol J. 1992. "Physician in Transition." *Holistic Medicine*, winter, 18–19.

Green, Jerry. 1978. "Contracts with Your Doctor?" *New Realities* 2(I):np.

———. 1985. "The Health Care Contract: A Model for Shared Responsibility." In *The New Holistic Handbook*, ed. Shepherd Blyss. New York: Viking Penguin. (Revised from *Somatics* 3[4], 1982.)

———. 1988. "Minimizing Malpractice Risks by Role Clarification." *Annals of Internal Medicine*, August, 234–237.

Greenberg, Michael. 1990. *Off the Pedestal*. Elk Grove Village, Ill.: Making Medicine Work.

Greenwood, Michael, and Peter Nunn. 1992. *The Paradox of Healing*. Victoria, B.C.: Paradox.

Grossinger, Richard. 1982. *Planet Medicine*. Boulder, Colo.: Shambala.

Guo, David. 1989. "Medical Class Gets Apology for Lectures." *Pittsburgh Post-Gazette*, May 11.

Haas, Elson. 1981. *Staying Healthy with the Seasons*. Berkeley, Calif.: Celestial Arts.

———. 1992. *Staying Healthy with Nutrition*. Berkeley, Calif.: Celestial Arts.

Hahn, Robert A. 1985. "A World of Internal Medicine: Portrait of an Internist." In *Physicians of Western Medicine: Anthropological Approaches to Theory and Practice*, ed. Robert A. Hahn and Atwood D. Gaines. Boston: Reidel.

Hahn, Robert A., and Atwood D. Gaines, eds. 1985. *Physicians of Western Medicine: Anthropological Approaches to Theory and Practice*. Boston: Reidel.

Hall, J. A., D. L. Roter, and N. R. Katz. 1988. "Meta-Analysis of Correlates of Provider Behavior in Medical Encounters." *Medical Care* 26:657–675.

Hamilton, Ken. 1990. "Physician in Transition." *Holistic Medicine*, November, 8.

———. 1993. "Physician in Transition." *Holistic Medicine*, winter, 12–13.

Harder, Patty A. 1995. "From Quantity to Quality: A Dentist Goes Holistic." *Holistic Health News*. December 1.

Harkin, Tom. 1995. "The Third Approach." *Alternative Therapies*, March, 71.

Harman, Willis W. 1992. "Science and Metaphysics: The Union Whose Time Has Come." *Noetic Sciences Collection, 1980–1990*. Sausalito, Calif.: Institute of Noetic Sciences.

———. 1994. Address to the Institute for the Study of Consciousness in Berkeley, California. *Noetic Sciences Collection*. Unpublished.

Harner, Michael, ed. 1973. *Hallucinogens and Shamanism*. New York: Oxford University Press.

———. 1980. *The Way of the Shaman*. New York: Harper & Row.

Harris, Thomas. 1967. *I'm OK, You're OK*. New York: Harper & Row.

Harrison, Michelle. 1982. *A Woman in Residence*. New York: Random House.

Harwood, Michael. 1984 "The Ordeal: Life as a Medical Resident." *The New York Times Magazine*, June 3, 38–46, 70–82.

Hays, Bethany. 1992. "Physician in Transition." *Holistic Medicine*, spring, 18–20.

———. 1996. "Authority and Authoritative Knowledge in American Birth." *Medical Anthropology Quarterly* 10(2):291–294.

Henslin, J., and M. Biggs. 1971. "Dramaturgical Desexualization: The Sociology of the Vaginal Exam." In *Studies in the Sociology of Sex*, ed. J. Henslin. New York: Appleton-Century-Crofts.

Hochberg, Henry. 1990. "Physician in Transition." *Holistic Medicine*, July–August, 6–7.

Holmes, Rupert. 1996. Review of *Memory of Water*, by Michael Schiff. *Newsletter of the Monterrey Institute for the Study of Alternative Healing Arts*, January–March, 6–7. (Reprinted from *Network* 59 [December 1995].)

Hopkinson, K., A. Cox, and M. Rutter. 1981. "Psychiatric Interviewing Techniques III. Naturalistic Study: Eliciting Feelings." *British Journal of Psychiatry* 152:64–72.

House, James S., K. R. Landis, and D. Umberson. 1988. "Social Relationships and Health." *Science* 241:440–445.

Humiston, Karl. 1990. "Physician in Transition." *Holistic Medicine*, September–October, 4–7.

Huycke, L. I., and M. M. Huycke. 1994. "Characteristics of Potential Plaintiffs in Malpractice Litigation." *Annals of Internal Medicine* 120:792–798.

Illich, Ivan. 1976. *Medical Nemesis: The Expropriation of Health*. New York: Bantam.

Ivker, Robert. 1992. "Physician in Transition." *Holistic Medicine*, winter, 20–22.

Janiger, Oscar, and Philip Goldberg. 1993. "Daring to Be Different." *Hippocrates,* June, 42–48.

Johnson, Kenneth C. 1997. "Randomized Controlled Trials as Authoritative Knowledge: Keeping an Ally from Becoming a Threat to North American Midwifery Practice." In *Childbirth and Authoritative Knowledege: Cross-Cultural Perspectives*, ed. Robbie Davis-Floyd and Carolyn Sargent. Berkeley and Los Angeles: University of California Press.

Johnson, Margaret P. 1997. "Visionaries." *Psychological Perspectives* 35:6–7.

Jones, H. Leonard Jr. 1991. "Physician in Transition." *Holistic Medicine*, February, 8–9.

Jordan, Brigitte. 1993. *Birth in Four Cultures: A Cross-Cultural Investigation of Childbirth in Yucatan, Holland, Sweden and the United States*. 4th ed., rev. and updated by Robbie Davis-Floyd. Prospect Heights, Ill.: Waveland.

Joy, W. P. 1979. *Joy's Way.* New York: P. Tarcher.

Kaiser, Leland R. N.d. "The Hospital as a Healing Community." Unpublished ms.

Katz, Pearl. 1981. "Ritual in the Operating Room." *Ethnology* 20(4):335–350.

Kaufman, Barry N. *Happiness Is a Choice*. New York: Fawcett/Columbine, 1991.

Keeler, George. 1990. "Physician in Transition." *Holistic Medicine*, May–June, 21–22; July–August, 12–13.

Khalsa, Gurudarshan Singh. 1990. "Physician in Transition." *Holistic Medicine*, March–April, 6, 28.

Kiecolt-Glaser, Janice K., and Ronald Glaser. 1991. "Stress and the Immune System: Human Studies." In *Annual Review of Psychiatry*, ed. A. Tasman and M. B. Riba. Washington, D.C.: American Psyciatric Press.

———. 1992. "Psychoneuroimmunology: Can Psychological Interventions Modulate Immunity?" *Journal of Consulting and Clinical Psychology* 60:569–575.

Kirkland, James, Holly F. Mathews, C. W. Sullivan III, and Karen Baldwin, eds. 1992. *Herbal and Magical Medicine: Traditional Healing Today*. Durham, N.C.: Duke University Press.

Kitzinger, Sheila. 1978. *Women as Mothers: How They See Themselves in Different Cultures*. New York: Random House.

Kleijnen, J., P. Knipschild, and G. ter Riet. 1991. "Clinical Trials of Homeopathy." *British Medical Journal* 302(6772):316–323.

Kleinman, Arthur. 1988. *The Illness Narratives: Suffering, Healing, and the Human Condition*. New York: Basic Books.

Konner, Melvin. 1987. *Becoming a Doctor: A Journey of Initiation in Medical School*. New York: Viking.

Kors, Alan C., and Edward Peters, eds. 1972. *Witchcraft in Europe, 1100–1700: A Documentary History*. Philadelphia: University of Pennsylvania Press.

Korten, David. 1995. "When Corporations Rule the World." *Noetic Sciences Review*, summer, 4–10.

Kubler-Ross, Elisabeth. 1969. *On Death and Dying*. New York: Macmillan.

———. 1975. *Death: The Final Stage of Growth*. New York: Simon and Schuster.

Kuhn, Thomas S. 1970. *The Structure of Scientific Revolutions*, 2d ed. Chicago: University of Chicago Press.

Kunisch, Judith. 1989. "Electronic Fetal Monitors: Marketing Forces and the Resulting Controversy." In *Healing Technology: Feminist Perspectives*, ed. Kathryn Strother Ratcliff. Ann Arbor: University of Michigan Press.

Kunnen, Albert. 1993. "Physician in Transition." *Holistic Medicine*, spring, 6–7.

Kupsinel, Roy. 1993. "Physician in Transition." *Holistic Medicine*, fall, 9–11.

Larson, E.J. "Scientists Are Still Keeping the Faith." *Nature*, April 3, 345.

Laughlin, Charles D., John McManus, and Eugene G. d'Aquili. 1990. *Brain, Symbol, and Experience*. New York: Columbia University Press.

Laule, Alice. 1991. "Physician in Transition." *Holistic Medicine*, fall, 6–7.

Lazare, A. 1973. "Hidden Conceptual Models in Clinical Psychiatry." *New England Journal of Medicine* 288:345–351.

Leach, Edmund. 1979. "Ritualization in Man in Relation to Conceptual and Social Development." In *Reader in Comparative Religion*. 4th ed. Edited by William A. Lessa and Evon Z. Vogt. New York: Harper & Row.

LeBaron, Charles. 1981. *Gentle Vengeance: An Account of the First Year at Harvard Medical School*. New York: Richard Marek.

Lee, Dorothy. 1950. "Codifications of Reality: Lineal and Non-Lineal." *Psychosomatic Medicine* 12 (May):89–97.

Leveno, K. J., F. G. Cunningham, S. Nelson, M. Roark, M. L. Williams, D. Guzick, S. Dowling, C. R. Rosenfeld, and A. Buckley. 1986. "A Prospective Comparison of Selective and Universal Electronic Fetal Monitoring in 34,995 Pregnancies." *New England Journal of Medicine* 315:615–619.

Levin, Jeffrey S., David B. Larson, and Christina M. Puchalski. 1997. "Religion and Spirituality in Medicine: Research and Education." *Journal of the American Medical Association* 278(9):792–793.

Ley, R. G. 1983. "Cerebral Laterality and Imagery." In *Imagery: Current Theory, Research, and Application*. New York: Wiley.

Lincoln, Bruce. 1981. *Emerging from the Chrysalis: Studies in Rituals of Women's Initiation*. Cambridge: Harvard University Press.

Lindsay, Cathy. 1990. "Physician in Transition." *Holistic Medicine*, January–February, 23.

Linfors, E. W., and F. A. Neelan. 1981. "Interrogation and Interview: Strategies for Obtaining Clinical Data." *Journal of the Royal College of General Practitioners* 31:426–428.

Litoff, Judy Barrett. 1978. *American Midwives, 1860 to the Present*. Westport, Conn.: Greenwood.

Loomis, Evarts. 1989. "Physician in Transition." *Holistic Medicine*, September–October, 6.

Lorber, Judith. "Good Patients and Problem Patients: Conformity and Deviance in a General Hospital." *Journal of Health and Social Behavior* 16:213–225.

Lyng, Stephen. 1990. *Holistic Health and Biomedical Medicine*. Albany: State University of New York Press.

McCombs, Ann, and Bob Anderson. 1996. "New Certifying Board on the Horizon." *Holistic Medicine*, winter, 5–7.

McGarey, Gladys T. 1995. "A Vision for the Future of Medicine." *Healthlinks*, summer–fall, 2.

McManus, John B. 1979. "Ritual and Human Social Cognition." In *The Spectrum of Ritual: A Biogenetic Structural Analysis*, ed. Eugene d'Aquili, Charles D. Laughlin, and John McManus. New York: Columbia University Press.

Malinowski, Bronislaw. 1954. "Magic, Science, and Religion." In *Magic, Science, and Religion and Other Essays*. New York: Doubleday/Anchor.

Manahan, Bill. 1988. "Physician in Transition." *Holistic Medicine*, November, 20–21.

———. 1989. "Physician in Transition." *Holistic Medicine*, January–February, 6–7.

Mander, Jerry. 1991. *In the Absence of the Sacred: The Failure of Technology and the Survival of the Indian Nations*. San Francisco: Sierra Club.

Martin, Emily. 1987. *The Woman in the Body*. Boston: Beacon.

Mendelsohn, Robert. 1979. *Confessions of a Medical Heretic*. New York: Warner.

———. 1981. *Mal(e) Practice: How Doctors Manipulate Women*. Chicago: Contemporary Books.

Merchant, Carolyn. 1983. *The Death of Nature: Women, Ecology, and the Scientific Revolution*. San Francisco: Harper & Row.

Miner, Horace. 1975. "Body Ritual among the Nacirema." In *The Nacirema: Readings on American Culture*, ed. James P. Spradley and Michael A. Rynkiewich. Boston: Little, Brown.

Moore, Sally Falk, and Barbara Myerhoff, eds. 1977. *Secular Ritual*. Assen, The Netherlands: Van Gorcum.

Myss, Carolyn. 1996. *Anatomy of the Spirit*. New York: Random House.

Naisbitt, John. 1980. *Megatrends: Ten New Directions Transforming Our Lives*. New York: Warner Books.

Needleman, Jacob. 1977. *A Sense of the Cosmos*. New York: Dutton.

Nelson, Craig S., et al. 1995. "Residents' Performance before and after Night Call as Evaluated by an Indicator of Creative Thought." *Journal of the American Osteopathic Association* 95(10):600–603.

Nolen, William A. 1979. "How Doctors Are Unfair to Women." In *Culture, Curers, and Contagion*, ed. Norman Klein. Novato, Calif.: Chandler and Sharp.

Northrup, Christiane. 1994. *Women's Bodies, Women's Wisdom*. New York: Bantam.

Oakley, Ann. 1980. *Women Confined: Towards a Sociology of Childbirth*. New York: Schocken.

———. 1984. *The Captured Womb: A History of the Medical Care of Pregnant Women*. New York: Basil Blackwell.

Office of Technology Assessment. 1978. "Assessing the Efficacy and Safety of Medical Technologies." Washington, D.C.: Office of Technology Assessment, U.S. Congress.

Ornish, Dean. 1990. *Dr. Dean Ornish's Program for Reversing Heart Disease: The Only System Scientifically Proven to Reverse Heart Disease without Drugs or Surgery*. New York: Random House.

Parsons, Talcott. 1951. *The Social System*. Glencoe, Ill.: Free Press.

Partington, Angela. 1994. *The Concise Oxford Dictionary of Quotations*. 3d. ed. New York: Oxford University Press.

Payer, Lynn. 1988. *Medicine and Culture: Varieties of Treatment in the United States, England, West Germany, and France*. New York: Holt.

Pauling, Linus. 1976. *Vitamin C, the Common Cold, and the Flu.* San Fancisco: Freeman.

Pelletier, Kenneth. 1977. *Mind as Healer, Mind as Slayer.* New York: Delacorte.

Peplau, H. E. 1952. *Interpersonal Relations in Nursing: A Conceptual Frame of Reference for Psychodynamic Nursing.* New York: Putnam.

Pert, Candace. 1993. "The Chemical Communicators." In *Healing and the Mind*, ed. Bill Moyers and Betty Sue Flowers. New York: Doubleday.

Perls, Frederick. 1969. *Gestalt Therapy Verbatim.* New York: Bantam.

Petry, Judith. 1992. "Physician in Transition." *Holistic Medicine*, fall–winter, 14–15.

Pollack, Ron. 1995. "Worthless Promises: Drug Companies Keep Boosting Prices." *Oakland Tribune*, July 7.

Prentice, A., and T. Lind. 1987. "Fetal Heart Rate Monitoring during Labor—Too Frequent Intervention, Too Little Benefit." *Lancet* 2:1375–1377.

Prigogine, Ilya. 1980. *From Being to Becoming.* San Francisco: Freeman.

Progoff, Ira. 1955. *Jung's Psychology and Its Social Meaning.* New York: Grove.

Puthoff, Hal. 1990a. "Everything for Nothing." *New Scientist* 26(July):52–55.

———. 1990b. "The Energetic Vacuum: Implications for Energy Research." *Speculations in Science and Technology* 13(4):247.

Ray, Paul H. 1996. "The Rise of Integral Culture." *Noetic Sciences Review*, spring, 4–15.

Remen, Rachel Naomi. 1992. "The Eye of an Eagle, the Heart of a Lion, the Hand of a Woman." *Noetic Sciences Review*, winter, 29–34.

———.1995. "The Healer's Art: Reclaiming the Heart of Medical Practice." Course syllabus, University of California, San Francisco School of Medicine (winter quarter).

———. 1996. *Kitchen Table Wisdom.* New York: Putnam.

Reynolds, Peggy, and George A. Kaplan. 1990. "Social Connections and Risk for Cancer: Prospective Evidence from the Alameda County Study." *Behavioral Medicine* 16(3):101–110.

Reynolds, Peter C. 1991 *Stealing Fire: The Mythology of the Technocracy.* Palo Alto, Calif.: Iconic Anthropology Press.

Roncalli, Lucia. 1997. "Standing by Process: A Midwife's Notes on Story-Telling, Passage, and Intuition." In *Intuition—The Inside Story: Interdisciplinary Perspectives*, ed. Robbie E. Davis-Floyd and P. Sven Arvidson. New York: Routledge.

Rogers, Sherry. 1994. "Confused! What about All Those Studies That Say I Shouldn't Take Vitamins?" *Townsend Letter*, August–September.

Rolde, Neil. 1992. *Your Money or Your Health.* New York: Paragon House.

Rooks, Judith. 1997. *Midwifery and Childbirth in America.* Philadelphia: Temple University Press.

Roman, Sanaya. 1989. *Spiritual Growth.* Tiburon, Calif.: Kramer.

Roter, D. L. 1989. "Which Facets of Communication Have Strong Effects on

Outcome: A Meta-Analysis." In *Communicating with Medical Patients*, ed. M. Stewart and D. Roter. London: Sage.

Roter, D. L., J. A. Hall, and N. R. Katz. "Relations between Physicians' Behaviors and Analogue Patients' Satisfaction, Recall, and Impressions." *Medical Care* 25:437–451.

Rothman, Barbara Katz. 1982. *In Labor: Women and Power in the Birthplace.* New York: Norton. (Reprinted in paperback as *Giving Birth: Alternatives in Childbirth* [New York: Penguin, 1985].)

Rubinstein, Robert A., Charles D. Laughlin, Jr., and John McManus. 1984. *Science as Cognitive Process: Toward an Empirical Philosophy of Science*. Philadelphia: University of Pennsylvania Press.

Rusk, Tom. 1993. *The Power of Ethical Persuasion*. New York: Penguin.

Saltzmann, Amy P. 1992. "Physician in Transition." *Holistic Medicine*, spring, 9–10.

Sandmire, H. F. 1990. "Whither Electronic Fetal Monitoring?" *Obstetrics and Gynecology* 76(6):1130–1134.

Schaef, Anne Wilson. 1987. *When Society Becomes an Addict*. San Francisco: Harper & Row.

———. 1992. *Women's Reality: An Emerging Female System in a White Male Society*. 3d ed. San Francisco: HarperCollins.

Schaef, Anne Wilson, and Diane Fassel. 1988. *The Addictive Organization.* San Francisco: Harper & Row.

Scheper-Hughes, Nancy, and Margaret Lock. 1987. "The Mindful Body: A Prologomenon to Future Work in Medical Anthropology." *Medical Anthropology Quarterly* 1(1):6–41.

Schmidt, Matthew, and Lisa Jean Moore. 1998. "Constructing a 'Good Catch,' Picking a Winner: The Development of Technosemen and the Deconstruction of the Monolithic Male." In *Cyborg Babies: From Techno-Sex to Techno-Tots*, ed. Robbie E. Davis-Floyd and Joseph Dumit. New York: Routledge.

Schroder, H. M., M. Driver, and S. Streufert. 1967. *Human Information Processing*. New York: Holt, Rinehart, and Winston.

Scully, Diana. 1980. *Men Who Control Women's Health: The Miseducation of Obstetrician-Gynecologists*. Boston: Houghton-Mifflin.

Selye, Hans. 1974. *Stress without Distress* New York: Signet.

Shaw, Nancy Stoller. 1974. *Forced Labor: Maternity Care in the United States.* New York: Pergamon.

Shealy, C. Norman, and Carolyn Myss. 1993. *The Creation of Health*. Walpole, N.H.: Stillpoint.

Shirokogoroff, Sergei M. 1935. *Psychomental Complex of the Tungus*. London.

Shy, Kirkwood, David A. Luthy, Forrest C. Bennett, Michael Whitfield, Eric B. Larson, Gerald van Belle, James P. Hughes, Judith A. Wilson, and Martin A. Stenchever. 1990. "Effects of Electronic Fetal Heart Rate Monitoring, as Compared with Periodic Auscultation, on the Neurologic

Development of Premature Infants." *New England Journal of Medicine* 322(9):588–593.

Siegel, Bernie. 1986. *Love, Medicine, and Miracles*. New York: Harper & Row.

———. 1995. "Everyday Miracles, an Interview with Bernie Siegel." *Common Ground* 86 (winter).

Smith, Murray E. G. 1994. "The Burzynski Controversy." *Townsend Letter*, April, 352–363.

Smith, Robert C. 1996. *The Patient's Story: Integrated Patient-Doctor Interviewing*. Boston: Little, Brown.

Smith, Robert C., et al. 1995a. "A Strategy for Improving Patient Satisfaction by the Intensive Training of Residents in Psychosocial Medicine: A Controlled, Randomized Study." *Academic Medicine* 70:729–732.

———. 1995b. "Improving Residents' Confidence in Using Psychosocial Skills." *Journal of General Internal Medicine* 10:315–320.

Smith, Robert C., and Ruth B. Hoppe. 1991. "The Patient's Story: Integrating the Patient- and Physician-Centered Approach to Interviewing." *Annals of Internal Medicine* 115:470–477.

Smith, Robert C., Alicia A. Marshall, Steven A. Cohen-Cole. 1994. "The Efficacy of Intensive Biopsychosocial Teaching Programs for Residents: A Review of the Literature and Guidelines for Teaching." *Journal of General Internal Medicine* 9:390–396.

Sperry, Roger W. 1974. "Lateral Specialization in Surgically Separated Hemispheres." In *The Neurosciences: Third Study Program*, ed. P. J. Vinken and G. W. Bruyn. Cambridge: MIT Press.

———. 1982. "Some Effects of Disconnecting the Cerebral Hemispheres." *Science* 217:1223–1226.

Spiegel, David. 1990. "Facilitating Emotional Coping during Treatment." *Cancer* 66:1422–1426.

———. 1993. "Social Support: How Friends, Family, and Groups Can Help." In *Mind-Body Medicine: How to Use Your Mind for Better Health*, ed. Daniel Goleman and Joel Gurin. Yonkers, N.Y.: Consumer Reports Books.

Spiegel, David, J. R. Bloom, H. C. Kramer, and E. Gottheil. 1989. "Effect of Psychosocial Treatment on Survival of Patients with Metastatic Breast Cancer." *Lancet* 2:888–891.

Sprenger, Jally, and George Deutsch. 1981. *Left Brain Right Brain*. San Francisco: Freeman.

Starhawk. 1989. *The Spiral Dance: A Rebirth of the Ancient Religion of the Great Goddess*. San Francisco: Harper & Row.

Starr, Paul. 1982. *The Social Transformation of American Medicine*. New York: Basic Books.

Stein, Howard F. 1990. *American Medicine as Culture*. Boulder, Colo.: Westview.

Stein, Leonard. 1967. "The Doctor-Nurse Game." In *Archives of General Psy-*

chiatry 16:699–703. (Reprinted in *Conformity and Conflict,* 4th ed., ed. James P. Spradley and David W. McCurdy [Boston: Little, Brown, 1980].)

Stoll, Walt. 1989. "Physician in Transition." *Holistic Medicine*, March–April, 10–11.

Sultanoff, Barry. 1993. "Physician in Transition." *Holistic Medicine*, winter, 6–11.

———. 1994. Letter to the Editor. *Townsend Letter* 130:483–484.

Sylvest, Vernon M. 1991. "Physician in Transition." *Holistic Medicine*, summer, 6–9.

Tannen, Deborah. 1995. *Talking from 9 to 5: How Women's and Men's Conversational Styles Affect Who Gets Heard, Who Gets Credit, and What Gets Done*. New York: Morrow.

Tao-Kim-Hai, Andre M. 1979 "Orientals Are Stoic." In *Culture, Curers, and Contagion*, ed. Norman Klein. Novato, Calif.: Chandler and Sharp.

Tap, Vincent, and Goppel, Marian. 1995. "Summary of a Report by the Health Council of the Netherlands on Alternative Modes of Treatment under Scientific Investigation." *Alternative Therapies* 1(2):5.

Thomasma, David C. 1995. "Toward a 21st Century Bioethic." *Alternative Therapies* 1 (March):74.

Tresolini, Carol P., and the Pew-Fetzer Task Force on Advancing Psychosocial Health Education. 1994. *Health Professions Education and Relationship-Centered Care*. San Francisco: Pew Health Professions Commission.

Turner, Victor W. 1967. *The Forest of Symbols*. Ithaca, N.Y.: Cornell University Press.

———. 1979. "Betwixt and Between: The Liminal Period in *Rites de Passage*." In *Reader in Comparative Religion*, ed. W. Lessa and E. Z. Vogt. 4th ed. New York: Harper & Row.

Tuscher, Richard A. 1992. "Physician in Transition." *Holistic Medicine*, summer, 10–11.

Tyler, Terry, and Gloria St. John. 1989. *MetaPhysicians' Tales*. Unpublished ms.

Vaccarino, J. M. 1977. "Malpractice—The Problem in Perspective." *Journal of the American Medical Association* 238:861–863.

Van Gennep, Arnold. 1966 (1908). *The Rites of Passage*. Chicago: University of Chicago Press.

Wagner, Marsden. 1997. "Confessions of a Dissident." In *Childbirth and Authoritative Knowledge: Cross-Cultural Perspectives*, ed. Robbie E. Davis-Floyd and Carolyn Sargent. Berkeley and Los Angeles: University of California Press.

Warter, Carlos. 1994. *Recovery of the Sacred*. Deerfield Beach, Fla.: Health Communications.

Weil, Andrew. 1988. *Health and Healing*. Boston: Houghton-Mifflin.

———. 1995. *Spontaneous Healing*. New York: Fawcett Columbine.

Wheatley, Margaret. 1992. *Leadership and the New Science: Learning about Organization from an Orderly Universe.* San Francisco: Berrett-Koehler.

White, Bowen. 1989. "Physician in Transition." *Holistic Medicine*, May–June, 14.

Whitfield, Barbara Harris. 1995. *Spiritual Awakenings.* Deerfield Beach, Fla: Health Communications.

Wilber, Ken. 1996. *A Brief History of Everything.* Boston: Shambala.

Williams, Redford B., J. C. Barefoot, R. M Califf, et al. 1992. "Prognostic Importance of Social and Economic Resources among Medically Treated Patients with Angiographically Documented Coronary Heart Disease." *Journal of the American Medical Association* 267:520–524.

Williams, Redford B., T. L. Haney, K. L. Lee et al. 1980. "Type A Behavior, Hostility, and Coronary Atherosclerosis." *Psychosomatic Medicine* 42:539–549.

Williams, Roger J. 1956. *Biochemical Individuality.* New York: Wiley.

———. 1959. *Alcoholism: The Nurtritional Approach.* Austin: University of Texas Press.

———. 1971. *Nutrition against Disease.* New York: Bantam.

Wilson, Jacqueline. 1990. "Physician in Transition." *Holistic Medicine*, July–August, 6–7.

Wiseman, Richard, and Marilyn Schlitz. 1998. "Experimenter Effects and the Remote Detection of Staring." *Journal of Parapsychology* 61(3).

Zerubavel, Eviatar. 1991. *The Fine Line: Making Distinctions in Everyday Life.* New York: Free Press.

Zola, Irving Kenneth. 1983. "The Case of Non-Compliance." In *Sociomedical Inquiries: Recollections, Reflections, and Reconsiderations.* Philadelphia: Temple University Press.

Index

About the Authors

Robbie Davis-Floyd, Ph.D., is a cultural anthropologist specializing in medical anthropology, ritual and gender studies, the anthropology of reproduction, and science and technology studies. A Research Fellow at the University of Texas at Austin, she lectures widely in these areas. She is the author of numerous academic articles and of *Birth as an American Rite of Passage* (1992). In 1993 she completed the updating and expansion of Brigitte Jordan's classic *Birth in Four Cultures*. Building on Jordan's work, she coedited *Childbirth and Authoritative Knowledge: Cross-Cultural Perspectives* (1997), which contains ethnography on birth in sixteen cultures. Her own contribution to that volume explores midwives' use of intuition in home birth, an interest that led her to coedit an interdisciplinary investigation of *Intuition: The Inside Story* (1997). Intrigued by anthropological analyses of the new reproductive technologies, she coedited *Cyborg Babies: From Techno-Sex to Techno-Tots* (1998). Her current research investigates the development of direct-entry midwifery in North America and the ongoing elaboration of new paradigms in business and health care.

Gloria St. John, M.B.A., has been involved in the business end of health care for twenty-five years. She has been a clinic and hospital adminstrator and a marketing and management consultant at the national level. She has worked with doctors in transition in virtually every professional setting. The author of dozens of articles on natural health subjects, she is currently editing a book on the natural treatment of arthritis, as well as several in the field of homeopathy. She has written two books on personal and spiritual growth and has taught and lectured on these subjects. She intends to pursue her deep interest in the human psyche through the practice of homeopathy, a vocation for which she is now training. Born and raised in Chicago, she lives in the San Francisco Bay area.